Handbook of
Psychopharmacology

Volume 2

Principles of Receptor Research

Handbook of
Psychopharmacology

Volume 2

Principles of Receptor Research

Edited by

Leslie L. Iversen
Department of Pharmacology
University of Cambridge

Susan D. Iversen
Department of Psychology
University of Cambridge

and

Solomon H. Snyder
Departments of Pharmacology and Psychiatry
The Johns Hopkins University
School of Medicine

PLENUM PRESS · NEW YORK AND LONDON

Library of Congress Cataloging in Publication Data

Main entry under title:

Handbook of psychopharmacology.

    Includes bibliographies and indexes.
    CONTENTS: v. 1. Biochemical principles and techniques in neuropharma-
cology.—v. 2. Principles of receptor research.—v. 3. Biochemistry of biogenic
amines.—v. 4. Amino acid neurotransmitters.
    1. Psychopharmacology. I. Iversen, Leslie Lars. II. Iversen, Susan D., 1940-
    III. Snyder, Solomon H., 1938-   [DNLM: 1. Psychopharmacology.
QV77 H236]
RC483.H36   615'.78   75-6851
ISBN 0-306-38922-3 (v. 2)

CONTRIBUTORS
TO VOLUME 2

P. CUATRECASAS, *Department of Pharmacology and Experimental Therapeutics and Department of Medicine, The Johns Hopkins University School of Medicine, Baltimore, Maryland*

M. D. HOLLENBERG, *Department of Pharmacology and Experimental Therapeutics and Department of Medicine, The Johns Hopkins University School of Medicine, Baltimore, Maryland*

A. S. HORN, *MRC Neurochemical Pharmacology Unit, Department of Pharmacology, University of Cambridge, Cambridge, England*

JOHN S. KELLY, *MRC Neurochemical Pharmacology Unit, Department of Pharmacology, Medical School, Cambridge University, Cambridge, England*

S. Z. LANGER, *Instituto de Investigaciones Farmacológicas, Consejo Nacional de Investigaciones, Cientificas y Técnicas, Buenos Aires, Argentina*

BRIAN MELDRUM, *Department of Neurology, Institute of Psychiatry, London, England*

R. D. MYERS, *Laboratory of Neuropsychology, Purdue University, Lafayette, Indiana*

PHILLIP G. NELSON, *Behavioral Biology Branch, National Institute of Child Health and Human Development, National Institutes of Health, Bethesda, Maryland*

BRUCE R. RANSOM, *Behavioral Branch, National Institute of Child Health and Human Development, National Institutes of Health, Bethesda, Maryland*

CONTENTS

CHAPTER 3

Electrical Recording of Brain Activity: The EEG and Its Value in
Assessing Drug Effects

BRIAN MELDRUM

CHAPTER 4

Neuropharmacological Responses from Nerve Cells in Tissue Culture

BRUCE R. RANSOM AND PHILLIP G. NELSON

CHAPTER 5

Biochemical Identification of Membrane Receptors: Principles and Techniques

M. D. HOLLENBERG AND P. CUATRECASAS

CHAPTER 6

Structure–Activity Relations for Neurotransmitter Receptor Agonists and Antagonists

A. S. HORN

CHAPTER 7
Denervation Supersensitivity
S. Z. LANGER

BLOOD–BRAIN BARRIER: TECHNIQUES FOR THE INTRACEREBRAL ADMINISTRATION OF DRUGS

R. D. Myers

1. INTRODUCTION

The greatest concern of the psychopharmacologist whose wish is to elucidate the properties of a given compound is its mode of action when administered by the systemic route. The basis for this is elementary. A drug that is prescribed to a patient ordinarily is taken orally or parenterally. For this reason, the vast majority of the research done on compounds that affect the central nervous system has utilized one or more of the systemic methods of administration. This having been said, there are five reasons why the logistics of this approach is not entirely coherent from a purely experimental—*not clinical*—standpoint.

First, the blood–brain barrier and the blood–cerebrospinal fluid barrier prevent a great number of compounds from entering the central nervous system. Therefore, even if the compound is synthesized within nerve tissue,

R. D. Myers ● Laboratory of Neuropsychology, Purdue University, Lafayette, Indiana. The research reported in this chapter has been supported over the years by National Science Foundation grant GB–24592 and U.S. Office of Naval Research Contract N 00014–67–A–0226–0003.

its peripheral administration would be experimentally fruitless. Although the nature of the exclusion afforded by these two barriers will be dealt with in the next section, generally speaking they do serve the brain and spinal cord in a protective capacity, without which the brain would be constantly subject to a plethora of chemical imbalances brought on by the constituents of circulating plasma.

Second, a drug given peripherally may exert a powerful effect on the autonomic nervous system. Because of the feedback to diencephalic and other central structures, the compound quite beguilingly may appear to act directly on some part of the brain. To illustrate, even though epinephrine does not readily penetrate the blood–brain barrier, the arousal and other behavioral changes following a systemic injection of this monoamine would lead one, as it has done so somewhat embarrassingly in the past, to a false conclusion about its "direct effect on the reticular activating system."

Third, a compound that circumvents the barriers of the brain may have an effect on neurons within the parenchyma which is diametrically opposite to that seen when the compound is given systemically. As an excellent example of this, the well-known paralytic action at the neuromuscular junction of intravenously injected curare is in marked contrast to curare's property of inducing electrical seizures when applied to the hippocampus.

Fourth, through the use of a systemic approach it is virtually impossible to ascertain the precise neuroanatomical locus of action of a compound that exerts a central effect.

Fifth, each major area of the brain and even the smaller subdivisions have a unique regional neurochemistry in terms of enzymatic, humoral, and other systems. What is often called the chemical anatomy of the brain is difficult to investigate by systemic means alone.

If one studies experimentally the response to a drug acting directly on a specific area of the brain, a somewhat more trenchant interpretation of its action can be put forward, and a set of inferences about its efficacy will thereby evolve.

2. CHARACTERISTICS OF THE BLOOD–BRAIN BARRIER

The blood–brain barrier operates at the level of the microcirculation in a highly selective fashion. A common misconception about this barrier is that its effectiveness in preventing substances from entering the brain depends solely on the size of a given molecule or some other physical or chemical characteristic. Actually, the factor of molecular weight in the case of an individual amino acid is unrelated to its facility of cerebral entry.

Another widespread misunderstanding is that the barrier is a passive anatomical filter. To illustrate this fallacy, the penetration of many lipid-insoluble solutes is uncommon, and according to Soloway (1958) the lipid solubility of a specific drug is a critical consideration. However, other substrates such as glucose and amino acids with a very low lipid solubility are nevertheless able to pass the blood–brain barrier. According to Oldendorf (1973a), an independent and saturable transport mechanism can now be demonstrated.

Several of the criteria for evaluating the flux of a substance between plasma and neural tissue have been discussed by Levin and Scicli (1969). In addition, the anatomy of the blood–CSF and blood–brain barrier has been the subject of vast speculation and elaborate ultrastructural evaluation (e.g., Livingston, 1960; Davson, 1963). Although the neuroglial processes may act as a sheath around the capillaries to filter the plasma, it is not yet clear that a unique structural element actually regulates the transport of substances between blood and brain. Even granting the possibility of such an ultrastructural filter, a chemical mechanism underlying the selectivity of penetration is an equally important possibility. For example, a difference of approximately 0.2 in the pH across the barrier is maintained so as to retard the transfer of OH^- and H^+ ions. Similarly, essential cations such as Na^+, K^+, Ca^{2+}, and Mg^{2+} are maintained in relative homeostasis within the brain parenchyma independent of the challenge of an excessive concentration of ions in the blood.

As Lajtha and others have shown, stereospecificity is also a vital hallmark of brain permeability (e.g., Lajtha and Toth, 1963; Nemoto and Sevringhaus, 1971). For example, the L-enantiomer amino acids are transported preferentially across the blood–brain barrier (Oldendorf, 1973a,b). In contrast, many D-enantiomer amino acids are taken up in very low amounts by the brain, probably because of their natural rarity in the organism.

Knowledge of whether the barrier is permeable to a given compound is essential, so that a misleading or fallacious interpretation of an experiment can be ruled out. For example, when the RNA in yeast or in an extract of brain homogenate is given intraperitoneally, an animal's memory is purportedly influenced. Yet such an influence is impossible since it is well known that the blood–brain barrier is impenetrable to RNA (Eist and Seal, 1965). Proteins such as cytochrome *c* also do not pass into the CSF across the choroid plexus or other region of leakage, probably because of an epithelial barrier (Milhorat *et al.*, 1973).

An understanding of the degree of influx of a compound into the brain may reveal important facts about its relative functional potency. In the case of heroin and morphine given intravenously, the former is taken up readily in the brain whereas the latter is not (Oldendorf *et al.*, 1972). The addict's preference for heroin could thus be related to the rapidity of entry of the particular narcotic.

2.1. Specific Activity of the Blood–Brain Barrier

In an elegant series of experiments, Crone (1961, 1965) and Oldendorf (1971) have independently characterized some of the features of the blood–brain barrier in terms of those substances that are capable of penetrating it. Both investigators analyzed a sample of venous blood collected from the brain for the content of the test substance almost immediately after it had been injected into the carotid artery. Negligible penetration during a single passage through the capillaries of inert ^{14}C-labeled polar substances was found. Table 1 shows the "uptake index" for urea, dextran, inulin, mannitol, and sucrose, which, in each case, was derived by comparing the uptake of the substance with the tritiated water reference since nearly all ^{3}H-water penetrates the cerebral capillaries.

A corresponding examination of the entry of the amino acids has shown that in the rat those that are nutritionally essential enter more freely than nonessential amino acids. As shown in Table 2, substances such as tyrosine that are not synthesized readily in the brain must therefore pass through the barrier. In general, the low rates of permeability of γ-aminobutyric acid (GABA), glutamate, and glycine may be related to their functional role as neurohumoral factors. This seems to be true also for certain of the amines, as shown in Table 3, in that minimal amounts of dopamine, norepinephrine, epinephrine, serotonin (5-HT), and histamine are taken up by cerebral tissue from the capillary network. Although the mechanism is not understood, it would seem that a precursor of a humoral substance, including a neurotransmitter, is readily exchanged between blood and brain.

TABLE 1

Uptake into the Brain During a Single 15-s Pass Through the Microcirculation Following a Rapid Injection into the Common Carotid Artery of ^{14}C-Labeled Inert Polar Substances Mixed with [3]HOH

	Injected concentration (mM)	Brain uptake index[a]
[3]HOH reference		100
Urea	0.020	2.37 ± 0.23
Dextran[b]	0.024	2.18 ± 0.36
Inulin	0.100	1.95 ± 0.38
Mannitol	0.024	1.94 ± 0.23
Sucrose	0.009	1.41 ± 0.47

From Oldendorf (1971).
[a] The brain uptake index is the percentage of the radioactivity remaining in the brain. Brain uptake index values are means ±SD. For each mean, $n = 3$.
[b] Mol wt 60,000.

TABLE 2

Uptake into the Brain of ^{14}C-Labeled Amino Acids

	Injected concentration (mM)	Brain uptake index[a]
^{3}HOH reference		100
Phenylalanine	0.003	55 ± 5
Leucine	0.008	54 ± 2
Tyrosine	0.006	50 ± 2
Isoleucine	0.008	40 ± 2
Methionine	0.021	38 ± 2
Tryptophan	0.022	36 ± 1
Histidine	0.008	33 ± 3
Arginine	0.008	22 ± 1.5
Valine	0.010	21 ± 2.5
Dopa	0.202	20 ± 1.4
Ornithine	0.006	18 ± 2.4
Lysine	0.008	16 ± 3.2
Cycloleucine	0.187	15.6 ± 0.1
Threonine	0.012	11.7 ± 0.37
Cysteine	0.067	8.1 ± 1.6
D-Tyrosine	0.002	8.1 ± 1.2
Serine	0.017	7.5 ± 0.52
DL-5-HTP	0.329	7.4 ± 0.84
Thyroxine	0.009	7.1 ± 1.1
Alanine	0.017	5.7 ± 0.51
Citrulline	0.022	5.2 ± 1.3
Asparagine	0.012	4.7 ± 0.52
AAIBA	0.156	3.3 ± 0.68
Proline	0.010	3.3 ± 0.35
Glutamic acid	0.010	3.21 ± 0.26
Aspartic acid	0.012	2.77 ± 0.79
Glycine	0.025	2.53 ± 0.21
GABA	0.762	2.2 ± 0.60

From Oldendorf (1971).
[a] Calculated as in Table 1. Values are means ±SD. For each mean, $n = 3$. Unless otherwise stated, all optically active amino acids are L-enantiomorphs.

Two crucial chemical phenomena seem to determine how readily a phenylethylamine substrate penetrates the brain. First, adding a methoxy group in the 3- and 4-positions or in the 3-, 4-, and 5-positions acts to lower the uptake of an amine into the brain. Similarly, attaching a hydroxyl group in the 3-position or the 3- and 4-positions lowers brain penetrability of the substance. Second, the decarboxylation of an amino acid, as in the reactions in which dopa is converted to dopamine, 5-hydroxytryptophan (5-HTP) to 5-HT, or histidine to histamine, serves to reduce the subsequent ingress of the substance from blood to brain.

TABLE 3

Uptake into the Brain of ^{14}C-Labeled Biogenic Amines

	Injected concentration (mM)	Brain uptake index[a]
^{3}HOH reference		100
β-Phenethylamine	0.346	67 ± 5
p-Methoxyphenethylamine	0.243	59 ± 2
Tryptamine	0.140	12.5 ± 3.2
3,4-Dimethoxyphenethylamine	0.134	11.7 ± 1.3
Glutamine	0.030	7.62 ± 0.39
Mescaline	0.276	5.6 ± 1.4
Norepinephrine	0.022	4.49 ± 1.3
Acetylcholine	0.023	4.5 ± 0.9
Dopamine	0.023	3.85 ± 0.38
Tyramine	0.029	3.07 ± 0.48
5-Hydroxytryptamine	0.022	2.63 ± 1.8
DL-Epinephrine	0.034	2.38 ± 0.11
Histamine	0.023	1.61 ± 0.36

From Oldendorf (1971).
[a] Calculated as in Table 1. Values are means ±SD. For each mean, $n = 3$.

In view of his findings, Oldendorf has made the cogent observation that a putative transmitter or other humoral factor which has a neuronal function is retained and localized in brain parenchyma. Therefore, the blood–brain barrier, in addition to its exclusion of plasma solutes, seems to restrict the passage of essential factors in the other direction, from brain to blood.

2.2. Breakdown of the Blood–Brain Barrier

There are several pathological conditions which disturb the integrity of the blood–brain barrier so severely that even molecules of protein may pass into the cerebral parenchyma (Brightman *et al.*, 1970). Surprisingly a substance such as penicillin, which is ordinarily excluded by the barrier, can like many other substances enter during a morbid change caused by a tumor or when the brain has been otherwise lesioned. Cerebral edema or other fulminating disease states such as lymphostatic encephalopathy can act to collapse the blood–brain barrier to Evans blue and Thorotrast. A deficiency of vitamin B in the diet can exacerbate the severity of pathological permeability (Földi-Börcsök and Földi, 1973). The integrity of the blood–brain barrier can also be lost as a result of a lesion produced by careless or damaging implantation of a cannula or other device into the brain parenchyma (Edvinsson *et al.*, 1971).

The evidence that a toxic chemical such as dimethylsulfoxide can break down the blood–brain barrier is subject to some debate (e.g., Kocsis *et al.*, 1968). However, it is clear that certain drugs such as chlorpromazine and nortriptyline can induce a selective change in the barrier's permeability. Pardridge *et al.* (1973) have shown that the penetrability of mannitol, inulin, and dopamine is enhanced substantially by these drugs in a dose-dependent fashion. This action may be due to an *in vivo* lysis of the plasma membranes of the endothelial cells in the brain's microvasculature.

Rapoport *et al.* (1971) have proposed that the blood–brain barrier can be broken down reversibly by the selective shrinkage of barrier cells, possibly the vascular endothelium, and the opening up of spaces between them. Electrolytes and nonelectrolytes that have a negligible lipid solubility may temporarily alter the barrier, whereas lipid-soluble nonelectrolytes can damage the barrier irreversibly (Rapoport *et al.*, 1972).

2.3. The Brain–CSF Barrier

The brain–CSF barrier has also been studied in great detail in many laboratories (see review of Cserr, 1971). Numerous factors are known to influence the bidirectional flux of a substance across the ependymal surfaces of the cerebral ventricles. Among these factors are active transport, passive diffusion, cation concentration, the level of pCO_2, the saturation of the transependymal transport mechanism, the gradient of osmotic tension, the rate of bulk formation of CSF, the morphology of the ependymal wall itself, the presence of certain drugs, and even the age of the animal (Lee and Olszewski, 1960; Fleischhauer, 1961; Davson and Pollay, 1963; Klatzo *et al.*, 1964; Ames *et al.*, 1965; Curl and Pollay, 1968; Levin and Sisson, 1972; Doggett and Spencer, 1972).

Of some interest is the fact that centrally active substances such as angiotensin II are able to pass into the CSF from the blood, but not into brain tissue (Volicer and Loew, 1971). Of course, the dynamics of the transport and exchange between the CSF and the brain of ions or molecules, including sodium, potassium, and glucose, can vary greatly (Brøndsted, 1970*a,b*; Davson and Welch, 1971). The phenomenon of the absorption or transport of substances from cerebrospinal spaces into the blood supply is equally remarkable. The clearance of compounds such as epinephrine, morphine, atropine, and metaraminol has been investigated extensively (Da Silva and Sproull, 1964; Albanus *et al.*, 1969; Wang and Takemori, 1972; Bass and Lundborg, 1973).

3. BYPASSING THE BLOOD–BRAIN BARRIER: PRINCIPLES

Numerous avenues are open to the investigator who wishes to circumvent the blood–brain barrier for one of the reasons alluded to in the first section of this chapter. But which approach should be taken? Probably the principal determinant is simply the question of the level of physiological resolution.

With respect to the theoretical aspects concerning a point of entry into the central nervous system, a wide spectrum of approaches is available, each with different probabilities of information yield. Clearly, the systemic route of administration of a drug that has an action on the nervous system is the most convenient and the most simple of approaches. A close intra-arterial injection given unilaterally into one of the vertebral arteries likewise can give indirect evidence of a central action of a compound, particularly if the latency of the response is compared with the interval required for the plasma to circulate. Nevertheless, the impossibility of anatomical localization in both instances is an inherent weakness.

As a first approximation of how a drug works, the brain may be approached from one of its two surfaces, inner or outer. As elaborated on by Feldberg (1963), the cortex comprises the chemically sensitive outer surface, whereas the ventricular lumen and cisterna magna comprise the equally sensitive inner surface. By placing either a tiny cotton pledget or a filter paper soaked in the drug on the surface of the cortex, a functional response of a given region may be examined quantitatively. As in the case of the spreading cortical depression produced by a concentrated solution of KCl applied locally, the wave of electrical negativity can be traced on a second-by-second basis.

By injecting a compound into the lateral, third, or fourth ventricle, one can examine the direct effect of the substance on the internal structures of the brain. In terms of this centrally induced response, a contrast is provided to that seen when the same substance is administered by a peripheral route.

The main criticism of either the cortical or ventricular mode of attack is the provisional nature of any anatomical interpretation made with reference to the efficacy of the compound. Given two vital factors—the dilution and the rapid diffusion—it is difficult to specify with precision the group of neurons affected by the test solution. What is worse, a chemical injected into the lateral ventricle may exert an effect totally opposite to that which occurs when the same compound is injected either into a portion of brain substance or into another portion of the ventricular lumen (see Myers, 1974).

The accurate microapplication of a compound to a specific structure in the brain of a number of different species has been made possible by the recent advent of relatively sophisticated infusion procedures and stereotaxic techniques. Following a microliter injection of a solution or the deposition of a compound in crystalline form in a given region, the regional pharmacology of a given structure such as the hypothalamus or the caudate nucleus can be examined. Moreover, if careful controls are exercised, a minute portion of brain tissue can be activated by a chemical in a way thought to simulate the circumscribed release of a humoral factor such as a neurotransmitter (*cf.* Myers, 1971). The three most widely used techniques, to be discussed in detail in the following section, involve localized injection of a solution, application of a chemical in solid form, and localized perfusion with push–pull cannulae.

A still finer-grained analysis is the technique by which a chemical is ejected onto the membrane of a single cell in the brain by iontophoresis through a micropipette (see Kelly, Chap. 2, this volume). When a three-, four-, or five-barreled array of micropipettes is lowered into a specific region, only a few neurons are exposed to a compound at a time. The compound under study is ejected during one interval, and, later, a second compound or control solution is ejected from another pipette. A third pipette is used as the recording electrode. The technique of iontophoresis offers the advantage of analysis of the sensitivity of a neuron to a specific substance; however, its very molecular nature limits rather severely the extrapolation of a given result. That is, the understanding of the relationship of the response of a single neuron may not apply to a chain of interrelated neurons.

In evaluating the procedure to use in relation to the pharmacological responsiveness of brain tissue, each of the techniques summarized in Table 4 has its strengths and weaknesses. In the final analysis, the decision to select

TABLE 4

Summary of Neuropharmacological Methods Currently Used to Bypass the Blood–Brain Barrier

Superficial application of chemical
  1. Cortical pledget, filter paper, crystals and salts
  2. Cortical superfusion
  3. Intracisternal injection (subarachnoid space)
  4. Intracortical microinjection (subarachnoid space)

Ventricular application of chemical
  1. Injection into the lateral ventricle, third ventricle, or fourth ventricle
  2. Chronic intraventricular infusion
  3. Perfusion of different parts of the cerebral ventricles

Application of chemical to brain parenchyma
  1. Crystalline substance deposited
  2. Crystals fused to needle that is removable
  3. Injection of microliter volume of drug solution
  4. Push–pull perfusion of drug solution
  5. Iontophoresis

one procedure over another depends principally on the level of resolution at which the problem is to be tackled. From a functional standpoint, the procedures of injecting a chemical directly into the brain parenchyma and of perfusing an isolated region of tissue provide two very powerful analytical tools. There are several reasons for this.

When the chemical sensitivity of a single structure in the central nervous system to an endogenous or exogenous substance is being considered, these two methods can enable one to ascertain the substance's site of action. Further, in determining whether a substance can stand up to the multi-pronged criteria for consideration as a transmitter, the possibility of assessing its "identical action" is very real. By means of a push–pull perfusion, substances in the perfusate can be collected for subsequent assay. Thereby, the difficult criterion of "collectibility of a transmitter" (Werman, 1972) may be met similarly.

Substances that are not found in synaptic vesicles or storage granules of a nerve but yet are manufactured in the body may have a distinct action on the neuron. For example, a large literature indicates that neurons may alter their firing rate in response to a local change in plasma constituents such as sodium, a steroid, an amino acid, a pyrogen, CO_2, glucose, a peptide, or other factor. Furthermore, a certain nucleus in one part of the brain may contain a large number of individual neurons that may sense or monitor osmotic tension of the blood, the temperature of the blood, and even the hydrostatic pressure. Other chemodetectors have been implicated in the monitoring of hormone levels insofar as their roles in elaborating a specific releasing factor in the hypothalamic–hypophyseal axis are concerned. Overall, then, the mimicry of synaptic activity in a large group of neurons is perhaps the principal objective of delivering a specific chemical to a structure in the brain.

4.   PHARMACOLOGICAL APPROACH TO THE INTERNAL OR EXTERNAL SURFACE OF THE BRAIN

The most straightforward approach to bypassing the blood–brain barrier involves either application of a drug to the cerebral cortex or its injection into the ventricular cavity. The main difference between these techniques is the totally different anatomical substrates which are affected by the chemical compound.

In this section, we will consider the methods for injecting or perfusing drugs onto the surface of the cortex or within the ventricular system. The details of surgical cannulation and the specific techniques for carrying out this sort of experiment are described by Bureš and Burešová (1972) and by Myers (1972).

4.1. Drugs Applied to the Surface of the Cortex

In order to overcome some of the disadvantages of an irreversible ablation of the cerebral cortex, a number of workers have attempted to produce a reversible lesion by applying a drug to a small area of tissue. An almost ideal technique for such an ablation is one that provides a fully reversible lesion and at the same time is controllable from a temporal standpoint.

Since Leão's (1944) discovery of the marked decrease of local electrical activity, termed "spreading depression," that follows an electrical or mechanical disturbance, Bureš and his coworkers have continued to study the effect of a concentrated solution of KCl on the cerebral cortex of the rat. A temporary functional ablation is produced, characterized by a disseminating wave of electrical negativity (Bureš and Burešová, 1972).

The solution is applied after the animal is prepared with a cylindrical cup cemented to the skull. After a trephine opening is made with a dental bur, a cotton sponge soaked in saline is inserted and a cap is screwed onto the cup. For applying the drug topically, the cap is simply removed and either a small circle of filter paper or a cotton pledget saturated with KCl or other drug solution is applied to the surface of the dura. When an animal such as a rat is to be used for a long-term experiment, a microinjection technique has been found to be equally suitable. In this case, a guide cannula is inserted about a millimeter below the skull and a microinjection needle is lowered through the guide so that it passes 0.5–1.5 mm below the pia–arachnoid membrane. After a volume of 0.5 μl of a drug is infused, the solution spreads up to the surface of the cortex, disperses there, and exerts an effect. The main advantage of this technique is that the danger of infection in the chronic preparation is reduced considerably (Bureš and Burešová, 1972).

Another notable use of placing a drug onto cortical tissue has been to examine how a toxic material evokes the development of an epileptogenic focus. In this case, a compound such as alumina cream, penicillin, or crystalline cobalt is inserted into the trephine hole and a piece of gelfoam is then placed over the compound, after which the skin is sutured so that the animal can be maintained chronically. The simplicity of this procedure makes it very useful for investigating the mechanisms of a seizure focus in a large number of animals.

In general, much of the pharmacological and endocrinological research involving the topical application of a drug to the cerebral cortex has been devoted to the study of the effects of functional decortication on memory consolidation and other phenomena of learning and retention. The process of transfer of training from one cerebral hemisphere to the other with a reversible "split-brain" preparation and the stages of recovery following a unilateral or bilateral decortication produced by KCl have been widely scrutinized.

4.2. Administration of a Drug into the Cerebral Ventricles

Perhaps the most complete documentation of experiments on the action of compounds injected into the cerebral ventricles is that of Feldberg (1963). In an extraordinary account of his experiments, Feldberg presents the philosophy, the technique, and a vivid description of many fascinating experiments which opened up whole new vistas in CNS physiology.

The procedure for making an acute injection into a cerebral ventricle or the cisterna magna not only will depend on the species but also will vary according to the site of injection. In every case, the stereotaxic landmarks must be determined before the surgery is undertaken. Ordinarily, a stainless steel needle is simply inserted stereotaxically into the ventricular lumen or cisterna magna, and the injection made. This procedure has been utilized by many investigators in the examination of abnormal electrical potentials, respiratory physiology, and cardiovascular function.

To follow a specific action of a particular drug over a long period of time requires the repeated injection of a solution into the ventricular lumen. A permanent cannula such as that devised by L. Collison (see Feldberg, 1963), or a modification thereof, is most essential. A special feature of this cannula is the side opening, which prevents damage to the choroid plexus when it is implanted.

In order to eliminate any possible effect of the biologically active fluid (Feldberg *et al.*, 1970) always present in the hub and tube of the Collison cannula, an open-ended guide tube can be implanted at the surface of the ventricle or just above the lumen itself (Myers, 1971). As shown in Fig. 1, an inner injector cannula is inserted through this guide to a depth at which the solution will flow in readily without any evidence of back pressure greater than that produced by the CSF. By this procedure, the probability is much greater that only the drug contained in the solution will be dispersed in the ventricular cavity. A cannula through which an injection into the cisterna magna can be made repeatedly in the conscious cat has also been devised (Feldberg *et al.*, 1970).

A difficulty with the permanently implanted cannula is the ever-present question of its patency. Should it become blocked, the injected fluid will simply pass upward around the external surface and into the subarachnoid space along the surface of the cortex. Confusing and perhaps misleading results are then obtained. Therefore, several basic adaptations of the single-cannula technique have been advanced. The multiple cannulation procedure for a chronic preparation has a distinct advantage in that the animal does not have to be eliminated from the investigation should an occlusion take place in one cannula. Instead, a contralateral or other cannula can be used and the animal can be retained in one's study.

Today, many types of experiments are carried out in which the ventricular approach is successful. Many pharmaceutical houses have set up

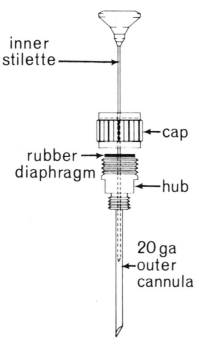

FIG. 1. A modified Collison cannula, in which the threaded segment at the base of the hub permits the cannula to be screwed into the skull. The inner stylet (shown) or injector cannula is lowered through the holes in the top surface of the cap. A rubber diaphragm, cut from the septum of a gas chromatograph, is inserted between the cap and the Collison hub to maintain a fluid- and airtight seal. From Myers (1971).

laboratories in which autonomic, cardiovascular, or other drugs are given by the ventricular route in order to examine their generalized action on the central nervous system. Other important areas of research include studies of endogenous factors present in the brain, blood-borne factors such as angiotensin, and essential cations. In addition, the ventricular route is now being used extensively for labeling the stores in neurons that contain biogenic amines so that the rate of amine synthesis, release, and turnover can be examined. The function of these same neurons can also be impaired by a partially selective lesioning agent such as 6-hydroxydopamine or 5,6-dihydroxytryptamine administered by way of the ventricular route or cisterna magna (Breese, Chap. 7, Vol. 1). Altogether, the ventricular route is probably the most advantageous with respect to administering a compound continuously via a chronic infusion system (Myers, 1963). This permits continual dispersion of a drug, and, if a small volume is delivered, toxic side reactions do not arise.

Frequently, any criticism of an experiment which utilizes ventricular injection dwells on one point: the question of anatomical localization.

However, if a small volume is injected in a lateral ventricle, the contralateral ventricle and other parts are not reached by the drug, at least in a concentration which would be pharmacologically active. As a first step, therefore, the ventricular approach is a most utilitarian one. Time and again, an experimental result based on this technique has led to an important discovery about the action of a given compound. Although a substance can have a different effect at a site in brain tissue, the ventricular approach nevertheless provides a provisional scaffolding of neuropharmacological information (Myers, 1974).

4.3. Perfusion of Brain Surfaces

Two principles are involved in the perfusion of the cerebral cortex or the ventricular cavity. First, such a perfusion offers a unique way for maintaining an aberrant concentration of a drug or other chemical compound; thus an interval sufficiently long is provided so that a detailed experimental analysis can be undertaken. Second, the humoral activity of a very small portion of exposed cortex can be assayed by collection of the substance contained in the perfusate.

4.3.1. Superfusion of the Cortex

In the cortex superfusion procedure, a physiological solution is washed over a restricted region of the cortex in order to bathe the neurons in that area with the perfusion medium. As shown in Fig. 2, a superfusion chamber is a hollow cylinder, either screwed or cemented to the skull after a trephine opening has been made. For the chronic preparation, the cylinder usually rests very lightly on the surface of the pia–arachnoid membrane. After the dura mater has been dissected away, a tight-fitting cap is screwed onto the cylinder so that a sterile preparation is maintained. A superfusion reservoir can be constructed from teflon, nylon, or stainless steel.

The specific procedure for perfusion will depend on the scientific question that is raised. Ordinarily, aseptic precautions are taken in the case of the chronic preparation. Further, a single-channel infusion pump, which provides a constant rate of inflow, delivers the solution containing the test drug, and the outflow is provided by the negative pressure of gravity. A cortical electrode can be placed inside the reservoir so that the changes in electrical potential that may arise during the superfusion can be monitored. If an anticholinesterase such as neostigmine is added to the perfusion medium, a change in the quantum release of acetylcholine from the surface of the cortex can be detected.

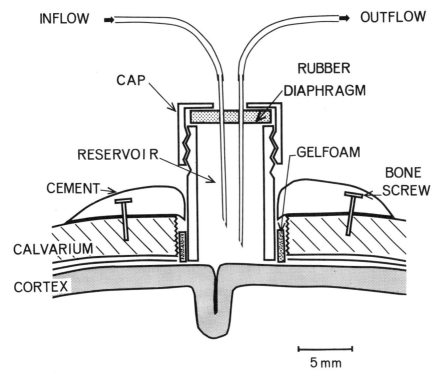

FIG. 2. Diagram of a stainless steel reservoir shown resting on the surface of the cerebral cortex. The dura mater has been excised to the edge of the craniotomy hole. Note that gelfoam is placed between the bone and the external wall of the reservoir in order to prevent the cranioplast cement from coming in contact with the bone or pia–arachnoid layer. By maintenance of equal rates of inflow and outflow, the cortex is bathed with the perfusion fluid without danger of a compression lesion. From Beleslin and Myers (1970).

4.3.2. Perfusion of the Cerebral Ventricles

Ventricular perfusion affords several advantages over a simple injection of a drug into the ventricle. First, by using cannulae implanted in an array as shown in Fig. 3, a regional perfusion of rather remarkable precision can be accomplished. For example, when the perfusion is restricted to the anterior horn of a lateral ventricle, a compound can penetrate the ependymal wall and affect such structures as the caudate nucleus, the septum, and the olfactory gray matter. Similarly, perfusion of the inferior horn will enable the drug to reach the amygdala and a large portion of the hippocampus. By such a regional perfusion, a relatively quantitative estimate may be obtained pertaining to the anatomical locus of an effect of the compound under scrutiny.

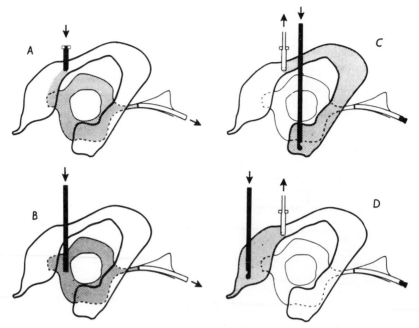

FIG. 3. Diagrams of the arrangement for perfusing the third ventricle (A, B) or the inferior (C) or anterior (D) horn of the left lateral ventricle of the anesthetized cat. From Feldberg and Myers (1966).

If the procedure is to be used for an analysis of the acute effect of a drug, then the principal consideration is once again the selection of accurate stereotaxic coordinates, which will, of course, depend on the species and the size of animal. When the preparation is tested repeatedly, each solution and the cannulae, glassware, and syringes must be rendered pyrogen free. Usually, a single set of these materials is assigned to a given animal to prevent immune responses from occurring. The chronically prepared animal can be used as its own control since the ventricular cavities can be tapped repeatedly. Furthermore, the walls of the cerebral ventricles will continue to retain their sensitivity to a drug for many weeks if the perfusions are repeated at 2- to 3-day intervals.

Just as we have seen with the cortical superfusion procedure, a distinct advantage of ventricular perfusion lies in the attainment of a steady-state change in the concentration of the drug or other chemical. As long as careful monitoring of pressure, occlusion, edema, and localized hemorrhage is maintained, the experiment can be completed without difficulty. Again, if an inner cannula is lowered through a permanently implanted guide tube, the chemical milieu of the ventricle can be repeatedly sampled by means of regional perfusion (Myers et al., 1971a). Figure 4 shows the cannula configuration for a monkey.

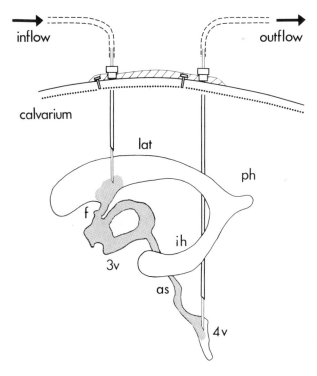

Fig. 4. Diagram in the sagittal plane, of the perfusion from the
left lateral ventricle to the fourth ventricle. Shaded area indicates
the path which perfusate may take between the two cannulae.
Abbreviations: as, aqueduct of Sylvius; f, foramen of Monro; ih,
inferior horn of lateral ventricle; lat, lateral ventricle; ph,
posterior horn of lateral ventricle; 3v, third ventricle; 4v, fourth
ventricle. From Myers *et al.* (1971a).

Certain very elaborate systems for perfusing the ventricles of large
animals have been developed by Pappenheimer *et al.* (1962), Ashcroft *et al.*
(1968), and others. With these systems, the pressure of the cerebrospinal
fluid can be continuously monitored and the inflow regulated by the volume
of outflow. In addition, it is possible to recirculate CSF by means of a
peristaltic pump. Fluid collected from the cisterna is returned to the lateral
ventricle.

Finally, the sites reached by the drug or from which a neurally active
substance is released can be verified anatomically by switching the perfusion
medium from the artificial CSF to a solution such as bromophenol blue.
When this dye is perfused at the same rate as the original perfusate, it is
taken up evenly by the cerebral parenchyma. If left in contact with the tissue
for 30 min or longer, deep blue staining of all the structures occurs.

Following the blunt dissection of the cerebrum with a spatula and scalpel, the anatomical region of perfusion can be verified readily. After sufficient practice, the entire ventricular cavity of a cerebral hemisphere can be laid open with a single stroke of a scalpel blade.

5. DRUGS ADMINISTERED TO THE BRAIN PARENCHYMA

As is described in the *Handbook of Drug and Chemical Stimulation of the Brain* (Myers, 1974), well over a thousand studies have been published in which a drug or other chemical was applied directly to the brain parenchyma. This procedure is now widely used among behavioral physiologists, endocrinologists, neuropharmacologists, and other scientists who are interested in altering the chemical milieu of a distinct structure in the brain. The rationale for this is essentially threefold. First, the concentration of a substance occurring naturally in that structure can be artificially elevated by injecting it at a concentration higher than normal. Second, substances including peptides and steroids that are synthesized systemically can be tested for the possibility of action on a specific part of the brain. Third, a drug with a suspected central action can be tested at different sites in order to ascertain whether or not it has such an action and, if so, which region is affected.

The underlying principle of each of the techniques to be described revolves about neuroanatomical specificity. That is, a chemical analysis of individual anatomical regions is the hallmark of the field of chemical stimulation. Largely as a result of the morphological mapping of responses to a given compound, it is now certain that neurons in the forebrain and midbrain contain (1) membranes that are sensitive to a chemical, (2) specialized receptors which recognize the presence of the molecule of a specific class of substances, (3) a mechanism whereby a group of cells is able to be excited or inhibited in synchrony, and (4) a selectivity which enables some neurons within the structure to be excited while others remain at a resting discharge rate.

5.1. Injection of Solution

At present, there are more than two dozen kinds of cannulae and/or cannula systems that have been devised for the delivery into tissue of a chemical in solution (see Myers, 1974, for review). One reason this procedure is selected so often is that a number of controls can be used. If the volume of a solution injected is sufficiently small, one can specify the following with some precision: (1) the local site of action, (2) the dose of the

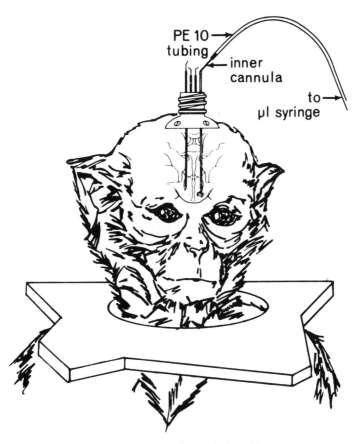

FIG. 5. Rhesus monkey acclimated to a primate chair and implanted chronically with a bilateral array of 22-gauge outer microinjection cannulae with tips resting in different regions of the hypothalamus. The 28-gauge inner injector cannula, which is attached to a microliter syringe via PE 10 tubing, is lowered to a depth 1 mm below the outer cannula. Injection of a chemical in solution in a volume of 0.5–1.0 μl enables precise localization of the chemical agent. From Sharpe and Myers (1969).

chemical which acts at a site, (3) the pH of the substance, (4) the temperature, (5) the osmolarity, and (6) the extent of diffusion. Figure 5 recapitulates diagrammatically the method itself.

The validity of any interpretation about the morphological specificity of a chemical's action depends entirely on histological localization of the site of injection. As one can readily imagine, if a volume greater than 2 or 3 μl is infused, the solution simply takes the path of least resistance and enters the ventricle or subarachnoid space. Unfortunately, hundreds of research reports are based on experiments in which a volume greater than 1.0 or 2.0 μl of solution was delivered. Even today, after all of the published cautions about the devastating effect of a large volume, some research workers continue to use necrotizing, disseminating, and nonlocalizable injection volumes.

When a microliter or less is infused, it is possible to map anatomically the specific sites of action of a given substance. This has been done repeatedly and with great success in many laboratories throughout the world (see Myers, 1974). However, any conclusion to be drawn about a research finding will depend on the punctiliousness with which each anatomical control is undertaken. For example, it is essential that a representative histological map of sections be constructed which displays the cannula track and the cytology of the locus of injection. Further, it is necessary to inject substances at other anatomical loci to rule out the possibility of irritation or nonspecificity. It is likewise essential to verify the extent of diffusion. Employing either a dye known to have some affinity for cerebral tissue (bromophenol blue) or a radioactive tracer is the most straightforward procedure (Myers, 1966; Myers, *et al.*, 1971a) (Fig. 6).

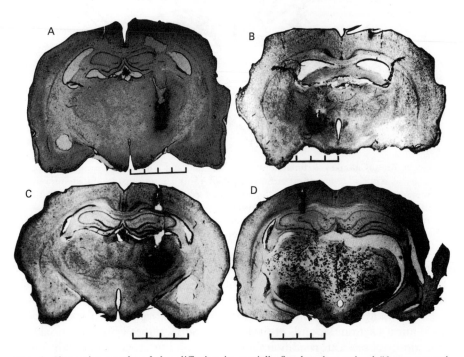

FIG. 6. Photomicrographs of dye diffusion in partially fixed and unstained 50-μm coronal sections of rat brain. (A) Evans blue, 0.5 μl at the border of the ventral thalamic nucleus and medial lemniscus. (B) Picric acid, 1.0 μl into the dorsolateral area of the hypothalamus. (C) Bromophenol blue, 2.0 μl into the lateral nuclear mass of the thalamus. (D) Evans blue, 3.0 μl into the ventral thalamic nucleus just dorsal to the zona incerta. Scale is in millimeters. From Myers (1966). Magnification ×5.

Ideally, the chemical is delivered in a balanced physiological salt solution with care being taken to bring the solution as close as possible to the level of isotonicity. The use of a carrier vehicle such as 0.9% NaCl as a control solution is not recommended simply because this salt causes marked changes in an animal's temperature, water intake, and even emotional state when it is delivered at certain sites in the diencephalon (Veale and Myers, 1971).

Another important aspect in this field is the imperative usage of a dose–response analysis. Although this is a complicated issue, suffice it to say that there are many examples in the physiological literature which show that a low dose of a compound injected at a site will evoke a specific response whereas a high dose will block the reaction. Such a blockade may be due to a regional hyperpolarization, a total swamping of the receptor sites, or some other local effect inhibiting the response. For example, the frequently used cholinomimetic carbachol can evoke a focal seizure when applied to neurons in the brain stem.

Finally, if one wants to make some functional sense of the reaction to a specific chemical compound, it is helpful to know how a pharmacological antagonist will alter the response. Notwithstanding the artificiality of the agents that are now used peripherally to block the autonomic ganglia, the use of the same antagonist may aid in the delineation of the role of a given chemical in an anatomical pathway. Clearly, the exclusive use of a synthetic agonist and antagonist in some combination for chemical stimulation is illusory and misleading.

5.2. Depositing a Chemical in Crystalline Form

Largely because of the unphysiological concentration and level of tonicity, some pharmacologists deprecate the use of crystals or salts of a compound that are deposited directly into the brain parenchyma. However, the use of a chemical in solid form is justified on three premises. First, it is the only recourse when a virtually insoluble substance such as a steroid hormone is to be examined. Second, some chemical compounds diffuse to a lesser degree than a liquid when placed in the brain parenchyma; hence anatomical localization is, in some instances, more feasible. Third, it is more convenient insofar as benchwork preparation is concerned than the injection of a solution (albeit convenience and science have no relationship).

A number of clever procedures for cannulation have been developed including those for (1) delivering crystals at different depths, (2) ejecting a pellet at any time in the course of an experiment, and (3) fusing crystalline hormone to different-size chemitrodes. A crude way of specifying the dose of crystal has been designated as the "one-tap or three-tap" method (see Myers, 1974, for review).

A number of vehicles have been employed for the delivery of a solid chemical to brain tissue. To prevent the rapid dissolution of a steroid, the compound can be dissolved in cocoa butter, which has a convenient melting point of 35°C, agar, paraffin wax, talc, gum arabic, or phenol. In addition, to prevent the crystalline material from being dislodged as it is lowered to a target site, a film of saturated sucrose or other material can be applied at the cannula tip. Eserine has been used frequently as a capping over an implant of acetylcholine to prevent its metabolic degradation.

Five general problems arise when a solid chemical is delivered to brain tissue. First, it is virtually impossible to render a crystal or pellet pyrogen free, since many of the commonly used test substances degrade on prolonged heating. Second, because osmotic tension and pH cannot be controlled, substances of equal physical characteristics must be tested. Third, with repeated usage, the cytology of the target site will change because of necrosis and hence affect the dissolution of the crystal when it touches the brain tissue. Fourth, a definitive dose–response curve is almost impossible to obtain with a crystalline implant. Therefore, in a test in which a pharmacological antagonist should be matched quantitatively against the corresponding agonist, the crystalline implant will yield great variability. Fifth, with the use of an unbuffered chemical, there is probably a greater danger of affecting the closely knit network of capillaries as well as the membrane structure of neurons and neuroglia contiguous to the implant.

5.3. Isolated Perfusion with Push–Pull Cannulae

A principal limitation of any procedure in which a chemical is applied to one of the surfaces of the brain or directly into the interstitial space pertains to the duration of stimulation and its control. That is, the rate of dissolution, penetration into tissue, and metabolic degradation will determine the temporal course of the chemical's action. Moreover, in contrast to the electrical stimulation of a punctate region, a so-called chemical stimulus cannot be turned off or on at the experimenter's discretion. The technique of perfusing an isolated portion of cerebral tissue within a circumscribed structure may go far to resolve these difficulties.

There are several clear-cut advantages of the procedure of push–pull perfusion as summarized by Myers (1972). Since the solution is drawn off at the same rate as it is perfused or pumped in, the stimulating characteristics of the drug can be determined quickly. Second, a chemical or a drug can be maintained at a very precise and usually quite low concentration because the neurons are bathed continuously during perfusion. Third, the extent of diffusion can be delimited equally as well as the concentration of the chemical. Fourth, tests have shown that 85–95% of the constituents delivered in the push perfusate are recovered in the pull effluent.

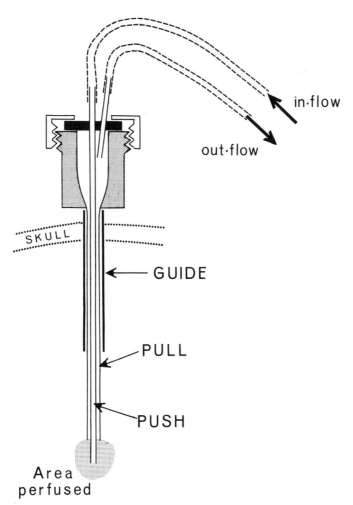

FIG. 7. Position of the push–pull cannulae after being lowered into a permanently implanted guide tube. Perfusate from the push syringe is pumped into the inflow tube through the inner push cannula to the tip, where a spherical area of tissue (1.5 mm diameter) is perfused (shading). The perfusate is immediately withdrawn, at the same flow rate, into the space between the push and pull cannulae and thence into the body of the pull cannula. In the outflow tube, the perfusate flows back into the pull syringe. The diagram is not to scale because of the smallness of some of the parts. From Myers (1970).

Generally, the push–pull cannula assembly is constructed in a concentric manner (Myers, 1967), as shown in Fig. 7. That is, the smaller push cannula rests inside the pull cannula, which has a much larger inside diameter, thus providing a clear passageway for withdrawal of the effluent. The alternative cannula configuration is the side-by-side version pioneered by Delgado (1966), in which the push and pull tubes are cemented together in parallel fashion with their tips adjacent to one another. However, the concentric cannula system is more widely used because the lesion produced by such a configuration is usually smaller, the localization is more circumscribed, and the changes of an occlusion are reduced (Myers, 1970).

By employing a removable push–pull cannula assembly, it is now possible to perfuse at different depths. Within a single guide tube, the raising or lowering of the cannulae to a different site will provide ordinarily a very satisfactory anatomical control. Such a removable push–pull cannula assembly has been used successfully for altering the cation levels in circumscribed regions of the diencephalon of the cat or monkey (see Myers, 1974). In addition to its usage for chemical stimulation, the push–pull perfusion method has been employed successfully for the collection of substances that are released by neurons in the mesencephalon and diencephalon, again in the cat or monkey (see Myers, 1972).

Finally, the large lesion normally produced in former times by any push–pull perfusion procedure has been largely if not entirely overcome by the use of a precision infusion withdrawal pump that is calibrated so that inflow and outflow volumes are identical. The procedure of using gravity for the pull side of the system, although inexpensive, is a weak tradeoff for the pump, particularly in view of the massive lesions ordinarily produced by unequal flow rates.

6. CONCLUDING COMMENT

A final thought pertaining to all of the methods for bypassing the blood–brain barrier is the persistent question about the high dose of a chemical that is usually required to evoke a specific response. This situation is particularly applicable to any experiment with a biogenic amine, in that the dose used frequently exceeds the amount of the substance found endogenously in the cerebral structure. Figure 8 provides one of several answers to this difficult question. Considering the fact that the specific receptors on the membrane that are sensitive to a given compound comprise a very tiny portion of all the anatomical elements, only a minute amount of the chemical would actually reach the target sites. The rest of the solution would disperse in the interstitial space and be lost among the glia, the capillaries, and the nonsensitive parts of the neurons. Altogether, the significant issue is always the magnitude of drug dose that alters the threshold of neuronal activity. Because of the current limitations of our chemical technology at the ultrastructural level, it is still impossible to specify this quantity in terms of nanograms per picogram of nerve receptor protein.

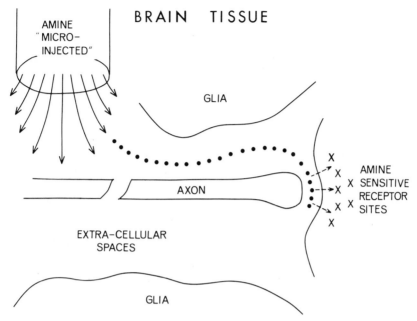

FIG. 8. A theoretical diagram to explain why a high pharmacological concentration of a neurotransmitter such as an amine is required to produce a physiological response, e.g., hyperthermia or hypothermia. When an amine is microinjected into brain tissue, it diffuses in every direction throughout the extracellular fluid spaces onto glia and around axons and other nerve processes. Only the smallest fraction of the amine reaches (• • •) the amine-sensitive receptor sites at a postsynaptic membrane to activate a neuron involved in a specific physiological system, e.g., a thermoregulatory function. From Myers (1974).

7. REFERENCES

ALBANUS, L., AQUILONIUS, S.-M., SUNDWALL, A., and WINBLADH, B., 1969, The fate of intracerebroventricular injection of atropine and methylatropine in relation to their pharmacological effects, *Acta Pharmacol. Toxicol.* **27**:81–96.

AMES, A., III, HIGASHI, K., and NESBETT, F. B., 1965, Relation of potassium concentration in choroid-plexus fluid to that in plasma, *J. Physiol.* **181**:506–515.

ASHCROFT, G. W., DOW, R. C., and MOIR, A. T. B., 1968, The active transport of 5-hydroxyindol-3-ylacetic acid and 3-methoxy-4-hydroxyphenylacetic acid from a recirculatory perfusion system of the cerebral ventricles of the unanaesthetized dog, *J. Physiol.* **199**:397–425.

BASS, N. H., and LUNDBORG, P., 1973, Postnatal development of mechanisms for the rapid efflux of primary amines from the cerebrospinal fluid system of the rat: Elimination of [³H]metaraminol following intrathecal infusion, *Brain Res.* **53**:399–411.

BELESLIN, D. B., and MYERS, R. D., 1970, A technique for repeated superfusion or withdrawal of fluid from the exposed cerebral cortex of a conscious animal, *Physiol. Behav.* **5**:1173–1175.

BRIGHTMAN, M. W., KLATZO, I., OLSSON, Y., and REESE, T. S., 1970, The blood–brain barrier to proteins under normal and pathological conditions, *J. Neurol. Sci.* **10**:215–239.

BRØNDSTED, H. E., 1970a, Transport of glucose, sodium, chloride and potassium between the cerebral ventricles and surrounding tissues in cats, *Acta Physiol. Scand.* **79:**523–532

BRØNDSTED, H. E., 1970b, Exchange of glucose between plasma, brain extracellular fluid and cerebral ventricles in cats and effects of intraventricular acetazolamide and insulin, *Acta Physiol. Scand.* **80:**122–130.

BUREŠ, J., and BUREŠOVÁ, O., 1972, Inducing cortical spreading depression, in: *Methods in Psychobiology*, Vol. 2 (R. D. Myers, ed.), pp. 319–343, Academic Press, London.

CRONE, C., 1961, *Om Diffusion of nogle organiske Non-elekrolytter fra Blod til Hjernevaev*, Munksgaard, Copenhagen. [In Danish, with summary in English.]

CRONE, C., 1965, Facilitated transfer of glucose from blood into brain tissue, *J. Physiol.* **181:**103–113.

CSERR, H. F., 1971, Physiology of the choroid plexus, *Physiol. Rev.* **51(2):**273–311.

CURL, F. D., and POLLAY, M., 1968, Transport of water and electrolytes between brain and ventricular fluid in the rabbit, *Exp. Neurology* **20(4):**558–574.

DA SILVA, F. H. L., and SPROULL, D. H., 1964, Systemic absorption of adrenaline from the cerebral fluid spaces of the cat., *J. Physiol.* **171:**494–503.

DAVSON, H., 1963, The cerebrospinal fluid, *Ergebn. Physiol.* **52:**20–73.

DAVSON, H., and POLLAY, M., 1963, Influence of various drugs on the transport of ^{131}I and PAH across the cerebrospinal-fluid–blood barrier, *J. Physiol.* **167:**239–246.

DAVSON, H., and WELCH, K., 1971, The permeation of several materials into the fluids of the rabbit's brain, *J. Physiol.* **218:**337–351.

DELGADO, J. M. R., 1966, Intracerebral perfusion in awake monkeys, *Arch. Int. Pharmacodyn. Ther.* **161:**442–462.

DOGGETT, N. S., and SPENCER, P. S. J., 1972, Ouabain and the onset of the blood–brain barrier in neonate chicks, *Nature* **237:**513–514.

EDVINSSON, L., NIELSEN, K. C., OWMAN, C., and WEST, K. A., 1971, Alterations in intracranial pressure, blood–brain barrier, and brain edema after sub-chronic implantation of a cannula into the brain of conscious animals, *Acta Physiol. Scand.* **82:**527–531.

EIST, H., and SEAL, U. S., 1965, The permeability of the blood–brain barrier (BBB) and blood–cerebrospinal fluid barrier (BLB) to C^{14} tagged ribonucleic acid (RNA), *Am. J. Psychiat.* **122:**584–586.

FELDBERG, W., 1963, *A Pharmacological Approach to the Brain from Its Inner and Outer Surface*, Edward Arnold, London.

FELDBERG, W., and MYERS, R. D., 1966, Appearance of 5-hydroxytryptamine and an unidentified pharmacologically active lipid acid in effluent from perfused cerebral ventricles, *J. Physiol.* **184:**837–855.

FELDBERG, W., MYERS, R. D., and VEALE, W. L., 1970, Perfusion from cerebral ventricle to cisterna magna in the unanaesthetized cat: Effect of calcium on body temperature, *J. Physiol.* **207:**403–416.

FLEISCHHAUER, K., 1961, Regional differences in the structure of the ependyma and subependymal layers of the cerebral ventricles of the cat, in: *Regional Neurochemistry* (S. Kety and J. Elkes, eds.), pp. 279–283, Pergamon Press, London.

FÖLDI-BÖRCSÖK, E., and FÖLDI, M., 1973, Permeability of the blood-brain-barrier in lymphostatic encephalopathy combined with complex vitamin B deficiency: The protective effect of vitamin (factor) P treatment, *Experientia* **29:**985–987.

KLATZO, I., MIQUEL, J., FERRIS, P. J., PROKOP, J. D., and SMITH, D. E., 1964, Observations on the passage of the fluorescein labeled serum proteins (FLSP) from the cerebrospinal fluid, *J. Neuropathol. Exp. Neurol.* **23:**18–35.

KOCSIS, J. J., HARKAWAY, S., and VOGEL, W. H., 1968, Dimethyl sulfoxide: Breakdown of blood–brain barrier? *Science* **160:**1472–1473.

LAJTHA, A., and TOTH, J., 1963, The brain barrier system. V. Stereospecificity of amino acid uptake, exchange and efflux, *J. Neurochem.* **10:**909–920.

LEÃO, A. A. P., 1944, Spreading depression of activity in the cerebral cortex, *J. Neurophysiol.* **7**:359–398.

LEE, J. C., and OLSZEWSKI, J., 1960, Penetration of radioactive bovine albumin from cerebrospinal fluid into brain tissue, *Neurology* **10**:814–822.

LEVIN, E., and SCICLI, G., 1969, Brain barrier phenomena, *Brain Res.* **13**:1–12.

LEVIN, E., and SISSON, W. B., 1972, The penetration of radiolabeled substances into rabbit brain from subarachnoid space, *Brain Res.* **41**:145–153.

LIVINGSTON, R. B., 1960, Cerebrospinal fluid, in: *Medical Physiology and Biophysics*, 18th ed. (T. C. Ruch and J. F. Fulton, eds.), pp. 889–902, Saunders, Philadelphia and London.

MILHORAT, T. H., DAVIS, D. A., and LLOYD, B. J., Jr., 1973, Two morphologically distinct blood–brain barriers preventing entry of cytochrome *c* into cerebrospinal fluid, *Science* **180**:76–78.

MYERS, R. D., 1963, An intracranial chemical stimulation system for chronic or self-infusion. *J. Appl. Physiol.* **18**:221–223.

MYERS, R. D., 1966, Injection of solutions into cerebral tissue: Relation between volume and diffusion, *Physiol. Behav.* **1**:171–174.

MYERS, R. D., 1967, Transfusion of cerebrospinal fluid and tissue bound chemical factors between the brains of conscious monkeys: A new neurobiological assay, *Physiol. Behav.* **2**:373–377.

MYERS, R. D., 1970, An improved push–pull cannula system for perfusing an isolated region of the brain, *Physiol. Behav.* **5**:243–246.

MYERS, R. D., 1971, Methods for chemical stimulation of the brain, in: *Methods in Psychobiology*, Vol. 1 (R. D. Myers, ed.), pp. 247–280, Academic Press, London.

MYERS, R. D., 1972, Methods for perfusing different structures of the brain, in: *Methods in Psychobiology*, Vol. 2 (R. D. Myers, ed.), pp. 169–211, Academic Press, London.

MYERS, R. D., 1974, *Handbook of Drug and Chemical Stimulation of the Brain*, Van Nostrand Reinhold, New York.

MYERS, R. D., YAKSH, T. L., HALL, G. H., and VEALE, W. L., 1971a, A method for perfusion of cerebral ventricles of the conscious monkey, *J. Appl. Physiol.* **30**:589–592.

MYERS, R. D., TYTELL, M., KAWA, A., and RUDY, T., 1971b, Micro-injection of ^{3}H-acetylcholine, ^{14}C-serotonin and ^{3}H-norepinephrine into the hypothalamus of the rat: Diffusion into tissue and ventricles, *Physiol. Behav.* **7**:743–751.

NEMOTO, E. M., and SEVERINGHAUS, J. W., 1971, The stereospecific influx permeability of rat blood–brain barrier (BBB) to lactic acid (LA), *Clin. Res.* **19**:146 (abst.).

OLDENDORF, W. H., 1971, Brain uptake of radiolabeled amino acids, amines, and hexoses after arterial injection, *Am. J. Physiol.* **221**:1629–1639.

OLDENDORF, W. H., 1973a, Carrier-mediated blood–brain barrier transport of short-chain monocarboxylic organic acids, *Am. J. Physiol.* **224**:1450–1453.

OLDENDORF, W. H., 1973b, Stereospecificity of blood–brain barrier permeability to amino acids, *Am. J. Physiol.* **224**:967–969.

OLDENDORF, W. H., HYMAN, S., BRAUN, L., and OLDENDORF, S. Z., 1972, Blood–brain barrier: Penetration of morphine, codeine, heroin, and methadone after carotid injection, *Science* **178**:984–986.

PAPPENHEIMER, J. R., HEISEY, S. R., JORDAN, E. F., and DOWNER, J. deC., 1962, Perfusion of the cerebral ventricular system in unanaesthesized goats, *Am. J. Physiol.* **203**:763–774.

PARDRIDGE, W. M., CRAWFORD, I. L., and CONNOR, J. D., 1973, Permeability changes in the blood-brain barrier induced by nortriptyline and chlorpromazine, *Toxicol. Appl. Pharmacol.* **26**:49–57.

RAPOPORT, S. I., HORI, M., and KLATZO, I., 1971, Reversible osmotic opening of the blood–brain barrier, *Science* **173**:1026–1028.

RAPOPORT, S. I., HORI, M., and KLATZO, I., 1972, Testing of a hypothesis for osmotic opening of the blood–brain barrier, *Am. J. Physiol.* **223**:323–331.

SHARPE, L. G., and MYERS, R. D., 1969, Feeding and drinking following stimulation of the diencephalon of the monkey with amines and other substances, *Exp. Brain Res.* **8:**295–310.

SOLOWAY, A. H., 1958, Correlation of drug penetration of brain and chemical structure, *Science* **128:**1572–1574.

VEALE, W. L., and MYERS, R. D., 1971, Emotional behavior, arousal and sleep produced by sodium and calcium ions perfused within the hypothalamus of the cat, *Physiol. Behav.* **7:**601–607.

VOLICER, L., and LOEW, C. G., 1971, Penetration of angiotensin II into the brain, *Neuropharmacology* **10:**631–636.

WANG, J. H., and TAKEMORI, A. E., 1972, Studies on the transport of morphine out of the perfused cerebral ventricles of rabbits, *J. Pharmacol. Exp. Ther.* **181:**46–52.

WERMAN, R., 1972, CNS cellular level: Membranes, *Ann. Rev. Physiol.* **34:**337–374.

2

MICROIONTOPHORETIC APPLICATION OF DRUGS ONTO SINGLE NEURONS

John S. Kelly

1. INTRODUCTION

To many of us, the ultimate test of transmitter identity is the demonstration that a putative transmitter substance when applied to a single neuron has the ability to mimic the effects of the naturally occurring transmitter. It follows, therefore, that a great deal of ingenuity has been devoted to developing techniques which leave the neural elements of the tissue intact and yet allow test substances to be applied directly onto the neurons for which they are believed to have an affinity. Ideally, the application should be restricted to the postjunctional receptors, or at least to the synaptic regions of the neuron thought to be operated by the transmitter under study. Often, however, we are content to apply our substances into the rough vicinity of the neuron, perhaps as much as 30–60 μm from the neural membrane. This technique also has an attraction for pharmacologists since substances thought to act in a specific fashion at a particular synapse can be tested directly for their ability to antagonize, potentiate, or mimic the actions of the naturally occurring transmitter. This chapter is therefore primarily concerned with the techniques used to eject pharmacologically active agents into the extracellular space of neurons with fine glass microelectrodes (Fig. 1).

John S. Kelly●M.R.C. Neurochemical Pharmacology Unit, Department of Pharmacology, Medical School, Cambridge University, Cambridge, England

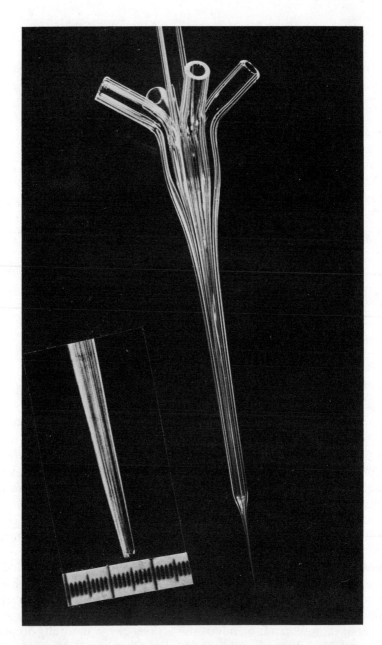

Fig. 1. Five-barreled microelectrode pulled from glass blank prepared by Wesley Coe Ltd., Cambridge, England. The insert is a photomicrograph of the microelectrode tip and a graticule scale showing 2-μm graduations.

2. BASIC PRINCIPLES

Since the basic principles and the techniques used in microiontophoresis have changed very little since the early review by Curtis (1964), and the latest technical innovations have been described in reviews by Krnjević (1972), Bloom (1974), and Kelly *et al.* (1975) and in an account of a symposium edited by Bradley *et al.* (1974), I will confine myself to restating the basic principles and drawing attention to some of the difficulties which can easily be overlooked when discussing the outcome of experiments based on microiontophoresis.

Although strictly speaking the term "microiontophoresis" should be restricted to the use of current of the appropriate polarity to eject a substance as ions from the tip of fine microelectrodes filled with a concentrated solution of the substance in an ionized form (Curtis, 1964), I, like many others, will use it to describe all techniques which involve the ejection of substances such as drugs and dyes from fine microelectrodes. Habit rather than prejudice has prevented me from adopting the term "microelectrophoresis," which Curtis has suggested avoids the impression that only ionized substances can be ejected from microelectrodes. Nevertheless, most drugs ejected from a microelectrode are ionized and are forced from the tip of the microelectrode by the passage of current in the appropriate direction. Accordingly, cations flow out through the tip of the microelectrode when the current is said to be "positive"; i.e., the inside of the electrode is made positive with respect to the extracellular medium, and current in the reverse direction (negative) causes anions to leave the microelectrode. Only rarely have I heard the "positive" and "negative" currents referred to as "cationic" and "anionic," as they were named by Curtis (1964). A potential of opposite polarity must also be used to prevent the efflux of ions from the microelectrode when it is not in use. This potential and the resultant current are also known by a variety of names, and although "retaining current" is preferred by Curtis (1964), the terms "backing" and "braking" are often used for these voltages or currents. Although it is customary to discuss the mechanisms involved in iontophoretic ejection before those involved in spontaneous release, recent developments that have shown these processes to interact make it more convenient for me to discuss them in the reverse order.

2.1. Spontaneous Efflux of Active Material from Microelectrodes

Although the spontaneous leakage of active materials from microelectrodes has always been recognized as an undesirable feature of the technique, it has often been disregarded on the basis that the leakage is eliminated by the application of a "retaining current," i.e., a voltage or current of opposite polarity to that used to eject the active ion from the electrode (Curtis, 1964). Although there is no doubt that the spontaneous efflux of material from the electrode tip can be effectively controlled by "retaining currents," it now appears that these currents do not simply counteract the diffusional forces but effectively denude the fluid inside the electrode tip of their active content. Only by the creation of a pool of extremely dilute solution immediately inside the tip can the retaining current offset the continuous flow of fluid from the tip of the electrode caused by the hydrostatic pressure created by the column of fluid standing in the vertically held microelectrode. Although, in general, the existence of a pool of inert liquid inside the tip of the microelectrode is of little conse-quence, it can under certain experimental situations become excessively large and cause the amount of active ions released by subsequent applica-tions of iontophoretic current to be reduced to a negligible amount (Bradshaw et al., 1973b).

2.1.1. Bulk Flow

The actual importance of bulk flow, the flow caused by hydrostatic pressure, was first emphasized by Krnjević et al. (1963b), who found that in the absence of a retaining current the spontaneous efflux of acetylcholine from a large number of microelectrodes was correlated with the resistance of the microelectrodes measured in megohms (Fig. 2). Furthermore, the experimental results fitted a theoretical curve which related the diffusional release to only two parameters, the concentration of acetylcholine in the microelectrodes and the physcial shape of the microelectrode tips. On this basis, they suggested that the spontaneous efflux of acetylcholine from a microelectrode was not only the result of a diffusion of ions from the highly concentrated solution within the electrode out into the external medium devoid of such ions but also the result of bulk flow from the tip of the electrode.

The theory therefore declared that the rate of spontaneous release (Q) from a microelectrode tip is the sum of two components, Q_D and Q_F, the rates of diffusion and bulk flow, respectively:

$$Q = Q_D + Q_F \tag{1}$$

By making rather simple assumptions about the shape of the electrode tip and characterizing it in terms of r_i, the radius of the opening at the tip, and θ, the angle of taper, Q_D should be directly proportional to the concentration (C_i) and diffusion coefficient (D) of the solution inside the shaft of the microelectrode:

$$Q_D = C_i D \pi \tan \theta r_i \tag{2}$$

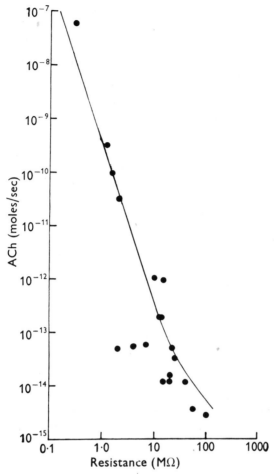

FIG. 2. Spontaneous flux of acetylcholine from micro-pipettes with different electrical resistances, plotted on log-log paper. Points are experimental observations, while line gives values predicted theoretically by equation (4) from the tip resistances. From Krnjević et al. (1963b).

The same assumptions about shape also allowed Krnjević et al. (1963b) to show the bulk flow to be proportional to the hydrostatic pressure (p^*) and inversely proportional to the viscosity (η) of the solution inside the tip of the electrode:

$$Q_F = C_i\, 3\pi \tan \theta p^* r_i^3 (8\eta)^{-1} \tag{3}$$

Therefore,

$$Q = \pi \tan \theta C_i [Dr_i + 3p^* r_i^3 (8\eta)^{-1}] \tag{4}$$

Unfortunately, r_i, the internal radius of the orifice immediately inside the tip, cannot be measured directly and an estimate must be made from measurements of the microelectrode resistance based on the assumption that the resistance (R) is proportional to the specific resistivity of the solution (ρ_i) contained in the microelectrode and inversely proportional to the internal diameter of the tip (r_i):

$$R = \rho_i(\pi \tan \theta r_i)^{-1} \qquad (5)$$

When the appropriate values of ρ_i, and θ for electrodes containing 3 M acetylcholine were substituted in equation (5), it simplified to

$$r_i = 3.09(R)^{-1} \qquad (6)$$

It appears, therefore, that both on theoretical grounds by inspection of equations (4) and (6) and on experimental grounds (Fig. 2) the spontaneous efflux of material from microelectrodes increases extremely rapidly as the internal radius of the tip increases. Indeed, even relatively small-tipped electrodes with orifices of between 0.03 and 0.3 μm and containing 3 M solutions will release spontaneously 0.05–5.0 pmol/s. However, this release will not, as often stated in the literature (Clarke et al., 1973; Bradshaw et al., 1973b), be solely a consequence of diffusion, but will also be the result of bulk flow. Krnjević et al. (1963b) suggested that the release due to bulk flow will often exceed the release by diffusion when the internal radius of the tip exceeds 0.125 μm and will account for over 90% of the release when the tip exceeds 0.4 μm. Surprisingly enough, the majority of studies on the release of radioactively labeled compounds from microelectrodes in the absence of a retaining current have ignored this distinction between diffusion and bulk flow. Clearly, the use of double isotope labeling techniques could resolve this problem by simultaneous measurement of the release of the test substance and labeled water. Lacking this information, we must assume that in the absence of a retaining current the average microelectrode with an internal tip diameter of between 0.03 and 0.3 μm will release material from its tip at a rate equivalent to an ejection of between 0.02 and 2×10^{-12} liter/s of the solution with which its shaft is filled. This theoretical value derived from equation (4) is in relatively good agreement with the experimental values given in Table 1 for a variety of substances and microelectrodes. The low spontaneous efflux reported by some authors is a direct consequence of the dilute solutions with which their microelectrodes were filled.

Unfortunately, the majority of workers mentioned in Table 1 did not report a value for the spontaneous release observed from their microelectrodes in the absence of a retaining current. Clarke et al. (1973), for instance, only mentioned in passing that the spontaneous release from some microelectrodes containing relatively low concentrations of [23]NaCl was

TABLE 1

Iontophoretic Release of Test Substances

Substance	Concentration (M)	pH	Polarity of ejecting current[a]	Transport number	Spontaneous release (pmol/s)	Reference
A. Model substances						
[24Na]Sodium chloride	1.65×10^{-1}			0.27–0.36	high	Clarke et al. (1973)
[14C]Sucrose	0.32 + 0.2 mM NaCl			70.4	0.016–2.43	Krnjević and Whittaker (1965)
B. Putative transmitters						
Acetylcholine	3.0			0.42	0.02–0.48	Krnjević et al. (1963b), Curtis (1964)
Acetylcholine	1.0			0.3–0.5		Curtis (1964)
[Me-3H]Acetylcholine	5.5×10^{-2}			0.24[b] 0.48[b]	0.002[b] 0.005[b]	Bradley and Candy (1970)
β-Alanine	2.0	3.0		0.3–0.6		Curtis (1964)
ω-Aminocaprylic acid	2.0			0.3–0.6		Curtis (1964)
[3H]Cyclic AMP				0.048		Shoemaker et al. (1974)
Cystathione	1.1×10^{-1}			0.3		Werman et al. (1966)
Epinephrine acid tartare	1.75	3–4		0.21	0.5–6.0	Krnjević et al. (1963a)
GABA	1.0×10^{-1}			0.3		Werman et al. (1966)
[2,3-3H]GABA	1.0	2.5	+ve	0.223	0.001	Obata et al. (1970)
		7.0	+ve	30.0		
		12.0	−ve	0.039		
[3H]GABA	5.0×10^{-1}	1.4	+ve	0.135		Zieglgänsberger et al. (1974)
		5.9	+ve	0.695		
		12.7	−ve	0.024		Werman et al. (1966)
[3H]Glycine	1.0×10^{-1}			0.5		
[3H]Glycine	5.0×10^{-1}	2.3	+ve	0.281		Zieglgänsberger et al. (1974)
		6.9	+ve	0.152		
		9.6	−ve	0.074		

TABLE 1 (continued)

Substance	Concentration (M)	pH	Polarity of ejecting current[a]	Transport number	Spontaneous release (pmol/s)	Reference
[³H]Glycine + phosphate buffer	5.0 × 10⁻¹	2.2	+ve	0.283		Zieglgänsberger et al. (1974)
		6.7	+ve	0.531		
		9.5	−ve	0.132		
L-Glutamic acid	2.0	8.0		0.3–0.6		Curtis (1964)
DL-[3-³H]Glutamate	0.1–1.0	8.5–9.0	−ve	0.2–0.5		Zieglgänsberger et al. (1969)
DL-[3-³H]Glutamate	1.0	7.0	−ve	0.126	0.01	Obata et al. (1970)
5-Hydroxytryptamine	1.3 × 10⁻¹	3–4		0.14	0.01–0.03	Krnjević et al. (1963a)
[³H]-5-Hydroxytryptamine creatine sulfate				0.18[b] 0.31[b]	0.003[b] 0.033[b]	Bradley and Candy (1970)
[³H]-5-Hydroxytryptamine creatine sulfate	2.5 × 10⁻²					
[³H]-5-Hydroxytryptamine creatine sulfate	5.0 × 10⁻²	4.0		0.22		Haigler and Aghajanian (1974)
[³H]Leucine	1.0	2.5	+ve	0.242		Zieglgänsberger et al. (1974)
		5.9	+ve	0.231		
		9.7	−ve	0.033		
Norepinephrine	1.7	3–4		0.34	0.01–0.02	Krnjević et al. (1963a)
DL-[7-³H]Norepinephrine hydrochloride		5.5		0.09[b] 0.19[b]		
[7-³H]Norepinephrine	3.0 × 10⁻²				0.005	Bradley and Candy (1970)
DL-[¹⁴C]Norepinephrine bitartrate	3.0 × 10⁻¹			0.05–0.30	0.008	Hoffer et al. (1971)
	5.0 × 10⁻¹					
PGE₁	2.0 × 10⁻²	3.0		0.17	0.024	Bradshaw et al. (1973b)
	3.0 × 10⁻²	7.0–7.5		0.033	0.0003	
	0.53–1.0	7.0–7.5		0.069	0.0014	

[5,6-³H]PGE₁	1.0	7.0–7.5		0.223[b]	Coceani and Viti (1972)
Substance P	7.0×10^{-3}	5–7	+ve	0.16	Krnjević and Morris (1974)
C. Antagonists					
[³H]Atropine	1.0×10^{-2}	3.7	+ve	0.13	Zieglgänsberger et al. (1974)
	2.0×10^{-1}			0.12	
[³⁵S]Chlorpromazine	2.0×10^{-2}	4.2	+ve	0.087	Zieglgänsberger et al. (1974)
[¹⁴C]Curare	5.0×10^{-3}	4.5	+ve	0.056	Zieglgänsberger et al. (1974)
	2.0×10^{-2}			0.162	
[³H]Decamethonium	1.0×10^{-2}	4.2	+ve	0.132	Zieglgänsberger et al. (1974)
	2.5×10^{-1}			0.137	
[¹⁴C]Imipramine	2.0×10^{-3}	4.5	+ve	0.046	Zieglgänsberger et al. (1974)
[³H]Haloperidol	6.7×10^{-3}	4.2	+ve	0.068	Zieglgänsberger et al. (1974)
[³H]Levallorphan	1.1×10^{-2}	4.4	+ve	0.074	Zieglgänsberger et al. (1974)
	1.1×10^{-1}	4.4	+ve	0.087	
D-[³H]Lysergic acid diethylamide	1.5×10^{-2}			0.02	Bradley and Candy (1970)
[³H]Lysergic acid diethylamide	0.01–0.10			0.0023	Haigler and Aghajanian (1974)
				0.0145	
				0.0025	
Strychnine hydrochloride	saturated			0.5	Curtis (1964)

[a]Polarity of ejecting current quoted when of particular interest.
[b]Microelectrodes fabricated from two different designs—note that the higher transport number is correlated with a higher spontaneous release.

sufficiently large to dwarf the amount released by an iontophoretic current of 20–40 nA.

2.1.2. Limitation of Spontaneous Efflux by Retaining Currents

Only fairly recently have radioactively labeled substances been used to show that retaining currents can effectively reduce the spontaneous efflux of material from the tip of a microelectrode. However, even this simple statement has been contested. For instance, Obata *et al.* (1970), who reported the spontaneous release of γ-aminobutyric acid (GABA) from some of their microelectrodes to be as low as $0.5–30.0 \times 10^{-14}$ mol/s, found that the spontaneous release continued unaltered even in the presence of retaining currents as high as 5000 nA. Only with larger-tipped electrodes, whose spontaneous release was 2 orders of magnitude greater, was the release abolished by retaining currents of the size normally employed.

More recently, Bradshaw *et al.* (1973*b*) embarked on a much more detailed study of the effects of retaining currents using microelectrodes containing 0.02 M [^{14}C]norepinephrine. The spontaneous release in the absence of retaining currents was approximately 0.024 pmol/s (i.e., 2×10^{-12} liter/s) and this could be effectively controlled by the use of relatively small retaining currents. However, all retaining currents of sufficient strength to limit spontaneous release interfered with subsequent release by iontophoresis. Although, as shown in Fig. 2, a retaining current of 25 nA reduced the release to less than 10% of the spontaneous level, further increases in current by as much as fourfold did not abolish the remaining release. However, during the use of higher retaining currents the subsequent release by iontophoretic pulses of constant amplitude and duration was decreased (Fig. 3). Only when both the amplitude of the retaining current and the interval between iontophoretic pulses were held constant did the release by constant iontophoretic pulses remain constant (Fig. 3C–D). However, the retaining current had to be discontinued for some time before the maximum iontophoretic release could be achieved (Fig. 3F).

Although Bradshaw *et al.* (1973*b*) explained their results in terms of a model based solely on diffusion and omitted any reference to bulk flow, their description probably does reflect the qualitative changes which occur inside the tip of the microelectrode during the passage of a retaining current. Following the immersion of the microelectrode tip in the external medium, a concentration gradient is established between the solution in the microelectrode and the external medium. In the steady state, the diffusional release which occurs as a result of this concentration gradient in the microelectrode tip will, at least in part, be limited by the entry of water into the tip in reponse to the high osmotic pressure within the concentrated solution in the shaft of the microelectrode tip and this will dilute the fluid of the tip and decrease the amount of active material released both by diffusion and by bulk flow. Even

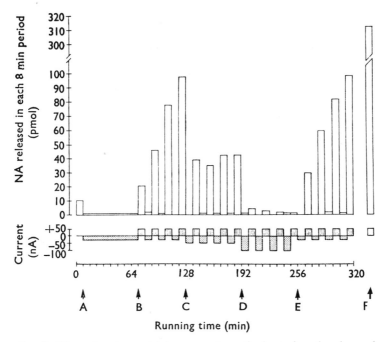

FIG. 3. Effect of various retaining currents on the iontophoretic release of norepinephrine (NA) from four barrels of a multi barreled micropipette. Lower graph shows the iontophoretic current applied to each of the four NA-containing barrels. Retaining currents are shown below the line and ejecting currents above the line. Upper graph shows the release of NA during each 8-min period of sample collection. Ejecting and retaining currents were applied alternately and the parameters (intensity and duration) of the ejecting pulses were kept constant throughout the study. Changes in the parameters of the applied currents are indicated by capital letters under the time base. After a prolonged application of retaining current (A–B), successive ejecting pulses (B–C) evoked progressively greater outputs. Increases in the intensity of the retaining current reduced the amount of NA released by the ejecting pulse (C–D, D–E). Restoration of the original retaining current (E) was followed by progressively increasing outputs. Control (output during an ejection pulse not preceded by a retaining pulse) is shown at the right of the figure (F). From Bradshaw *et al.* (1973*b*).

the smallest retaining current will presumably reduce the concentration of material inside the microelectrode tip and effectively create an interphase of dilute solution between the fluid inside the microelectrode and the external medium, whose magnitude will depend on both the amplitude and the duration of the retaining current. Eventually, the tip of the microelectrode will be effectively depleted of active material and the spontaneous release will cease, regardless of whether it is the result of diffusion or of bulk flow. However, a substantial depletion of active material from the tip will delay the

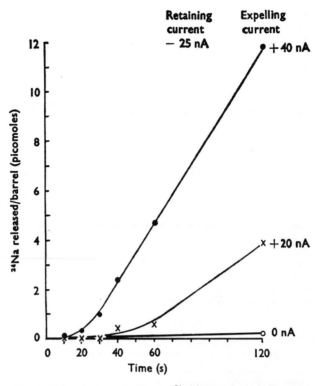

FIG. 4. Delayed onset of release of $^{24}Na^+$ into rat cerebral cortex *in vitro* following a prolonged application of retaining current for 60 s. Each point is the mean release per barrel from five barrels of a glass micropipette due to the passage of +40 nA (●), +20 nA (×), or 0 nA (○) through each barrel for the time shown. Before each period of release, a retaining current of −25 nA was passed through each barrel for 60 s. There was no detectable release of $^{24}Na^+$ during the passage of retaining current. From Clarke *et al.* (1973).

onset of release during subsequent applications of iontophoretic current (Fig. 4) (Clarke *et al.*, 1973), and the total amount released during each application will be diminished, as discussed earlier and shown in Fig. 3 (Bradshaw *et al.*, 1973*b*).

2.1.3. Conclusion

Spontaneous efflux from microelectrodes is in general a result of bulk flow rather than simple diffusion. Bulk flow can be reduced to a minimum by reducing the size of the microelectrode tip to the smallest compatible with release during microiontophoresis and by filling the shaft of the microelectrode with relatively dilute solutions. Although the remaining release can be effectively controlled by retaining currents, the possibility must be considered that even the smallest retaining current can delay or reduce the amount of material released by a subsequent application of iontophoretic current.

2.2. Release of Ionized Substances During Passage of Iontophoretic Current

As stated earlier, the passage of current through a fine-tipped microelectrode causes ions of appropriate polarity to leave the microelectrode at a rate determined by the current, I; i.e., the total quantity of ions moving *in* and *out* of the electrode (Q) obeys Faraday's law:

$$Q = It(F)^{-1} \qquad (7)$$

Q will be in microcoulombs (μC) where I is the current in nanoamperes (nA), t the time in seconds, and F the constant 96,500.

2.2.1. Transport Number

In practice, it appears that not all of the current flowing through the tip of the microelectrode can be accounted for by summing the number of charged ions which flow in and out of the tip on the basis of equation (7), and the term "transport number" has been introduced to describe the proportion of the total charge passed through the microelectrode carried by the particular ion under study. Although the earlier reports (*cf.* Curtis, 1964) all suggested that the passage of acetylcholine, GABA, and glutamate from conventional microelectrodes containing high concentrations of fully ionized solutions was extremely efficient and the "transport number" for these substances appeared to be near the optimal value 0.5, these workers stressed the need for caution when applying the values they had observed *in vitro* to the experimental situation. Somehow, in a manner which is not at all clear from the early literature, it became generally accepted that even with microelectrodes which seemed to pass current reliably the transport number varied not only with the physical characteristics of the solutions they contained but also from microelectrode to microelectrode in a totally unpredictable manner to the extent that each microelectrode was regarded as having its own peculiar transport number. This inability to predict the actual amount of substance passed by any one microelectrode in response to a given current application has led to the practice of expressing the dosages used during microiontophoresis in terms of the total charge passed through the microelectrode in μC or nA and seconds. Although this empirical approach has been deplored on the basis that it disguises one of the inherent difficulties of the technique, it does appear to work in practice and may even be justified by the observations that show the response of many neurons to be linearly related to either the current or the log of the current used to eject the test substance into their immediate neighborhood.

Although in theory the introduction of ^{3}H- and ^{14}C-labeled compounds has now made it relatively simple to determine for each individual microelectrode the exact relationship between the amplitude of the applied current and the amount of release (Gent *et al.*, 1974), this approach at the moment appears to be unnecessary in view of the problems that will be discussed later. The linear relationship between the rate of release by microiontophoresis and the amount of current passed was first established many years ago by Krnjević and his colleagues using the time-honored techniques of bioassay for acetylcholine and fluorescence spectroscopy for the amines (Krnjević *et al.*, 1963*a,b*). However, the use of radioactive materials not only gives much more accurate results but in addition allows the release to be measured into small cubes of brain tissue rather than small vessels containing artificial extracellular medium. Although, in general, most of the studies agree that the release from any given microelectrode is linearly related to the current passed, the actual rate of release appears to vary from microelectrode to microelectrode in a totally unpredictable way (Fig. 5). Indeed, the amount of release appears to bear no obvious relationship to the external diameter of the tip, the microelectrode resistance, or even the rate of spontaneous release which occurs in the absence of a retaining current (Hoffer *et al.*, 1971; Bradshaw *et al.*, 1973*b*). However, in two independent studies which compared two groups of microelectrodes prepared by different techniques the efflux of material was greater on average from the group of electrodes which showed the higher rate of spontaneous efflux (Bradley and Candy, 1970; Coceani and Viti, 1972).

Since it is impossible to generalize further on the basis of the relatively few reports published to date, the transport numbers obtained in several of these studies are shown in Table 1. Although the majority of these studies were straightforward and the reliability of the values shown in Table 1 is beyond doubt, a few studies were complicated by a number of rather unpleasant phenomena which must be mentioned. Hoffer *et al.* (1971), for instance, found the release of [^{3}H]norepinephrine into small cubes of brain tissue to be reduced to approximately 50% of that into small vessels containing physiological solutions. Clarke *et al.* (1973) found no such difference when using ^{23}NaCl as a model putative transmitter. However, norepinephrine appears at best to be the most unpredictable of all the commonly tested putative transmitters. Both Krnjević *et al.* (1963*a*) and Hoffer *et al.* (1971) found that a relatively high proportion of their microelectrodes failed to release detectable amounts of norepinephrine even though they appeared to pass adequate amounts of current. Indeed,

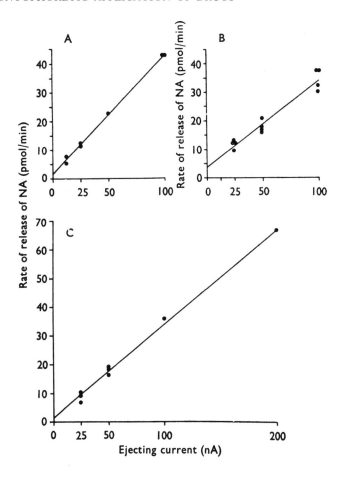

FIG. 5. Relationship between the intensity of the ejecting current and the rate of release of norepinephrine (NA) from three micropipettes (all four barrels). The rate of release was linearly related to current intensity over a wide range of intensities (+12.5 to +200 nA). (A) Calculated regression line: $y = 1.623 + 0.414x$. (B) Calculated regression line: $y = 3.690 + 0.308x$. (C) Calculated regression line: $y = 0.832x$. From Bradshaw *et al.* (1973*b*).

those that failed to release norepinephrine appeared to be identical in every respect to those that did. Although at first sight the existence of "rogue" microelectrodes which appear adequate in that they pass the normal amount of current yet do not pass norepinephrine is extremely disturbing, Hoffer *et al.* (1971) go on to reassure us by stating that these electrodes could be identified during the passage of the expelling current by the marked

increase in the high-frequency noise which contaminated electrical recordings made from an adjacent barrel of the same microelectrode filled with
NaCl.

Presumably, this noise would make these microelectrodes unusable in
practice and they would therefore be rejected, on a different basis. However,
this may not always be the case and the possibility arises that some of the
microelectrodes considered adequate in the past, not only on account of
their tip size and resistance but also because of their ability to pass current,
do not release adequate amounts of active material. Indeed, this very
possibility has now been raised by Bloom *et al.* (1974) to interpret the failure
of others (Godfrained and Pumain, 1972; Lake and Jordan, 1974) to
confirm Bloom's observation that the vast majority of cerebellar Purkinje
cells are as readily depressed by iontophoretic cyclic AMP as they are by
amines. Shoemaker *et al.* (1974) found that [^{3}H]cyclic AMP of high specific
activity was apparently reproducibly released during less than one-third of
the tests they carried out. There was a marked variation not only from
microelectrode to microelectrode but also in the amount passed from the
same microelectrode on different occasions even when the same amount of
current was generated either by the same device or by another based on a
different electronic principle.

Furthermore, Bloom *et al.* (1974) suggest that their findings are in
keeping with their experience of *in vivo* testing of hundreds of neurons in
the cerebellum and other regions of the brain, and they are therefore
prepared to state quite categorically that "many iontophoretic pipettes do
not deliver cyclic AMP despite the effective passage of controlled constant
current." Although at present it is difficult to envisage what is happening
within the tips of these "rogue" microelectrodes, both Krnjević *et al.* (1963a)
and Hoffer *et al.* (1971) have suggested that the tips might be blocked by a
semipermeable membrane which allows the passage of only a small number
of positively charged ions present in the aqueous solution without allowing
norepinephrine to escape. Clearly, if such membranes can form across the
opening of microelectrodes tested strictly *in vitro*, even greater numbers of
such membranes may be expected to form *in vivo*, where the microelectrode
is continually pushed down through millimeters of tissue containing all
manner of membranes. Experience suggests that many of these membranes
appear to be ideally suited for plugging the tips of microelectrodes. On the
other hand, Krnjević *et al.* (1963a) have also suggested that when the lumen
of a microelectrode is substantially occluded the current flows along the
inner surface of the glass by surface conductance. Presumably, cations such
as sodium and potassium are held in this layer by fixed charges belonging to
the surface of the glass (Davies and Rideal, 1961).

Although, as mentioned earlier, the majority of reports confirm that for
any one microelectrode the rate of release is directly proportional to the
amplitude of the ejecting current and the rate of release is assumed to be

constant throughout a particular current application, Clarke *et al.* (1973) have suggested that this *in vitro* finding is an oversimplification. In their experience, the rate of release takes some time to build up after the onset of the current and with moderate currents this lag phase may be as long as 1 min (Fig. 4). Furthermore, since ejections with the lower currents appear to take even longer to reach a constant level, the total amount of release evoked by different currents at the end of constant short applications of the order of 20 s will deviate significantly from that predicted by Faraday's law. Although they did not examine the effect of different retaining currents in detail, it is clear from their paper that this effect can be overcome by reducing the magnitude of the retaining current used during the preceding 60 s (see Section 2.1.2).

Presumably, it follows from the work of Bradshaw *et al.* (1973*b*) discussed earlier that the duration of the retaining current is critical and that the uncommonly long intervals of 60 s used by Clarke *et al.* (1973) between each application of ejecting current may have exaggerated the slow onset of each ejection phase.

It appears, therefore, that even small retaining currents not quite large enough to bring about a rapid cessation of the spontaneous efflux will, when applied for moderately long intervals, interfere with the subsequent release of substances by microiontophoresis. Presumably, at the onset of the current ejection only a fraction of the current flow is carried by the ions released from microelectrode into the medium, while the rest of the current flow brings about the reversal of the dilution within the tip of the microelectrode caused by the retaining current. Clearly, this work also suggests that when the length of the ejection phase is relatively short (perhaps less than 30s) compared to the duration of the retaining current not only will the onset of release be slowed but also the total amount released will be reduced and will no longer be linearly related to the amplitude of the current.

2.2.2. Conclusions About the Ejection of Substances from Microelectrodes by Microiontophoresis

Much more is known about the amounts of substances passed from microelectrodes by current than is apparent from the continued use of nanoamperes to describe the magnitude of an application of substance to a single cell by microiontophoresis. However, the use of nA as a parameter to measure release can be justified on the basis that the amount of material released from a particular microelectrode by a particular current application is determined not only by the amount of current passed but also by the physical properties of the microelectrode and the solution it contains. In addition, the previous history of the microelectrode with respect to both the intensity and the duration of retaining currents may well prove to be of extreme importance. It should, however, be stressed that many of the recent papers drawing attention to the effects of retaining currents on subsequent release by microiontophoresis ignore the possibility that one of the functions of the retaining current is to denude the microelectrode tip of ions so that the material released by bulk flow is inactive. Tip dilution may therefore be a necessary evil. I would like to suggest that most of the early workers were well aware of the slow onset of release at the beginning of each microiontophoretic application and arranged their experiments accordingly. Furthermore, as will be seen in the rest of this chapter, most of those workers interested in the speed with which microiontophoretically released substances evoke an effect on a nearby neuron avoid most of these difficulties by using extremely short pulses of current to eject instantaneous boluses of the substance from the tip of the microelectrode (Del Castillo and Katz, 1955; Krnjević and Phillis, 1963; Krnjević and Miledi, 1958; Gottesfeld *et al.*, 1972).

2.3. Electro-osmosis

As stated earlier, this chapter is mainly concerned with the release of fully ionized solutions by microiontophoresis. However, it is perhaps worthwhile to draw attention to the release of solution which will occur when a cationic potential is applied to an electrode containing a nonionized solution of a substance by a process known as "electro-osmosis." This flow of solution from the tip of the microelectrode appears to be the result of an interaction between the mobile charges in the thin layer of liquid which come into intimate contact with the inner surface of the glass wall of the microelectrode near its tip and the glass wall itself. Since the glass is usually negatively charged, outward flow occurs when a positive current is passed. Under normal circumstances, this flow appears to be important only when the electrode tip is extremely small and the number of cations in the bulk flow of solution is very low. Under these conditions, M_0, the magnitude of flow from the tip of the electrode, is said to be dependent on C, the concentration of the solution in the electrode, μ, the electro-osmotic mobility of the solution, ρ_i, the specific resistivity of the solution, and I, the current (Krnjević *et al.*, 1963a):

$$M_0 = C\mu\rho_i I \tag{8}$$

However, the electro-osmotic mobility of this solution can be determined only with great difficulty and one must resort to approximation of values by measuring the electromobility of small particles of ground-up microelectrode in the test solution (Davies and Rideal, 1961). In practice, the release by electro-osmosis from the ionized solution has been shown to be extremely small. For instance, Krnjević *et al.* (1963b) calculated that less than 11% of the release seen during microiontophoresis from electrodes containing 3 M acetylcholine could be accounted for by electro-osmosis. However, the release by electro-osmosis from nonionized solutions by currents of the magnitude commonly used during microiontophoresis can be extremely large. For instance, when Krnjević and Whittaker (1965) used currents of approximately 60 nA (1.20 μC) they found the release of ^{14}C-labeled sucrose to be of the order of 2.2×10^{-6} ml/μC, i.e., a flow rate approaching 2.8×10^{-9} liter/s, even though this rate falls rather short (56%) of the values predicted by equation (8) (cf. Krnjević and Whittaker, 1965, p. 305). Although it is often suggested that the electro-osmotic release in some microelectrodes is related to the current passed, Krnjević and Whittaker (1965) found that the maximal amount of release usually occurred with currents of approximately 60 nA. (The microelectrodes had relatively large tips—about 20 μm—compared to those described in Table 1.) Even with the best of their microelectrodes, however, release tended to fail after a few minutes of current passage, as the resistance of the microelectrodes increased. Although this increase in resistance often reversed spontaneously, there was always an upper limit to the amount of current passed by a particular microelectrode regardless of the size of the voltage applied. More recently, Obata et al. (1970) have shown the rate of release of GABA from a neutral solution in which GABA is thought to be in the zwitterionic form to be at a somewhat lower rate of 0.31×10^{-9} liter/μC, i.e., 30 pmol/μC. Although this value is at least 1 order of magnitude smaller than that found for sucrose by Krnjević and Whittaker (1965), Obata et al. (1970) made no attempt to compare the physical characteristics of the two solutions and thought that some of the decrease may have been due to the presence of approximately 2.5 mM GABA chloride in their solutions. Although it is always stated that the presence of ions will drastically reduce the release by electro-osmosis (presumably by reducing the thickness of the electrical double layer near the inner surface of the glass) Obata et al. (1970) found the release to remained relatively high (10 pmol/μC) even when 0.1 M NaCl was added to the solution. Indeed, release exceeded that expected to occur when the same current is passed through an electrode containing an ionized GABA solution of the same concentration (cf. Table 1).

2.4. Microinjection

Another approach to the problem of applying nonionizable substances to neurons is the use of microinjection, i.e., the application of pressure to the microelectrode. Although the most convenient method of applying pressure is said to be the use of compressed air at known pressure (Krnjević and Phillis, 1963; Krnjević and Whittaker, 1965; Curtis, 1964; Krnjević et al., 1963b), many more sophisticated systems are available (Brooks et al., 1957; Keynes, 1964; Kopac, 1964; Grundfest et al., 1954; Caldwell et al., 1960;

Chambers and Kopac, 1950). Unfortunately, pressure is not the only factor controlling the release of solution from the microelectrode when the tip is as fine as those used in conjunction with single-unit electrical recording. Clearly, from our early discussion on bulk flow (equation 3) both the shape and the internal diameter of the microelectrode tip, as well as the viscosity of the solution, are of great importance. Indeed, quite small changes in the internal diameter of the microelectrode tip cause large changes in the rate of flow generated by a particular intensity of pressure. Presumably, therefore, the great variability of the release reported by most authors can be explained in terms of partial plugging of their microelectrode tips by particulate matter in the filling solutions or perhaps more likely by components of the tissue through which microelectrodes were pushed.

Since the release during an application of pressure is essentially a method for increasing the bulk flow from the tip of the microelectrode, the actual amount of fluid forced from the tip by any particular pressure can be calculated from equation (3) derived by Krnjević et al. (1963b). Indeed, Krnjević et al. (1963b) verified this equation by demonstrating that a pressure of approximately 140 mm Hg will release a 3 M solution of acetylcholine at a rate of approximately 1 pl/s. This value is in good agreement with their measurements on the physical characteristics of the 3 M acetylcholine solution, and the size and shape of their microelectrode tips. Krnjević and Phillis (1963) also used microinjections in vivo to show that excitant and depressant amino acids are just as effective when applied by means other than microiontophoresis, which may cause negative or positive current to pass through the tissue in the vicinity of the neuron under study.

Obata et al. (1970) studied the release of [³H]GABA and glutamate from microelectrodes containing 1 M solutions and showed the average release from nine microelectrodes to be 3.95 pmol/s when the pressure was 400 mm Hg. Since inside the microelectrode this amount of GABA was contained in a volume of about 4 pl, this value is in extremely good agreement with the value of 1 pl/s obtained by Krnjević et al. (1963b) using one-third the pressure. Like Krnjević et al. (1963b), they found the amount released by a particular pressure to be extremely variable. In general, however, it does appear that the amount of nonionized substance released from a microelectrode is proportional to the pressure, and that some degree of quantification may be possible by monitoring the pressure and using microelectrodes with the same tip diameter. Earlier, I mentioned the difficulties involved in measuring the internal diameter of the microelectrode tip and described in detail how Krnjević et al. (1963b) had drawn attention to the correlation between spontaneous release and microelectrode tip resistance, and I suggested that microelectrode resistance might be an adequate measure of the internal diameter of the microelectrode tip. However, an increase in bulk flow through the electrode tip provoked by an application of pressure leads to a reduction in the apparent resistance of the tip (Bingley, 1965;

Rubio and Zubieta, 1965), and the magnitude of this change in resistance should be related to the rate of injection. In practice, however, Firth and De Felice (1971) were unable to discover a simple relationship between the changing resistance of the microelectrode and the pressure applied. Although they suggested that their difficulties were in part the result of technical problems, they felt that the standard theory may well need revision. However, their calculations based on the standard theory predicted that the volume of fluid ejected from their electrode tips by a particular pressure would be almost identical to that determined directly by Krnjević *et al.* (1963*b*) and Obata *et al.* (1970). They also showed that the application of negative pressure caused large increases in resistance which could be the result of a decrease or even a cessation of bulk flow. The use of negative pressure to reduce spontaneous release of nonionizable substances is extremely pertinent since the spontaneous efflux cannot be controlled by the use of retaining currents. Interestingly enough, they also drew attention to the possibility that the movement of fluid inside the tip of the microelectrode under the influence of a pressure gradient might cause the mobile layer of ions on the surface of the glass to be dragged along, resulting in the generation of a current (Rutgers, 1940). This "streaming" current of potential, which must contribute to the tip potential of microelectrodes under normal pressure (Adrian, 1956), could be used to measure the surface charge on the glass. This method could be extremely useful in calculating some of the physical constants of solutions and microelectrode glass that are required to determine the electro-osmotic flow (*cf.* equation 8). This notion is perhaps more than a far-fetched fancy, since workers in other fields have already attempted to use changes in the electro-osmotic tip potential and resistance to measure the resistivity and pressure of the fluid inside cells and tissue spaces (Lavallee, 1964; Schanne *et al.*, 1966; Weiderhelm *et al.*, 1964). Unfortunately, all of these studies have been carried out using microelectrodes containing concentrated solutions of electrolytes such as potassium chloride and the influence of pressure on microelectrodes containing nonelectrolytes may turn out to be a completely different problem, even though it may be amenable to the same theoretical treatment.

3. DISPERSAL OF IONTOPHORETICALLY APPLIED SUBSTANCES WITHIN THE BRAIN

Although in the previous section it was suggested that the iontophoretic current forces an appreciable amount of ionized material to leave the microelectrode and enter the tissue, the dispersal of the ejected ions within the tissue is thought to occur solely by diffusion. In other words, the voltage difference necessary to generate the current flow arises solely within the microelectrode and potentials of only a few millivolts occur in the brain tissue, presumably only within a few micrometers of the microelectrode tip (Curtis *et al.*, 1960). Even slightly larger voltages of the order of, say, tens of millivolts would facilitate the movement of ions only in the immediate vicinity of the microelectrode tip (say, 4μm) and would be unlikely to influence ion movements over the distances of $10-100 \mu$m which often separate the microelectrode tip from the neuron under study.

3.1. Theoretical Curves Based on Models of Diffusion

Unfortunately, even if we do assume that ions leave the ejection site by diffusion there is no simple method of determining the resultant concentrations which develop in the immediate vicinity of the neuron under study. Although in the future this problem may be resolved by autoradiography (Globus *et al.*, 1968; Schubert *et al.*, 1972), fluorescent microscopy (Bunney *et al.*, 1973), or, as we will discuss later, the use of ion- and drug-sensitive microelectrodes, at present our only resort is to use the theoretical curves based on well-established models of diffusion described by Crank (1957) and Carslaw and Jaeger (1959). In this respect, however, the users of iontophoresis may well be no worse off than any other pharmacologist, since there is little reason to believe that the concentration of drug in the immediate vicinity of the receptors on the surface of neurons in the central nervous system is related in any simple manner to the concentration of the substance in the arterial blood or even in brain tissue itself. Thus all investigators ought to be aware of the factors which, at least in part, may influence the concentration of substances at a particular site within the brain tissue (*cf.* review by Pappenheimer, 1953; Thron, 1974). However, approaches quite different than those described here are available for the situation where low concentrations of substances are added to incubations of brain homogenates and tissue slices *in vitro* (Neame and Richards, 1972).

3.1.1. Diffusion Theories

On purely theoretical grounds, Jaeger and others (Crank, 1957; Carslaw and Jaeger, 1959; Del Castillo and Katz, 1955; Jaeger, 1965; Waud, 1968) have evolved equations which allow the diffusion of drugs through the tissues to be described in terms of the concentration (C) of the drug at any particular radial distance (r) from the microelectrode tip at a particular time (t) provided that it is assumed that the spread of the substance is solely by diffusion and that the material is being liberated continuously from a point source into an infinite homogeneous volume at a constant rate (q):

$$C = q(4\pi Dr)^{-1} \operatorname{erfc} r[2(DT)^{1/2}]^{-1} \tag{9}$$

where D is the diffusion coefficient of the substance and erfc is the "error function complement," a convenient mathematical device which allows many problems in diffusion to be resolved by reading the value of an "error function" from tables in one of the standard works (Crank, 1957; Carslaw and Jaeger, 1959). Later, however, Jaeger (1965) modified the general equation to fit the special case in which the material is not released continuously but ceases after a definite time t_1, perhaps long before an approximation to the steady-state situation can be established:

$$C = q(4\pi Dr)^{-1}[\text{erfc } r[2(DT)^{1/2}]^{-1} - \text{erfc } r\{2[D(t - t_1)]^{1/2}\}^{-1}] \qquad (10)$$

This is of particular relevance because iontophoresis often involves the application of drugs intermittently for fixed intervals of, say, 10 s, which are much shorter than the 100 s which may be required to reach the equilibrium condition (Fig. 5).

Since equations (9) and (10) involve both space and time—r, t, and t_1—it is extremely difficult to illustrate the results in a general fashion and it is therefore necessary to calculate curves of special numerical interest. For instance, Curtis et al. (1960) with the help of Jaeger calculated typical concentration curves based on the assumptions that the ejection current is 100 nA passing continuously for a time t (i.e., t and t_1 have the same value), the apparent transport number (n) of the ionized substance and the microelectrode tip has the optimal value of 0.5, the valency (z) is equal to 1, and the diffusion constant (D) equals 1×10^{-5} cm²/s:

$$C = 8.25 \times 10^{-6} \, nI(zDr)^{-1}\{\text{erfc } (r \times 10^{-4})[2(Dt)^{1/2}]^{-1}\} \qquad (11)$$

They also suggest that when $r \times 10^{-4}$ is not greater than $2(Dt)^{1/2}$, erfc approaches unity and equation (11) can be replaced by an approximation which is correct to within 5% and avoids reference to the error function tables:

$$C = 8.25 \times 10^{-6} \, nI(zDr)^{-1}\{1 - 5.85 \times 10^{-5}r[(Dt)^{1/2}]^{-1} + 1.61 \times 10^{-9}r^2(Dt)^{-1}\} \qquad (12)$$

As suggested earlier, Fig. 6 shows that current applications of nearly 100 s are required to insure that both the substance concentration and the spread within the tissues are maximal—i.e., a steady-state situation is reached where C varies inversely as the diffusion coefficient (D):

$$C \propto 1/D \qquad (13)$$

However, Curtis et al. (1960) suggested that changes in D, the diffusion coefficient, and z, the valency, are relatively unimportant and that in most

m-moles/L

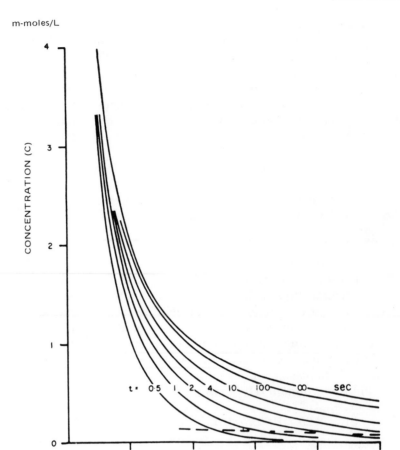

FIG. 6. Concentration (ordinate) in millimoles, of a univalent ion of diffusion coefficient $1 \times 10^{-5}\ cm^2/s$ and transference (transport) number 0.5 at a distance $r\ \mu m$ (abscissa) from the tip of an electrode when passed by an iontophoretic current of 100 nA. The different curves indicate concentration–distance relationships at the indicated times after the beginning of the iontophoretic current. From Curtis *et al.* (1960).

instances (within a factor of about 2) the concentration of a substance in the tissue at any particular distance from the microelectrode tip can be assumed to be independent of whether it is uni- or bivalent and whether or not it is charged or loses its charge on passing into the tissue. For instance, it is convenient to iontophorese both GABA and glycine from acid solutions as univalent cations, although on entering the tissue, which is at neutral pH, they both presumably lose protons and become zwitterions without charge.

In conclusion, it therefore appears that in most situations the maximal concentration of a drug at any particular point in the tissue is dependent on the duration of the iontophoretic current application, and for relatively short periods of less than, say, 200 s will continue to rise as long as material continues to be ejected from the electrode. However, it must be stressed that this assumes that the brain tissue behaves like an infinite sea of 0.9% saline and that no mechanism exists for the sequestration or inactivation of the diffusing substance. For instance, Curtis *et al.* (1960) have derived equations to deal with the special case where cholating agents are released by iontophoresis and act by complexing with the calcium present in the brain tissue. As we will see later, it may be possible to evolve models which take more account of both the known structure and function of the brain with respect to the diffusion of drugs (see Section 3.2).

3.1.2. Electrical Model of Diffusion

Although the equations just examined are perfectly adequate and can be used to make all the predictions described above, they are undoubtedly far too cumbersome to allow the average worker in the field to quickly estimate the concentration of substance that might be in the vicinity of the neurons under study. This is particularly true when the response of the neurons is extremely sensitive to small variations in the duration of short applications of current lasting less than, say, 30 s. Unfortunately, even for those well versed in mathematics the outcome of equations containing "error functions" is not only difficult to foresee but also extremely awkward to explore with a digital computer. Thus it has been suggested by Waud (1968) that these equations are much more readily understood when simulated by an electrical analogue which can be constructed from simple components readily available in most neurophysiology laboratories or by relatively simple analog computers.

In the electrical model, the spread of substance from the point source is likened to the flow of current along an electrical network made up of a chain of resistors and capacitors; i.e., the material flows out radially from a central small sphere surrounded by a series of concentric shells each represented by a single resistor in series and a capacitor in parallel. However, the values of the components do not remain constant but are varied so that the "resistance" to flow between neighboring shells falls off as the distance of the shells, i.e., the number of shells from the center, while the "capacity" of each shell in the series rises as the square of the distance.

In practice, therefore, the model can be built from a chain of real capacitors and resistors arranged so that the relationship between r, the radial distance from the tip of the electrode, and t, a particular instant in real time, is

$$r = t(RCD)(\Delta r)^{-2} \tag{14}$$

TABLE 2

Values of R and C for a Network[a] to Simulate Diffusion from a Point Source of a Substance with $D = 3 \times 10^{-6} cm^2/s$

Radius of shell midpoint (μm)	C (pF)	R (MΩ)
1	35	95
2	128	26
3	282	11.8
4	505	6.06
5	790	4.22
6	1130	2.95
7	1540	2.16
8	2015	1.65
9	2545	1.31
10	3140	1.068
11	3810	0.875
12	4520	0.738
	(μF)	
15	0.036	2.32
20	0.063	1.32
25	0.098	0.845
30	0.140	0.592
35	0.193	0.431
40	0.251	0.332
45	0.320	0.260
50	0.390	0.214
55	0.475	0.175
60	0.568	0.146
70	1.86	0.280
100	16.5	0.505
150	35.6	0.234
200	63	0.132

From Waud (1968).
[a]Circuit:

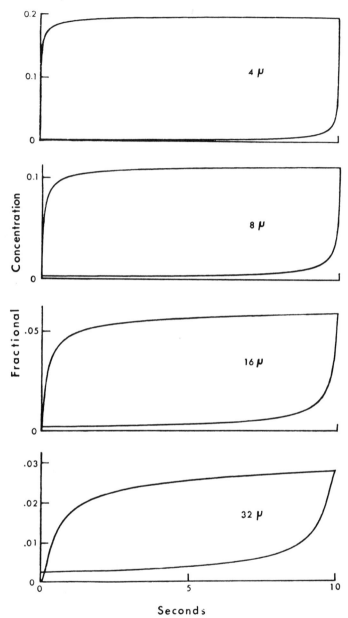

FIG. 7. Computed concentration at various distances from a point source of 10 s duration. $D = 10^{-5}$ cm^2/s. Panels from above downward represent events 4, 8, 16, and 32 μm from origin. Ordinate, concentration relative to that at origin; abscissa, time in seconds. Rise of concentration was recorded from left to right (upper curves); then point source was terminated and fall in concentration was recorded from right to left. From Waud (1968).

where Δr is the width of the shell to be represented by a given resistor (R) and capacitor (C) pair. Indeed, Waud (1968) has published a table (Table 2) of the resistor and capacitor values necessary to construct such a network which divides the radial distance into 1-μm units and assumes that the diffusion coefficient of the substance (D) is 3×10^{-6} cm²/s. The concentration of substance at a given point r is then obtained by applying the substance as a voltage pulse to the beginning of the chain where r equals zero and recording the potential wave at the appropriate point in the chain. Figure 7 shows the results that were obtained by Waud (1968) at four different distances along the chain when the application of substance was 10 s in duration. These are of particular interest since it is clear that with such a pulse the steady state is reached asymptotically, and that even when the microelectrode is placed as close as 8 μm from the cell almost 1 s is required for the fast phase of the rise in concentration. At a more realistic distance of 32 μm, considerable time is required for the concentration to reach a maximum. On the same graph is shown the speed with which the concentration falls off with time at the end of each application. This rapid decline in concentration at the end of the pulse explains why the return of excitation at the end of a GABA pulse seems so much more abrupt than the onset of inhibition. Without such an analogue model, these curves must be calculated from a variant of equation (10) where t_1, the duration of the drug application, is used as the basic unit of time and all the other times are expressed as (n) multiples of t_1. The concentration (C_{nt_1}) at any point in time (nt_1) after the end of the drug application is then expressed as a fraction of the concentration (C_{t_1}) at the end of the drug application at time t_1 and is given by the equation

$$(C_{nt_1}) \cdot (C_{t_1})^{-1} = [\![\mathrm{erfc}\ r[2(nDt_1)^{1/2}]^{-1}$$
$$- \mathrm{erfc}\ r\{2[(n-1)Dt_1]^{1/2}\}^{-1}]\!] \cdot \{\mathrm{erfc}\ r[2(Dt_1)^{1/2}]^{-1}\}^{-1} \qquad (15)$$

In conclusion, therefore, it appears from the use (Waud, 1968) of a simple electrical model that even if the iontophoretic ejection of substances were perfected to a level where they could be effectively ejected into the tissue without the apparent delay caused by a dilution inside the tip (Section 2.2) the onset of the response of a neuron would be considerably delayed by the simple process of diffusion.

In the past, Paton and Waud (1964) made extensive use of the electrical model to measure the actual time taken for drug–receptor interactions by comparing the rate with which block occurs at the neuromuscular junction during iontophoresis of tubocurarine with the rate that might be expected to occur solely due to the diffusion time.

3.1.3. Instantaneous Release from a Point Source

Although the experimental situation just described is the one most commonly encountered, it is much easier, in practice, to investigate the special case where all of the ejected substance (M) is assumed to be liberated instantaneously from the tip of the electrode (i.e., r and t both equal zero). Only in this situation is it possible to visualize the concentration (C) of the ejected substance at a point some distance from the tip of the microelectrode (r) rising slowly to a maximum value (C_{max}) and then subsequently falling off toward zero, i.e., as a monophasic wave of drug diffusing out from the microelectrode tip into the tissue. Therefore, at any given point r the concentration C at time t is given by the equation (cf. Del Castillo and Katz, 1955; Crank, 1957; Carslaw and Jaeger, 1959)

$$C = M[8(\pi Dt)^{3/2}]^{-1}e^{-r^2/4Dt} \tag{16}$$

The maximum concentration (C_{max}) reached at r is given by

$$C_{max} = M(8r^3)^{-1}(6/\pi)^{3/2}e^{-3/2} = 0.0736M(r^{-3}) \tag{17}$$

and occurs at a time (t_{max}):

$$t_{max} = r^2(6D)^{-1} \tag{18}$$

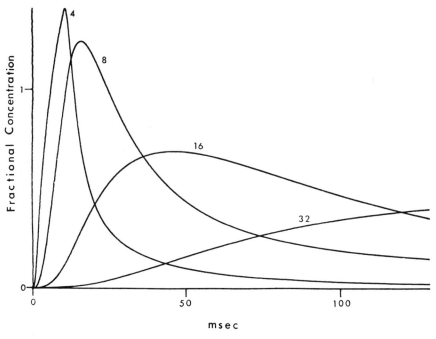

FIG. 8. Computed concentrations at various distances from a point source of 10 ms duration. $D = 10^{-5}$ cm^2/s. Figures beside curves give distance from point source in micrometers. Ordinate, concentration relative to that at origin $\times 10^4$ for curve 32; $\times 4 \times 10^4$ for 16; $\times 1.6 \times 10^3$ for 8; 6.4×10^3 for 4. Abscissa, time in milliseconds. From Waud (1968).

Although I have selected Fig. 8 (from Waud, 1968) to illustrate the theoretical time course with which the concentration of a substance in the tissue might be expected to rise at different distances from the electrode tip, Del Castillo and Katz (1955) had shown very much earlier that similar curves (Fig. 9) could be obtained experimentally by recording the response of the postsynaptic membrane of the neuromuscular junction to acetylcholine released from a microelectrode some distance away. Since variations in both the amount of acetylcholine released and the distance between the point of acetylcholine release and the recording site caused predictable changes in

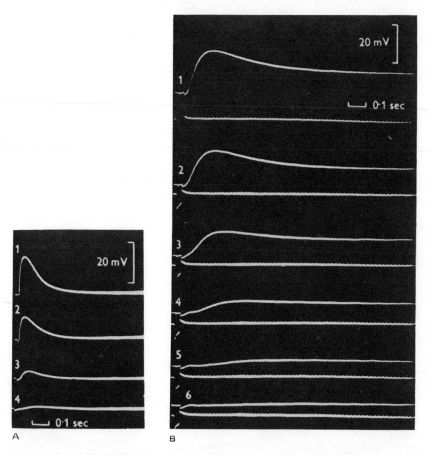

FIG. 9. Acetylcholine potentials from a single end plate. (A) Effect of varying the distance between "source" and "receptor." The potentials were due to a brief outward pulse (about $0.13\,\mu A \times 0.54\,ms = 7 \times 10^{-11}$ C). Between records 1 and 4, the acetylcholine pipette was moved 17 μm away from·the muscle surface. (B) Effect of position of the acetylcholine pipette, at another end plate. Outward pulse, shown in lower traces, of about 4.8×10^{-10} C. Pipette was displaced 44 μm between records 1 and 6. From Del Castillo and Katz (1955).

the amplitudes and time courses of the postsynaptic responses (Fig. 9), they were able to suggest that the shape of the response curves was solely dependent on the speed with which acetylcholine diffused through the extracellular fluid and that the interaction between acetylcholine and the receptor could be assumed to occur instantaneously. Although the simplicity of these fundamental experiments is often overlooked, they are undoubtedly the basis of the belief that *the instantaneous amplitude of the postsynaptic response is directly proportional to the drug concentration at the receptors.* Although further debate about the many other factors which may influence both the amplitude and time course of the postsynaptic response is beyond the scope of this chapter, it should be mentioned that measurements of spike frequency, membrane potential, and conductance may all prove in the long run to be rather inadequate measures of the postsynaptic response. Presumably, many of these problems could be overcome if it were possible to record directly the electrical activity of the individual receptors, perhaps in the same way as the activity of the acetylcholine receptors at the neuromuscular junction has become amenable to investigation by high-gain recordings of "shot noise" from the membrane (Katz and Miledi, 1972, 1973; Anderson and Stevens, 1973).

Although the experiments of Del Castillo and Katz (1955) clearly established the validity of the diffusion equations for microiontophoresis carried out on the surface fibers of frog muscle bathed in extracellular fluid, the possibility must be considered that substances ejected into the brain are unable to diffuse freely and that barriers exist between the electrode tip and the receptors on the neuron under study. The nature of these barriers is difficult to define since morphological studies show the true extracellular space to be extremely small, and functional studies suggest that a considerable proportion of the brain is composed of astroglia, which appears relatively accessible to several ions thought to be extracellular markers (De Robertis and Gerschenfeld, 1961). It is of interest, therefore, that the experiments of Del Castillo and Katz (1955) have in essence been repeated within the brain (Krnjević and Phillis, 1963; Gottesfeld *et al.*, 1972). Indeed, they also showed the maximum response of the neuron under study to occur at a time when the glutamate concentration in the vicinity of a neuron situated some 30 μm away from the microelectrode tip should be approaching a maximum. For instance, Krnjević and Phillis (1963) found the peak excitation evoked by a glutamate pulse to occur with a latency of 300 ms and were thus able to calculate the effective concentration in the vicinity of the neuron to be 0.14 mM and the diffusion distance (l) between the tip of the microelectrode and the neuron under study to be 30 μm,

$$l = (6Dt)^{1/2} \tag{18}$$

by assuming that their electrodes could instantaneously release approximately 5×10^{-14} mol of glutamate and that the diffusion coefficient for glutamate in brain is 5×10^{-6} cm²/s. From a series of such calculations, Krnjević and Phillis (1963) were able to suggest that the effective concentration of glutamate required to excite individual neurons always fell within a narrow range around about 0.1 mM and the calculated diffusion distance was always small enough to fall within the range of distances over which multibarreled electrodes might be expected to record action potentials of a reasonable amplitude.

Although the absolute values calculated by Krnjević and Phillis (1963) are highly speculative, the consistency of their data obtained from a number of different neurons, each thought to lie at a different distance from the tip of the microelectrode, is in keeping with the view that glutamate released from a microelectrode into the brain spreads freely through the tissue at a speed that approaches the diffusion rate of glutamate in water.

More recently, Herz *et al.* (1969) were able to confirm this view in a much more exacting study in which a pair of multibarreled microelectrodes were mounted side by side so that their tips were separated by a known distance of between 12 and 300 μm. The spike activity recorded from nonspontaneously active neurons by one electrode during the application of glutamate from the other and the inhibition of spontaneously firing neurons by GABA released by the opposite electrode were used as a measure of amino acid diffusion between the two microelectrodes. Like Krnjević and Phillis (1963), they found a strong correlation between their data obtained from dose–response curves and curves computed from the diffusion equation (12). The coefficient of diffusion for the amino acid was estimated to be approximately 1×10^{-5} cm²/s and the minimum effective concentration of glutamate appeared to be approximately 0.25 mM. They also confirmed the suggestion of Krnjević and Phillis (1963) that optimal conditions occur for electrical recording when the multibarreled microelectrode and the neuron under study lie approximately 20–30 μm apart. Unfortunately, placement of the electrodes farther apart than a few tens of micrometers produced erroneous results; the apparent spread of glutamate was much faster than that likely to be achieved by simple diffusion. Clearly, these results must have been caused by an excitatory interaction between two neurons mediated by a short-axoned pathway perhaps containing one or more intervening synapses (*cf.* Biscoe and Curtis, 1967; Curtis and Felix, 1971; Kelly and Renaud, 1974).

3.2. Tissue Uptake Mechanisms and Drug Redistribution

Although the experiments described in the previous section suggest that glutamate and GABA can spread considerable distances in the brain by diffusion, this may well be an oversimplification. The possibility must arise that the tissue around the tip of the microelectrode can sequester the ejected material. Indeed, it is becoming more and more difficult to ignore the evidence which suggests that the majority of neurotransmitters can be taken up by nerve terminals (Iversen, 1971) and glial cells (Schon and Kelly, 1974) and the evidence which suggests that the penetration of drugs such as local anesthetics into nerve cells (Ritchie and Greengard, 1966) is dependent on their state of ionization and in turn on their lipid solubility. It therefore seems reasonable to suppose that the concentration of a substance released by microiontophoresis in the immediate vicinity of the neuron under study is unlikely to be determined solely by diffusion and may well be dependent on either the presence or the absence of active uptake systems for the substance in question or its lipid solubility. It should be remembered that most of the substances ejected from microelectrodes are in a highly ionized form only by virtue of the acid or alkaline content of the electrode and that the buffering capacity of the tissue will tend to reverse this situation so that the lipid solubility of the free base will determine the redistribution of the substances between the aqueous and lipid phases of the environment.

A theoretical approach to this problem was explored by Krnjević and Lisiewicz (1972), who were attempting to determine whether the amount of calcium injected inside a neuron in order to elicit a detectable response was compatible with the known volume of the neuron and the ability of intracellular organelles to actively take up calcium. They drew attention to the relatively simple hypothesis that at some particular radial distance from the electrode tip (r_0) the efflux from the microelectrode will exactly match the ability of the tissue to sequester the injected material and the concentration of substance in the tissue will be zero. Just as before (equation 16), the flux (F) of substance passing through the tissue at any particular point r from the tip of the electrode can be calculated from the diffusion equation:

$$F = -4\pi r^2 D(dt/dr) \tag{19}$$

However, at distance r_0 mentioned above, the concentration will never rise above zero and dt/dr will also equal zero due to the activity (a) of some process in the tissue which inactivates the substance released:

$$r_0 = [3F_0(4\pi a)^{-1}]^{1/3} \tag{20}$$

This equation can be arranged in a way which makes the activity (a) of the uptake process look as if it could be measured by microiontophoresis:

$$a = 3F_0(4\pi r_0^3)^{-1}$$

By assuming F_0 to be the minimum calcium application required to affect the neuronal membrane and the diameter of the average motoneuron to be 20–30 μm, Krnjević and Lisiewicz (1972) were able to suggest that an injection of 20 fmol/s of calcium into a motoneuron would be inactivated by an uptake process with a capacity of 320 nmol/cm/s.

Although in general the usefulness of this method is restricted by our inability to measure the distance r_0 between the microelectrode tip and the receptor sites on the neuron under study, a certain amount of information could be obtained by comparing the minimal effective dose of two substances released onto the same neuron from separate barrels of the same electrode. However, the significance of the difference between these two values would be somewhat ambiguous since this value is often taken to be a measure of the difference in sensitivity of the postsynaptic membrane for the two substances under test and any effect due to inactivation by the intervening tissue is ignored. A number of authors have, however, reported an increase to occur in the postsynaptic sensitivity to certain putative transmitters when the tissue surrounding the microelectrodes is treated with substances known to inhibit the reuptake in question (Curtis et al., 1970; Gottesfeld et al., 1972; Bradshaw et al., 1973a; Segal and Bloom, 1974).

In conclusion, the effect of reuptake and redistribution of substances injected into the brain by microiontophoresis is an unknown quantity which at present does not seem amenable to direct experimentation. Even more difficult is the possibility that the effects of sequestration of substances into special tissue compartments may be offset in part by the "preferred diffusional pathway" for certain substances being restricted to a very small proportion of the total brain volume. This in itself could cause the concentration of the injected substance at a given distance from the microelectrode tip to be anything from 3 to 20 times greater than that predicted by the diffusion equations, which assume the brain to consist of a homogeneous medium of 0.17 mM NaCl. On the other hand, enhancement of diffusion by a restriction in the extracellular space will not occur and may even change to a hindrance if the width of the diffusional space is reduced to the dimension that might occur in synaptic clefts. Indeed, simple curves are available to describe the diffusion of transmitter substances within the cleft (Eccles and Jaeger, 1957; Jaeger, 1960). Clearly, the problem can never be resolved by the use of mathematical devices and must eventually be tackled directly by means of histochemical or autoradiographic techniques, or the use of ion- or drug-sensitive probes. Since many of the problems discussed throughout this chapter could be resolved by the use of drug-sensitive probes with fast response times, it is encouraging to see so many accounts of the use of ion-sensitive electrodes (Walker, 1971; Krnjević and Morris, 1972; Kříž et al., 1974; Prince et al., 1973; Thomas, 1974) and the development of miniature electrodes containing substrate-specific enzymes (Gough and Andrade, 1973). However, both of these approaches might be too sophisticated. A recent report has shown that the spread of adrenergic neurotransmitters, their metabolites, and many psychoactive drugs in the brain can be followed in vivo by the use of voltammetric electrodes (cf.

McCreery *et al.*, 1974). Perhaps an even more direct approach will be possible following the development of microscintillation techniques; for instance, Caldwell and Lea (1973) have prepared a microelectrode capable of determining the radioactive flux of ^{14}C-labeled glycine inside a single squid giant axon.

4. CONCLUSIONS

The introduction of radioactively labeled compounds has allowed many authors to investigate the iontophoretic release of ionized substances from their microelectrodes. Indeed, the *in vivo* results published by many of these authors (Table 1) are in keeping with the two main prejudices held by the majority of workers in this field:

1. The release from the majority of microelectrodes is linearly related to the amount of current passed.
2. The actual amount of material released by a particular current varies from microelectrode to microelectrode and from substance to substance in a quite unpredictable way.

Although the effects of this variability can usually be overcome, it makes the interpretation of negative results extremely difficult. This is particularly true of negative results obtained with both putative transmitters and antagonists whose transport numbers are less than 10% of those usually obtained with the more commonly used agonists (*cf.* Table 1).

Our present knowledge of the release of nonionizable substances by "iontophoretic currents" is in all probability too scanty to lead to any definite conclusions. However, it is worth mentioning that the basic principles predict that the release will be of significance only when the internal diameter of the microelectrode tip is small, and the results to date suggest that maximal release is attained with relatively low levels of current. Although the initial amount of material released by these small currents is often fairly large, perhaps 60 times greater than that expected from an ionized solution, the release can rarely be maintained at this level for more than a few minutes without the resistance of the electrode increasing and the release dropping to a relatively low level.

Although the use of pressure to release the materials from microelectrodes has always appeared an attractive proposition, the technique has never really become widely used. This is perhaps not surprising since again most of the available data suggest that there is a marked variability in the amount of material that can be ejected from a particular microelectrode.

Since it is now possible to determine the exact amount of material that will be released by a particular electrode by iontophoresis, it is rather disappointing to report that we have almost no knowledge of the concentration gradient of the ejected substance in the surrounding brain tissue. Although a number of authors have found that the duration of the delay between the ejection of glutamate or GABA and the onset of excitation or inhibition is similar to that predicted by models of diffusion, the assumptions involved seem to be quite unreasonable. For instance, it is difficult to believe that all substances diffuse through the brain tissue at the same speed as they do through 0.9% saline and that their passage is quite unimpaired by the presence of neurons and glial cells. Furthermore, the possibility is ignored that certain components of the brain may actively accumulate the injected substance and that the water–lipid solubility of the substance may be the main determinant of its distribution in the brain. In all probability, only the introduction of small drug-sensitive probes will allow this problem to be tackled in a realistic manner.

ACKNOWLEDGMENTS

I am indebted to Mr. C. N. Rayner and Mr. G. Oaks for preparing the figures, Dr. P. M. Beart for reading the manuscript, and Mrs. Clara Catto for typing the final copy.

5. REFERENCES

ADRIAN, R. H., 1956, The effect of internal and external potassium concentration on the membrane potential of the frog muscle, *J. Physiol.* **133**:631–658.

ANDERSON, C. R., and STEVENS, C. F., 1973, Voltage clamp analysis of acetylcholine produced end-plate current fluctuation at frog neuromuscular junction, *J. Physiol.* **235**:655–692.

BINGLEY, M. S., 1965, The generation of potentials due to fluid flow and applied pressure, paper presented at the Society for Experimental Biology Conference, April 1965.

BISCOE, T. J., and CURTIS, D. R., 1967, Strychnine and cortical inhibition, *Nature* **214**:914–915.

BLOOM, F. E., 1974, To spritz or not to spritz: The doubtful value of aimless iontophoresis, *Life Sci.* **14**:1819–1834.

BLOOM, F. E., SIGGINS, G. R., and HOFFER, B. J., 1974, Interpreting the failure to confirm the depression of cerebellar Purkinje cells by cyclic AMP, *Science,* **185**:627–629.

BRADLEY, P. B., and CANDY, J. M., 1970, Iontophoretic release of acetylcholine, noradrenaline, 5-hydroxytryptamine and D-lysergic acid diethylamide from micropipettes, *Brit. J. Pharmacol.* **40**:194–201.

BRADLEY, P. B., ROBERTS, M. H. T. and STRAUGHAN, D. W., 1974, Recent advances in methods for studying the pharmacology of single cortical neurons. *Neuropharmacology* (Special Issue) **13**:401–573.

BRADSHAW, C. M., ROBERTS, M. H. T., and SZABADI, E., 1973a, Comparison of the effects of imipramine and desipramine on single cortical neurones, *Brit. J. Pharmacol.* **48**:358–359P.

BRADSHAW, C. M., ROBERTS, M. H. T., and SZABADI, E., 1973b, Kinetics of the release of noradrenaline from micropipettes; interaction between ejecting and retaining currents, *Brit. J. Pharmacol.* **49**:667–677.

BROOKS, V. B., CURTIS, D. R., and ECCLES, J. C., 1957, The action of tetanus on the inhibition of motor neurones, *J. Physiol.* **135**:655–672.

BUNNEY, B. S., WALTERS, J. R., ROTH, R. H., and AGHAJANIAN, G. K., 1973, Dopaminergic neurons: Effects of antipsychotic drugs and amphetamine on single cell activity, *J. Pharmacol. Exp. Ther.* **185**:560–571.

CALDWELL, P. C., and LEA, T. J., 1973, Use of intracellular glass scintillator for the continuous measurement of the uptake of ^{14}C-labelled glycine into squid giant axons, *J. Physiol.* **232**:4–5P.

CALDWELL, P. C., HODGKIN, A. L., KEYNES, R. D., and SHAW, T. I., 1960, The effects of injecting "energy-rich" phosphate compounds on the active transport of ions in the giant axons of *Loligo, J. Physiol.* **152**:561–590.

CARSLAW, H. S., and JAEGER, J. C., 1959, *Conduction of Heat in Solids*, 2nd ed., Oxford University Press, Oxford.

CHAMBERS, R. W., and KOPAC, M. J., 1950, in: *Handbook of Microscopical Technique*, 3rd ed., pp. 492–543, Harper, New York.

CLARKE, G., HILL, R. G., and SIMMONDS, M. A., 1973, Microiontophoresic release of drugs from micropipettes: Use of ^{24}Na as a model, *Brit. J. Pharmacol.* **48**:156–161.

COCEANI, F., and VITI, A., 1972, The release of prostaglandine E_1 from micropipettes *in vitro, Brain Res.* **45**:469–477.

CRANK, J., 1957, *The Mathematics of Diffusion*, Oxford University Press, Oxford.

CURTIS, D. R., 1964, Microelectrophoresis, in: *Physical Techniques in Biological Research,* Vol. V: *Electrophysiological Methods,* Part A (W. L. Natsuk, ed.), pp. 144–190, Academic Press, New York.

CURTIS, D. R., and FELIX, D., 1971, The effect of bicuculline upon synaptic inhibition in the cerebral and cerebellar cortices of the cat, *Brain Res.* **34**:301–321.

CURTIS, D. R., PERRIN, D. D., and WATKINS, J. C., 1960, The excitation of spinal neurones by the iontophoretic application of agents which cheolate calcium, *J. Neurochem.* **6**:1–20.

CURTIS, D. R., DUGGAN, A. W., and JOHNSTON, G. A. R., 1970, The inactivation of extracellularly administered amino acids in the feline spinal cord, *Exp. Brain Res.* **10**:447–462.

DAVIES, J. T., and RIDEAL, E. K., 1961, *Interfacial Phenomena*, Academic Press, New York.

DEL CASTILLO, J., and KATZ, B., 1955, On the localization of acetylcholine receptors, *J. Physiol.* **128**:157–181.

DE ROBERTIS, E., and GERSCHENFELD, H. F., 1961, Submicroscopic morphology and function of glial cells, *Int. Rev. Neurobiol.* **3**:1–65.

ECCLES, J. C., and JAEGER, J. C., 1957, The relationships between the mode of operation and the dimensions of the junctional regions at synapses and motor end-organs, *Proc. Roy. Soc. Lond. Ser. B* **148**:38.

FIRTH, D. R., and DE FELICE, L. J., 1971, Electrical resistance and volume flow in glass microelectrodes, *Can. J. Physiol. Pharmacol.* **49**:436–447.

GENT, J. P., MORGAN, R., and WOLSTENCRAFT, J. H., 1974, Determination of the relative potency of two excitant amino acids, *Neuropharmacology* **13**:441–447.

GLOBUS, A., LUX, H. D., and SCHUBERT, P., 1968, Somadendritic spread of intracellulary injected tritiated glycine in cat spinal motorneurones, *Brain Res.* **11**:440–445.

GODFRAIND, J. M., and PUMAIN, R., 1972, Cyclic AMP and noradrenaline iontophoretic release on rat cerebellar Pukinje neurons, *Arch. Int. Pharmacodyn. Ther.* **196**:131–132.

GOTTESFELD, Z., KELLY, J. S., and RENAUD, L. P., 1972, The *in vivo* neuropharmacology of amino-oxyacetic acid in the cerebral cortex of the cat, *Brain Res.* **42**:319–335.

GOUGH, D. A., and ANDRADE, J. D., 1973, Enzyme electrodes, *Science* **180**:380–384.

GRUNDFEST, H., KAO, L. Y., and ALTAMIRANO, M., 1954, Bioelectric effects of ions microinjected into the giant axon of *Loligo, J. Gen. Physiol.* **38**:245–282.

HAIGLER, H. J., and AGHAJANIAN, G. K., 1974, Lysergic acid diethylamide and serotin: A comparison of effects of serotinergic neurons and neurons receiving on serotinergic input, *J. Pharmacol. Exp. Ther.* **188**:688–699.

HERZ, A., ZIEGLGÄNSBERGER, W., and FÄRBER, G., 1969, Microelectrophoretic studies concerning the spread of glutamic acid and GABA in brain tissue, *Exp. Brain Res.* **9**:221–235.

HOFFER, B. J., NEFF, N. H., and SIGGINS, G. R., 1971, Microiontophoretic release of norepinephrine from micropipettes, *Neuropharmacology* **10**:175–180.

IVERSEN, L. L., 1971, Role of transmitter uptake mechanisms in synaptic transmission, *Brit. J. Pharmacol.* **41**:571–591.

JAEGER, J. C., 1965, Diffusion from constrictions, in: *Studies in Physiology, Presented to John C. Eccles* (D. R. Curtis and A. K. McIntyre, eds.), pp. 106–117, Springer, New York.

KATZ, B., and MILEDI, R., 1972, The statistical return of the acetycholine potential and its molecular components, *J. Physiol.* **224**:665–669.

KATZ, B., and MILEDI, R., 1973, The characteristics of "end-plate-noise" produced by different depolarizing drugs, *J. Physiol.* **230**:707–717.

KELLY, J. S., and RENAUD, L. P., 1974, Physiological identification of inhibitory interneurones in the feline pericuneate cortex, *Neuropharmacology* **13**:463–474.

KELLY, J. S., SIMMONDS, M. A., and STRAUGHAN, D. W., 1975, Microelectrode techniques, in: *Methods in Brain Research* (P. B. Bradley, ed.). pp. 333–377. Wiley, New York.

KEYNES, R. D., 1964, Addendum: Microinjection, in: *Physical Techniques in Biological Research*, Vol. V: *Electrophysiological Methods*, Part A (W. L. Natsuk, ed.). pp. 183–189. Academic Press, New York.

KOPAC, M. J., 1964, Micromanipulators: Principles of design, operation and application, in: *Physical Techniques in Biological Research*, Vol. V: *Electrophysiological Methods*, Part A (W. L. Natsuk, ed.). pp. 191–233. Academic Press, New York.

KŘÍŽ, N., SYKOVÁ, E., UJEC, E., and VJKLICKÝ, L. L., 1974, Changes of extracellular potassium concentration induced by neural activity in the spinal cord of the cat, *J. Physiol.* **238**:1–15.

KRNJEVIĆ, K., 1972, Microiontophoresis, in: *Methods in Neurochemistry* (M. Dekker, ed.), Pergamon Press, New York.

KRNJEVIĆ, K., and LISIEWICZ, A., 1972, Injection of calcium ions into spinal motorneurones, *J. Physiol.* **225**:363–390.

KRNJEVIĆ, K., and MILEDI, R., 1958, Acetylcholine in mammalian neuromuscular transmission, *Nature* **182**:805–806.

KRNJEVIĆ, K., and MORRIS, M. E., 1972, Extracellular K^+ activity and slow potential changes in spinal cord and medulla, *Can. J. Physiol. Pharmacol.* **50**:1214–1217.

KRNJEVIĆ, K., and MORRIS, M. E., 1974, An excitatory action of substance P on cuneate neurones, *Can. J. Physiol. Pharmacol.* **52**:736–744.

KRNJEVIĆ, K., and PHILLIS, J. W., 1963, Iontophoretic studies in neurones in the mammalian cerebral cortex, *J. Physiol.* **165**:274–304.

KRNJEVIĆ, K., and WHITTAKER, V. P., 1965, Excitation and depression of cortical neurones by brain fractions released from micropipettes, *J. Physiol.* **179**:298–322.

KRNJEVIĆ, K., LAVERTY, R., and SHARMAN, D. F., 1963a, Iontophoretic release of adrenaline, noradrenaline and 5-hydroxytryptamine from micropipettes, *Brit. J. Pharmacol. Chemother.* **20**:491–496.

KRNJEVIĆ, K., MITCHELL, J. F., and SZERB, J. C., 1963b, Determination of iontophoretic release of acetylcholine from micropipettes, *J. Physiol.* **165**:421–436.

LAKE, N., and JORDAN, L. M., 1974, Failure to confirm cyclic AMP as second messenger for norepinephrine in rat cerebellum, *Science* **183**:663–664.

LAVALLEE, M., 1964, Intracellular pH of rat atria muscle fibres measured by glass micropipette electrodes, *Circ. Res.* **15**:185–193.

McCREERY, R. L., DREILING, R., and ADAMS, R. N., 1974, Voltammetry in brain tissue: Quantitative studies of drug interactions, *Brain Res.* **73**:23–33.

MORGAN, R., VRBOVA, G., and WOLSTENCROFT, J. H., 1972, Correlation between the retinal input to lateral geniculate neurones and their relative response to glutamate and aspartate, *J. Physiol.* **224**:41P.

NEAME, K. D., and RICHARDS, T. G., 1972, *Elementary Kinetics of Membrane Carrier Transport*, Blackwell, Oxford.

OBATA, K., TAKEDA, K., and SHINOZAKI, H., 1970, Electrophoretic release of γ-aminobutyric acid and glutamic acid from micropipettes, *Int. J. Neuropharmacol.* **9:**191–194.

PAPPENHEIMER, J. R., 1953, Passage of molecules through capillary walls, *Physiol. Rev.* **33:**387–423.

PATON, W. D. M., and WAUD, D. R., 1964, A quantitative investigation of the relationship between rate of access of a drug to a receptor and the rate of onset or offset of action, *Arch. Exp. Pathol. Pharmacol.* **248:**124–143.

PRINCE, D. A., LUX, H. D., and NEHER, E., 1973, Measurement of extracellular potassium activity in cat cortex, *Brain Res.* **50:**489–495.

RITCHIE, J. M., and GREENGARD, P., 1966, On the mode of action of local anaesthetic, *Ann. Rev. Pharmacol.* **6:**405–430.

RUBIO, R., and ZUBIETA, G., 1961, The variation of the electrical resistance of micro-electrodes during the flow of current, *Acta Physiol. Latino-Am.* **11:**91–94.

RUTGERS, A. J., 1940, Streaming potentials and surface conductance, *Trans. Faraday Soc.* **36:**69–80.

SCHANNE, O. F., KAWATA, H., SCHAFER, B., and LAVALLEE, M., 1966, A study of the electrical resistance of the frog sartorius muscle. *J. Gen. Physiol.* **49:**897–912.

SCHON, F., and KELLY, J. S., 1974, Autoradiographic localization of (^{3}H)-GABA and (^{3}H)glutamate over satellite glial cells, *Brain Res.* **66:**275–288.

SCHUBERT, P., KREUTZBERG, G. W., and LUX, H. D., 1972, Use of microelectrophoresis in the autoradiographic demonstration of fiber projections, *Brain Res.* **39:**274–277.

SEGAL, M., and BLOOM, F. E., 1974, The action of norepinephrine in the rat hippocampus. I. Iontophoretic study, *Brain Res.* **72:**79–97.

SHOEMAKER, W. J., BALENTINE, L., HOFFER, B. J., SIGGINS, G. R., HENRIKSON, S., and BLOOM, F. E., 1974, in press, quoted from Bloom *et al.*, 1974.

THOMAS, R. C., 1974, Intracellular pH of snail neurones measured with a new pH-sensitive glass microelectrode, *J. Physiol.* **238:**159–180.

THRON, C. D., 1974, Linearity and superimposition in pharmacokinetics, *Pharmacol. Rev.* **26:**3–31.

WALKER, J. L., 1971, Ion specific liquid ion exchanger microelectrodes, *Anal. Chem.* **43:**89–92A.

WAUD, D. R., 1968, On diffusion from a point source, *J. Pharmacol. Exp. Ther.* **159:**123–128.

WEIDERHIELM, C. A., WOODBURY, J. W., KIRK, S., and RUSHMER, R. F., 1964, Pulsatile pressures in the microcirculation of frog's mesentery, *Am. J. Physiol.* **207:**173–176.

WERMAN, R., DAVIDOFF, R. A., and APRISON, M. H., 1966, The inhibitory action of cystathion, *Life Sci.* **5:**1431–1440.

ZIEGLGÄNSBERGER, W., HERZ, A., and TESCHENACHER, H., 1969, Electrophoretic release of tritium labelled glutamic acid from micropipettes *in vitro*, *Brain Res.* **15:**298–300.

ZIEGLGÄNSBERGER, W., SOTHMANN, G., and HERZ, A., 1974, Iontophoretic release of substances from micropipettes *in vitro*, *Neuropharmacology* **13:**417–422.

3

ELECTRICAL RECORDING OF BRAIN ACTIVITY: THE EEG AND ITS VALUE IN ASSESSING DRUG EFFECTS

Brian Meldrum

1. INTRODUCTION

The spontaneous and evoked electrical activity of the brain as recorded by means of macroelectrodes has been extensively investigated by psychopharmacologists (see bibliography by Fink, 1964). Used as an empirical tool, it can indicate the kind of behavioral effect a new drug will have in animals or man (e.g., Itil, 1973). However, with our present inadequate understanding of the relationship between electrochemical events at the cellular level and the gross electrical activity of the brain, it is rare that specific conclusions can be drawn about the mode of action of the drug. The problems are particularly severe when the spontaneous activity of the brain is studied by conventional EEG means alone. However, when activity in specific pathways is evoked either by focal electrical stimulation or by sensory stimulation in the appropriate modality, the possibility of correlating drug effects with cellular events is enhanced. In animal experiments, by the use of intracerebral electrodes to obtain focal recordings, we can approach the optimal situation whereby only one synapse intervenes between the pathway stimulated and

Brian Meldrum ● Department of Neurology, Institute of Psychiatry, London, England

the neurons producing the potential we are recording. This offers the possibility of direct correlation with microelectrode studies. However, even in such a situation there are often inadequately identified variables such as drug-induced changes in background excitation or inhibition or in feedback mechanisms so that any direct action of the systemically administered drug on the synapse studied is difficult to identify.

As psychopharmacologists using macroelectrode recording as a tool, we thus have two obligations. First, we must make the most appropriate use of available procedures. It is hoped that the brief review of techniques given in the first half of this chapter will help those more expert in other fields to avoid elementary errors (e.g., recording the EEG at such a slow speed that epileptic activity cannot be distinguished from slow-wave sleep).

The second obligation is to clarify the relationship between the action of drugs at the molecular or cellular level and their effects on cerebral electrical activity and behavior. The second half of this chapter gives only an elementary introduction to this topic. A fuller account will require more fundamental neurophysiological knowledge combined with further progress in the areas covered elsewhere in this volume.

2. SELECTION OF ANIMAL SPECIES

The choice of animal for EEG drug studies depends on the objective of the research program. Rats, rabbits, cats, monkeys, and baboons are commonly employed, but for some studies in psychopharmacology it is essential to use human volunteers or patients. Rats are cheap, and genetically homogeneous samples can be selected; they resist infection and tolerate chronic electrodes and cannulae well. They are relatively easy to train to lever-push for food rewards, so simple behavioral assessments can be made concurrently. Several atlases of the rat brain are available (König and Klippel, 1963; Wünscher et al., 1965; Pellegrino and Cuchman, 1967; Sherwood and Timiras, 1970; Albe-Fessard et al., 1966), and the aminergic pathways have been particularly well described (Fuxe, 1965; Hillarp et al., 1966). However, the brain and skull are relatively small, making regional EEG studies difficult. The rabbit and the cat have larger brains and are easy to handle. Stereotaxic atlases are available for both animals (Jasper and Ajmone-Marsan, 1954; Monnier and Gangloff, 1961; Snider and Niemer, 1961; Verhaart, 1964). An "EEG atlas" for pharmacological research in the rabbit has been produced (Longo, 1962), and there is an extensive literature on the neurophysiology and neuropharmacology of the cat. Both rabbits and cats spend a large proportion of the day dozing or sleeping so that assessment of drug-induced changes in EEG pattern has to take account of variations associated with spontaneous fluctuations in the state of arousal. Surgical simplification of the nervous system can obviate this problem, but many drug effects are then lost (see Section 3). There are clear species differences in drug responsiveness between cats and primates, the best known being the excitatory action of morphine in cats (Brooks *et al.*, 1941).

The cerebral anatomy of monkeys and baboons corresponds closely to that of man. Stereotaxic atlases are available for rhesus monkeys, *Macaca mulatta* (Snider and Lee, 1961); squirrel monkeys, *Saimiri sciureus* (Emmers and Akert, 1963); and baboons, *Papio papio* (Riche *et al.*, 1968) and *Papio cynocephalus/anubis* (Davis and Huffman, 1968). They can be trained to perform a wide variety of tasks and they also show complex social behaviors. Disadvantages include the high cost of purchase and maintenance, difficulties in handling the larger animals, and the high spontaneous incidence of disease.

Among less commonly used species, the 1- to 5-day-old chick has the special advantage of a poorly developed blood–brain barrier so that the central effects of amino acids and drugs with low lipid solubility can be assessed (Key and Marley, 1962). The dog is occasionally used (see Pampiglione, 1963; Lucas *et al.*, 1974), but because of the anatomy of its skull and pericranial musculature scalp records are rarely satisfactory and the chronic implantation of electrodes is less easy than in the rabbit and cat.

Man is the only experimental animal available for studying the action of psychopharmacological agents on many subtle aspects of behavior. This is obvious for drugs distorting the sensorium and those modifying the use of language, but is also true for normal or pathological behavior patterns that are not easily reproduced in animals. The literature correlating drug-induced EEG changes with changes in awareness or behavior in volunteers and patients is very extensive and will not be reviewed here (but see Vols. 4 and 5). These studies show that psychopharmacological agents can be classified on the basis of their EEG effects in a way that corresponds closely to their clinical effectiveness (Borenstein *et al.*, 1965, 1970; Fink, 1969; Itil, 1973).

3. ACUTE EXPERIMENTS

A significant body of literature describes the effects of psychopharmacological agents on the EEG of rabbits and cats recorded in acute (nonrecovery) experiments. Recordings were, and often are, made with electrodes (phonograph needles) inserted by percussion into the exposed skull, or with ball electrodes in contact with the exposed pial surface of the brain under a pool of warm paraffin, or with deep electrodes inserted through a trephine hole or other traumatic skull opening.

Such experiments are conducted either under general anesthesia or during mechanical ventilation under peripheral muscular paralysis (induced by a neuromuscular blocking agent such as *d*-tubocurarine or gallamine triethiodide) or after partial surgical deafferentation of the higher centers of the brain as in the *encéphale* and *cerveau isolé* preparations (Bremer, 1943, 1952).

Drugs that produce general anesthesia modify the pattern of EEG activity and will complicate evaluation of the rather subtle effects of psychopharmacological agents. Although it is now customary to infiltrate pressure points and wound margins with local anesthetic agents, some workers prefer not to use paralyzed animals on ethical grounds. With adequate attention to the comfort of the animal, spontaneous fluctuations in level of arousal as indicated by the EEG are similar to those in the conscious animal. However, the fact that EEG changes cannot be correlated with drug-induced behavioral effects is a major disadvantage in these and other acute experiments.

EEG studies in rabbits and cats with transections at various levels in the brain stem have contributed significantly to our understanding of neurological mechanisms involved in arousal and the different stages of sleep (Bremer, 1952; Jouvet, 1969*a*). They have also given rise to some influential speculations about the major site of action of amphetamines, barbiturates, chlorpromazine, and other agents (see Sections 8 and 13). However, in this situation also, behavioral correlations of EEG changes cannot be studied. These considerations allied with the increasing cost of experimental animals and the advantages from the scientific point of view of using animals as their own controls have led to the widespread adoption of procedures for the chronic recording of the EEG.

4. CHRONIC IMPLANTATION OF ELECTRODES

It is possible to record the EEG in rats, rabbits, cats, and monkeys using either stick-on scalp electrodes or subdermal needle electrodes of the type routinely used in human electroencephalography. However, records obtained in this way in the conscious animal commonly show excessive movement artifacts and are contaminated with muscle action potentials. Thus most workers chronically implant recording electrodes, which, if intracranial, may be either epidural or intracerebral. Implantation always requires general anesthesia. In rats, rabbits, and cats, a high standard of cleanliness plus sterilization of instruments and the skin is usually adequate, but for primates full aseptic precautions with sterile drapes, surgical gloves, and gowns are usual. It is convenient to hold the head in a stereotaxic apparatus even when stereotaxic placement of electrodes is not required. Metal screws can be inserted directly into holes made by burrs or twist drills (in a dental drill), but when nylon or other insulating screws are used it is often necessary to thread the skull hole by means of a tap. Nylon screws inserted in this way and prepared with axial or para-axial holes provide a convenient mount for either epidural ball electrodes or deep "needle electrodes." Silver, nichrome, platinum, and stainless steel wires either are purchased with insulation (e.g., diamel-coated from Johnson Matthey) or can be insulated with varnish, epoxy resin, polyvinyl chloride tubing, or acrylic cement. Silver when chlorided is most suitable for epidural electrodes, but may have a local toxic action when they are intracerebral. Deep electrodes can be single (insulated except at the tip) for "monopolar" recording, or coaxial for bipolar recordings, or multiple with recording contacts exposed at different depths (e.g., as described by Ray et al., 1965b). Deep electrodes can be mounted in nylon or metal screws in the skull or in sockets with multiple sites (as in the system described by Monnier and Gangloff 1961, for the rabbit), or can be stereotaxically located and then fixed by the application of acrylic cement to the skull (in rats a cranked shaft to the electrode facilitates fixation by a thin layer of acrylic).

Electrodes can also be chronically implanted in the skull intramuscularly or subdermally to permit recording of the electro-oculogram (EOG), electromyogram (EMG), or electrocardiogram (ECG). Such simultaneous physiological monitoring greatly enhances the value of EEG records and is essential for studies of sleep and epilepsy.

It is often convenient to implant cannulae for drug administration either intravenously (femoral or jugular veins) or into one lateral ventricle (Feldberg, 1963).

Connection to EEG and other input leads is commonly provided by a miniature multisocket cemented to the skull, although in the rat isolated exposed metal contacts are sometimes employed. Such procedures allow repeated recordings to be made over periods of months or years.

The interval to be left between implantation and the first control recordings and drug tests varies with the species, the anesthetic used, the skill of the operator, and the observations to be made. In rats, cortical bruising or more severe traumatic lesions are not uncommon.

5. RECORDING PROCEDURES

5.1. Experiments in Animals with Chronic Implants

For each recording session, the animal with a chronic implant is placed in a suitably insulated chamber and connected to the EEG input leads. A variety of systems are employed to counterbalance the leads and keep them clear of the animal. Multicontact rotating connectors are advantageous, especially for cat studies. Monkeys and baboons can be seated in a primate chair which leaves them free to feed themselves and to perform motor acts appropriate to a discrimination task.

Several systems of telemetry are now available in which a preamplifier, FM transmitter, and battery are either mounted on the skull or held in a pack strapped to the trunk of the animal. This permits the animal to move freely within a recording cage or area. Equipment currently in use permits recording of two or four channels and under optimal conditions gives records comparable to those obtained with conventional leads and EEG amplifiers. With some systems, the signal varies according to the spatial relationship of the transmitter and aerial. Another disadvantage is that battery life is limited, and it is necessary to switch batteries.

5.2. Human Studies

The stick-on or needle electrodes routinely employed for scalp recording of the EEG in man require that the subject be sitting or lying in a relatively relaxed position. Free-range recordings using telemetry are valuable for the study of paroxysmal phenomena and sleep. Muscle potentials and movement artifacts reduce their value for drug studies where the major effects are changes in the proportion of fast or slow activities. There are several widely used conventional schemes for the siting of scalp electrodes (e.g., the "10-20 system," Jasper, 1958), which facilitate comparisons between results obtained in different laboratories.

5.3. Derivations

Potential differences can be recorded only between two sites. So-called monopolar recording involves the use of a neutral reference electrode or an average (Goldmann) reference. There is no truly neutral reference point, but an anteriorly or posteriorly placed skull electrode or an ear is sometimes selected. For an average reference recording, the potential difference between the selected electrode and all the other available electrodes connected together is recorded. A chain of electrodes with bipolar readings from successive pairs allows identification of the focal origin of discharges by inspection for phase reversal.

5.4. Amplifiers

Transient potential differences generated by the brain and recorded from the scalp or the cerebral surface have amplitudes up to $200 \mu V$ during normal physiological activity, but may exceed 1 mV during epileptic discharges. An AC recording system must first amplify this signal and then display it against time in a form that can be visualized and stored. Limitations of the representation of the changes in potential can be imposed by the amplifiers and by the recording system. Slow potential changes may be subject to loss or distortion according to the time constant selected for the AC amplifier. A time constant of 1 s is required for accurate presentation of the slow rhythmic activities of the EEG, but in practice 0.3 s is a compromise facilitating assessment of fast activities while still permitting appreciation of the slow rhythms. For slow potential shifts, such as the contingent negative variation (Walter *et al.*, 1964), very long time constants, e.g., 10 s, are required. Limitation on the recording of higher frequencies is imposed by the mechanical properties of the pen-writing system, which usually attenuates high frequencies, beginning in the range 70–100 Hz. Ink jet systems can write at frequencies of 200–400 Hz, but this requires very rapid paper speeds for full evaluation. Spontaneous rhythms in the cerebellum involve frequencies around 200 Hz (Adrian, 1935), but very few studies have been made on them. Very high frequency activity (more than 1000 Hz) can be recorded during epileptic seizures (Rodin *et al.*, 1971).

5.5. Paper Records

Measurement of physiological rhythmic activities is optimal recording at a paper speed of 3.0 cm/s. It is possible at 1.5 cm/s, but slower speeds cannot be used for this purpose. For recordings over several hours, the length of paper utilized makes reading and handling laborious.

5.6. Magnetic Tape Recording

For reproduction of the low-frequency components of the EEG, an FM recording system is required. However, with FM recording at slow tape speeds the high-frequency response is impaired; this is important when transients with high-frequency elements, such as evoked potentials, are being studied. Thus, in practice, the length of tape per spool and the upper frequency response required determine the duration of continuous recording obtained. Apart from the ease of storage and the possibility of replaying at different speeds to give better visualization on display tubes or paper records, the main advantage of recording the EEG on tape is to permit computer analysis of all or selected parts of the record. This usually requires a time channel or an accurate system of tape indexing that gives a visual display of the tape location being read. For many purposes, an event channel for indicating the occurrence of stimuli in evoked response studies and a voice channel are required. It may also be necessary to record physiological variables and behavioral responses. Thus 8 to 16 channels of FM or digital recording are commonly considered essential.

6. METHODS OF ANALYZING AND QUANTIFYING THE EEG

Each channel of the EEG has two coordinates, time and amplitude (potential difference). Visual inspection and measurement with rulers and grids permit the derivation of a variety of quantitative estimates. Much of the activity has the appearance of rhythmic waves of an approximately sinusoidal form. EEG studies in man have led to a classification of such rhythmic activities into frequency bands, or into periods when they occur as isolated waves (Storm van Leeuwen *et al.*, 1966). This classification has some physiological and pathological justification and is practically useful in describing the effects of drugs in man. "Delta" (δ) describes a rhythm below 4 Hz or a wave with a period greater than 0.25 s. "Theta" (θ) describes rhythms in the range 4–8 Hz (periods of 0.25–0.125 s). "Beta" (β) rhythms have a frequency greater than 13 Hz. "Alpha" (α) rhythm in adults is generally in the frequency range 8–13 Hz, but to be described as α-rhythm an activity must show both a predominantly posterior (occipital) distribution and a reactivity related to visual attention. Two other rhythmic activities are, like α-rhythm, defined according to their location and reactivity. The "mu" (μ) rhythm, at 7–11 Hz, occurs in relation to the motor cortex and has a nonsinusoidal form (arcade or comb pattern). It is associated with β-rhythm and is attenuated by actual or intended movement, especially of the hands. "Sigma" (σ) rhythm occurs in brief bursts, and has a frequency of about 14 Hz. It is prominent at the vertex and is characteristic of light to intermediate sleep. It is sometimes known as a "sleep spindle" because of the shape of its envelope.

In most animal studies, approximately pure sinusoidal rhythms do not make up a significant proportion of the record except during sleep and in a wide variety of pathological conditions, of which the most important are cerebral hypoxia and hypoglycemia. Theta rhythm recorded from the hippocampus in rats, rabbits, cats, and dogs can have a very "pure" form and shows clear correlations with processes of arousal, habituation, and conditioning (Parmeggiani, 1967; Lucas *et al.*, 1974). The effect of many drugs is to convert a background activity of a very mixed spectral composition into a pattern with one dominant frequency.

6.1. Hand Analysis

By adopting an arbitrary criterion of amplitude (e.g., 10 μV for α-rhythm) and selecting appropriate epochs (e.g., 60 or 100 s), it is possible to measure the "percent time" occupied by a given activity. Such an approach to quantification is very laborious. It can be confounded by the mixture of different activities and usually leaves much of the record unclassified. In a modified form, such eye-and-hand analysis is still widely practiced for sleep record analysis (see Section 10); however, soon after the introduction of the EEG into clinical medicine, mechanical and electronic means were sought for the quantitative analysis of the EEG.

6.2. Integration

By means of a rectifier plus condenser or equivalent arrangement, it is possible to obtain a value for the total cerebral electrical activity over a period which corresponds to the total area between the EEG trace and the pen zero line (Drohocki, 1948*a,b*). This operation can be conveniently performed by an analog computer. Digital systems permit a more sophisticated integration, which by squaring the successive amplitudes of the EEG and then summing the squares yields the variance of the signal. (The negative or positive amplitude of an EEG record is the difference between the signal and the mean or base line, Byford, 1965.)

These integration procedures apparently sacrifice all information about the frequency composition of the EEG record. However, the greater the proportion of large slow waves in the record, the greater the integrated value; thus there is a broad correlation between drowsiness or sleep and the integrated value. Integration procedures have been widely used in the assessment of drug effects (Dewhurst and Marley, 1965*a,b*; Finckh and Kugler, 1961; Goldstein *et al.*, 1963*a,b*; Murphree *et al.*, 1964). The measurements they provide facilitate determination of threshold doses and the duration of drug effects and permit comparisons between different doses and different drugs.

6.3. Frequency Analysis

In frequency analysis, the EEG is filtered to separate the activity into frequency bands. Two to five broad bands can be selected to correspond approximately to the frequency ranges used routinely in clinical EEG reporting. Bands 1–2, 2–4, 4–8, 8–16, and 16–32 Hz are mathematically convenient and have the practical advantage that comparable results can be obtained when magnetic tape records are replayed at different speeds. Alternatively, a large number of narrow bands can be selected; a frequency width of 1–3 Hz requires about 20 bands to cover the main physiological activities (1–33 Hz). Broad-band and narrow-band frequency analysis can now be very satisfactorily performed by means of electronic filters. By use of band-pass filters, the activity in any or all of the bands can be displayed polygraphically in real time using one pen per band. This may facilitate study of "masked" frequencies. However, most workers have chosen to quantify the data further by methods of integration (described above) using analog or digital computational devices. In wave analyzers of the Walter type

(Baldock and Walter, 1946; Shipton, 1961; Gay and Binnie, 1970), the activity in each narrow-frequency band is integrated during a brief epoch (10 s) and indicated by a series of pen deflections (the amplitude of each deflection corresponding to the integrated activity in a frequency band during a 10 s epoch).

Alternatively, a continuous plot can be made of activity in each of several broad-frequency bands by continuously integrating the square of the signal in that band (Byford, 1965). In a plot of this kind, the slope is proportional to the variance of the signal. The slope has a numerical value. Changes in the ratios between slopes of different frequency bands represent a very sensitive quantitative index of drug effects. Centrally acting drugs can readily be classified according to the doses enhancing fast or slow activities. Also, the times of onset and termination of drug action can be accurately determined. Because of its capacity to yield a fairly complex classification of psychotropic drugs, this procedure is superior to simple integrative procedures.

Frequency analysis involves a loss of much of the information in the original signal. In particular, sustained activity of low amplitude may not be differentiated from intermittent activity of higher amplitude. Small frequency shifts within a frequency band may also be ignored. This latter problem can be dealt with by spectral analysis.

6.4. Spectral Analysis

By means of relatively complex digital computational procedures (based on Fourier analysis of the waveform and calculation of the sine and cosine, (Matousek, 1973), it is possible to obtain graphic representations of the relative activity at different frequencies with a resolution much greater than 1 Hz. Recording such graphs with vertical displacement of successive traces corresponding to successive 20-s samples gives rise to a "compressed spectral array." In drug experiments, such an analysis and display permit ready appreciation of small frequency shifts in the dominant activities and also the times of appearance and disappearance of activities at particular frequencies. As with the broad-frequency-band signal variance plot of Byford, this procedure provides a graphic display on one sheet of paper of frequency data for an entire experiment (for one EEG channel). The results are mathematically less convenient but more detailed than those of the Byford procedure.

6.5. Correlation Procedures

In autocorrelation analysis statistical computational techniques are used to compare an EEG signal (considered as a time series) with itself displaced in time. The result is a type of spectral analysis that can be applied to epochs of various lengths.

Similar procedures can be used to give a comparison of one EEG signal with another recorded simultaneously from a different site. Such cross-correlation analysis provides important data when two signals are similar but have a phase or time lag. This may provide evidence about the site of origin or mode of spread of a particular discharge pattern. This technique has been applied to study of θ-activity in the limbic system during learning (Adey *et al.*, 1960), but is also relevant to studies on the spread of epileptic discharges.

7. SENSORY EVOKED RESPONSE ANALYSIS

In the EEG recorded at the scalp, responses to transient sensory stimuli tend to be obscured by the spontaneous or background activity. This is not always true for nonspecific responses occurring at the vertex following unexpected stimuli. However, evoked responses recorded over the primary receiving area following visual, auditory, or somatosensory stimulation in normal conscious subjects are generally smaller in amplitude than the background activity. The photographic superimposition of EEG traces on a cathode ray oscilloscope (Dawson, 1951) can aid the identification of elements common to a sequence of records following a stimulus.

By means of analog or digital computers, potential changes that are time-locked to a stimulus can be averaged and thus enhanced in relation to background activity, which does not have any constant relation to the occurrence of the stimulus. When the noise (background activity) is of similar amplitude and frequency distribution to the signal (evoked potential), the signal-to-noise ratio is enhanced according to the square root of N (N being the number of responses averaged). With averaging procedures, information about the variability of individual responses is lost. However, it is possible using a digital computer program to determine the standard deviation of a series of evoked potentials. Even this complex procedure does not answer many of the problems posed by the variability of evoked responses. The form of an evoked response and the latency of its various components can vary according to the number of stimuli in the sequence. They may also vary in relation to spontaneous changes in the background EEG activity (Kooi and Bagchi, 1964; Broughton *et al.*, 1965; Sato *et al.*, 1971). Information about variation in latency is lost on averaging; such variation may modify the average in exactly the same way as variation in amplitude.

Some of these problems can be resolved in animals with chronically implanted electrodes, where individual evoked responses can be measured and compared to computer-derived averages and assessed against the background EEG (Meldrum, 1966).

In chronic animal studies, it is important to record either from an epidural electrode or from a clearly defined depth. Many studies with "intracortical" electrodes are of little value because of the difficulty of identifying the successive components of the response in order to correlate them with other studies. A major advantage of animals with chronic implants is that recordings can be made simultaneously at various sites along the afferent pathway, thus facilitating the differentiation of "peripheral" and central drug effects (e.g., Vuillon-Cacciuttolo et al., 1973).

7.1. Visual Evoked Responses

Because of the need for a brief, precisely triggered stimulus, most early studies on averaged visual evoked responses employed a stroboscope flash as the stimulus. Responses differ markedly according to whether the eyes are open or closed. They also vary according to the time interval between flashes. Provided consistent recording electrode sites are chosen; comparable waveforms are seen in normal subjects. The flash-evoked responses can be modified by barbiturates, benzodiazepines, and lysergic acid diethylamide and other ergot alkaloid derivatives (Brown, 1969; Ebe et al., 1969; Vuillon-Cacciuttolo et al., 1973).

By use of a screen illuminated by a projector transient "meaningful" visual inputs or shifting checkerboard patterns can be provided. Few drug studies have yet been performed using these more sophisticated systems.

7.2. Somatosensory Evoked Responses

A brief shock (0.1–0.3 ms) to a peripheral nerve at the wrist or in the leg is the most commonly used stimulus for studying somatosensory potentials. In man, ring electrodes are used on the fingers and stick-on electrodes elsewhere. In animals, subdermal needle electrodes or fine wires are common. A piezoelectric crystal or other electromechanical device can be used to give a brief triggered mechanical stimulus to a fingernail.

Responses recorded over the primary receiving area show a consistent waveform and latency (see Regan, 1972) readily modified by centrally acting drugs (Allison et al., 1963).

7.3. Auditory Evoked Responses

Averaged scalp or extradural records of electrical activity following clicks or other brief auditory stimulation are difficult to interpret because of contamination, at short latency, by a "myogenic" component and, at longer latency, by the K-complex or nonspecific responses (Bickford *et al.*, 1964; Davis *et al.*, 1966). Also, the anatomical relationships of the primary receiving area add greatly to the difficulty of interpretation of records from surface electrodes.

8. FOCAL ELECTRICAL STIMULATION

Focal electrical stimulation is an important technique in EEG studies of drug action in two experimental contexts. One is the change in "background" EEG activity induced by brain stem or thalamic stimulation and the modification in these effects following drug treatment. The other is stimulation of identified pathways and recording of an evoked potential in order to assess the probable site or mode of action of a drug.

Details of appropriate stimulating electrodes and "stimulus parameters" are presented in the volume edited by Sheer (1961). The use of AC stimulating currents or of stimulus pairs (brief pulses alternately negative and positive) is important for avoiding both electrode polarization and local tissue damage.

The "activation" of the EEG (i.e., the replacement of mixed or slow background activities by irregular low-voltage fast activity) that results from electrical stimulation of the mesencephalic reticular formation (Moruzzi and Magoun, 1949; Rossi and Zanchetti, 1957) was the subject of much pharmacological research in the 10 years that followed its discovery. Modifications induced by atropine, barbiturates, and phenothiazines were described (Rinaldi and Himwich, 1955; Killam, 1957; Bradley and Key, 1958).

The effects of these drugs and of amphetamines and anticholinesterases were also studied in experiments combining transient sensory stimulation or brief shocks to afferent pathways, with recording of gross evoked potentials in the mesencephalic reticular formation (White and Rudolph, 1967). These and other experiments led to the hypothesis of a cholinergic cortical activating system originating at the mesodiencephalic level and an aminergic system operating through the cholinergic system and originating at a lower level in the brain stem. These concepts are discussed further in Section 13.

Focal electrical stimulation can produce abnormal EEG patterns, including several kinds of epileptic discharge. Rhythmic cortical spike-and-wave patterns can follow anterior thalamic stimulation in barbiturate-anesthetized cats (Jasper and Droogleever-Fortuyn, 1947).

The properties of afterdischarges following hippocampal stimulation in rats, rabbits, and cats are well documented and there is an extensive literature on their pharmacology (see review by Izquierdo and Nasello, 1972). Focal and generalized seizures following hypothalamic, septal, and neocortical stimulation are also well-defined phenomena, but their pharmacology has been less thoroughly explored.

Brief single stimuli given to thalamic relay nuclei or the lateral geniculate body can be used for studying early cortical responses (as described in Section 7). When the objective is to stimulate and record with one intervening synapse, the number of potential sites is very great but their selection is difficult. Detailed consideration of such results cannot be given here. However, it is important to remember that in the intact nervous system indirect effects are always possible. A minimal precaution is to record background EEG activity both at the cortex and at the "postsynaptic" site to identify any generalized effects of stimulation.

One special case where gross electrode recording and stimulation techniques have contributed to our understanding of synaptic mechanisms is the study of dorsal root potentials in the spinal cord. Changes in such potentials induced by barbiturates, benzodiazepines, picrotoxin, and drugs blocking the synthesis of γ-aminobutyric acid (GABA) can be correlated with changes in spinal reflexes and seizure thresholds (Bell and Anderson, 1972; Levy and Anderson, 1973; Hill et al., 1973; Schmidt, 1971). This has given an understanding of presynaptic inhibition that could not have been achieved by microelectrode recording alone.

9. ELECTROGENESIS OF THE EEG AND EVOKED POTENTIALS

Initial interpretations of the cellular events underlying the field potentials recorded by macroelectrodes were in terms of action potentials in nerve cell bodies and axons (Adrian and Matthews, 1934). As such events individually are very brief (durations of about 1 ms), the EEG was visualized as the algebraic sum or envelope of very many transient potentials which showed a limited amount of rhythmic phasing. This concept persists in the use of the terms "synchronized" and "desynchronized" to describe EEG appearances with regular high-voltage waves and those with low-voltage irregular patterns. However, once intracellular microelectrodes had revealed the time courses of postsynaptic inhibitory and excitatory potentials in neurons of the spinal cord (Eccles, 1953, 1957) and cortex (Phillips, 1956; Eccles, 1964), hypotheses explaining EEG and evoked potentials in terms of synaptic potentials became established (Towe, 1966).

A direct demonstration of the relationship between EEG potentials and neuronal transmembrane potentials is extremely difficult. A lissencephalic experimental animal is desirable because of the mathematical complexity of describing field potentials in a highly convoluted cortex. Intracellular recording from one large pyramidal neuron in the cerebral cortex of a cat has been technically possible for about 20 years. However, what is required is sampling of representative types of neurons, with recording of potentials in cell bodies and basal and apical dendrites. Another difficulty of interpretation is that the glial cells and the dendrites lying between the neuronal cell bodies in the third to fifth cortical layers and the pial surface act as a network of resistors and capacitors. This tends to filter out fast transients and to impose a phase lag on potential changes recorded at the surface that varies according to the frequency characteristics of the potential change. The electrical properties of these components can vary according to the past and present activity of the adjacent neurons. Dendritic membrane conductances change with neuronal activity. Concentrations of sodium and potassium in the extracellular fluid change with sustained neuronal activity, and this can modify glial cell membrane properties (Kuffler, 1967).

Using barbiturate-anesthetized or gallamine-paralyzed cats, Calvet *et al.* (1964) correlated cellular events and potential gradients at different cortical depths with macroelectrode surface potentials. Observed surface waves could be accounted for in terms of three dipoles—one superficial (cortical depth 0–500 μm, probably dendritic) giving surface-negative waves and two deeper dipoles with phase inversions at about 900–1000 μm one giving surface-positive waves and one giving surface-negative waves. The surface positive dipole is accompanied by an increase in cell firing rates and by depolarization of nerve cell body membranes deep in the cortex. The other deep dipole (surface negative) is associated with neuronal cell body hyperpolarization and a decrease in cell firing rates.

This simplified account appears to be broadly applicable to barbiturate spindles, to primary evoked potentials induced by afferent stimulation (including electrical stimulation of thalamic relay nuclei, Creutzfeldt *et al.*, 1966a), and to some epileptic discharges (Creutzfeldt *et al.*, 1966b). In the latter two situations, initially a number of pyramidal neuron cell bodies are depolarized relatively synchronously (associated with cell-body action potentials and a brief surface-positive wave). Secondarily, there is a negative wave with two or more components. One of these is related to electrotonic spread of depolarization into the superficial dendrites; the other is due to hyperpolarization of the cell body following inhibitory interneuron activity. In addition, Creutzfeldt *et al.* (1966a,b) identified a surface-positive wave related to deep inhibitory postsynaptic potentials.

Studies of the spontaneous components of the EEG in the unanesthetized cat show much less evidence of correlation between slow potentials recorded intracellularly and EEG records. A single neuron studied intracellularly over a 10-min period (Elul, 1972) shows brief episodes of close correlation with macroelectrode surface records and long periods with no correlation. Elul (1972) suggests that at any one time a relatively small proportion of neurons show similar synaptic potential changes and that the population that is thus synchronized is constantly varying, perhaps under thalamic control.

A study of intracellular potential changes in relay neurons of the ventrobasal nucleus of the cat thalamus has clearly established (Andersen *et al.*, 1964; Andersen and Sears, 1964; Andersen and Andersson, 1968) that spontaneous or stimulus-induced spindles recorded in the cerebral cortex during barbiturate anesthesia are driven or phased from the thalamus. Transient activity within thalamic relay neurons is followed by hyperpolarization of the soma membrane, due to inhibitory interneuron activity. The decline of this synaptic potential over a 100-ms period brings the relay neurons to an excitable state simultaneously. Their consequent synchronous firing induces both the rhythmic cortical activity and, by recurrent inhibition, repeated cycles of hyperpolarization in the thalamic neurons themselves. The clear evidence relating to barbiturate spindles in the cat (Andersen and Andersson, 1968) should not be taken as evidence that other rhythmic activities in the cortex are driven from subcortical pacemakers. Recurrent excitatory and inhibitory pathways exist within the cortex and may create the possibility of focal cortical phasing of activity. In this case, the period of the rhythm will depend on the time course of decay of synaptic potentials of the cortical neurons. The time course of decay of synaptic potentials in the spinal cord and thalamus can be modified by anesthetic agents, convulsant drugs, anticonvulsants, and psychotropic agents (Eccles, 1964; Schmidt, 1971; Hill *et al.*, 1973). Comparable actions probably occur at a cortical level. Studying correlations between actions of systemically applied drugs on synaptic potentials and on gross EEG rhythms may provide the understanding we seek of the cellular actions responsible for behavioral and EEG changes.

10. ASSESSMENT OF ALERTNESS, SEDATION, AND THE STAGES OF SLEEP

EEG recordings are commonly used for the continuous assessment of the level of wakefulness or sleep in man and animals. In an alert, tense human subject, the EEG shows predominantly low-voltage fast activity ("activated" or "desynchronized" EEG). Slight relaxation may be associated with the appearance of α-activity, during drowsiness θ-waves appear, in light sleep δ-waves are added to the θ-rhythm and spindles become prominent, and in deep sleep spindles disappear and irregular high-voltage δ-waves dominate the record. In all-night sleep EEG records, this slow-wave pattern is periodically interrupted by episodes of low-voltage fast activity associated with rapid eye movements (seen on the electro-oculogram) and the probability of dream recall (Dement and Kleitman, 1957). Subsequent studies (Jouvet, 1969a, 1972) have shown that slow-wave sleep and "paradoxical" or "rapid eye movement" (REM) sleep differ in many physiological respects.

Thus during REM sleep muscle tone is severely reduced (as shown by a "flat" EMG), tendon reflexes are absent, respiration is irregular in rhythm, cerebral blood flow is increased, arousal threshold is increased, and, in males, penile erection is commonly present. Slow-wave sleep is conveniently considered in terms of four levels which are somewhat arbitrarily defined by the proportion of θ- and δ-activity and of sleep spindles. Standardized criteria for "sleep staging" are given by Rechtshaffen and Kalès (1968). Automated procedures for this are now available (Frost, 1970; Galliard *et al.*, 1972). The study of sleep patterns in relation to psychopharmacology is further considered in Section 11.

Animals used for EEG studies in psychopharmacology show essentially the same stages of sleep and wakefulness as man, but a true α-rhythm is rarely prominent except in the anthropoid apes. They can of course be used for formal studies of sleep patterns and their modification by drugs as in man (see Section 11). However, all animals in chronic experiments show spontaneous cyclic fluctuations in the level of arousal. These fluctuations depend on a variety of factors including the time of day, the interval since feeding, the background level of lighting and noise, the presence of members of the same or other species (including "laboratory traffic"), and the familiarity of the surroundings. A large proportion of psychopharmacological agents induce either sedation or arousal. It is obvious that where such effects are to be assessed attention must be paid to the factors discussed and carefully controlled comparisons made with the effects of injection of saline or the drug carrier. Some quantitation is usually essential. Visual determination of the proportion of time occupied by different grades of EEG arousal is difficult and time consuming, so computer plotting of integrals of activity in different frequency bands may be advantageous.

Another procedure for assessing the degree of sedation is to deliver brief arousing stimuli (peripheral shock or loud noise) and to time the duration of EEG activation. The intensity and timing of such stimuli have to be adjusted in control tests to minimize the effects of habituation.

11. STUDY OF SLEEP PATTERNS

Whole-night or 24-hr EEG and polygraphic recordings of sleep patterns in chronically implanted cats and monkeys or in human patients or volunteers are now an important tool in psychopharmacological research. They provide a sensitive index of central drug actions and show some interesting correlations with subtle changes in psychopathology.

With proper experimental precautions, including 1 or 2 nights of preliminary recording to habituate the subject to the recording situation, a stable and consistent sleep pattern is shown (varying with species and with age). The latent interval from sleep onset to the first REM sleep episode is easily quantified and relatively constant. The duration of REM episodes increases progressively during the night. The total duration represents a constant proportion of the total sleep. The proportion of stage 4 sleep and its distribution between the first, middle, and last thirds of the night provide another index of drug action.

Barbiturates given in hypnotic doses decrease the proportion of REM sleep (and of sleep stages 3 and 4). Withdrawal produces a rebound, with an excess of REM sleep and of stage 3 and 4 sleep which persists for many nights (Ogunremi *et al.*, 1973). Benzodiazepine hypnotics also markedly reduce REM sleep (Kalès *et al.*, 1971; Gaillard *et al.*, 1973).

The reduction in REM sleep produced by three classes of drugs acting on normal or abnormal mood states is of great theoretical interest. These are monoamine oxidase inhibitors, tricyclic antidepressant drugs, and amphetamine and its derivatives (Akindele *et al.*, 1970; Dunleavy *et al.*, 1972; Lewis, 1970). In contrast, reserpine produces a marked enhancement of REM sleep (Hoffman and Domino, 1969). Control of the stages of sleep by a serotoninergic system originating in the nuclei of the median raphe and a noradrenergic system originating in the locus coeruleus has been proposed by Jouvet (1969*a,b*, 1972), but a completely consistent explanation of the drug effects in terms of these two systems has yet to be proposed.

12. ABNORMAL EEG RECORDS

12.1. Normal Rhythms Occurring Abnormally

An EEG record can be considered abnormal when certain normal rhythms are not present or when they are present but in unusual quantity or with an unusual distribution or unusual behavioral concomitants. Thus the activated EEG seen after amphetamine is abnormal because of the absence of slower rhythms. Similarly, the all-night sleep EEG after a monoamine oxidase inhibitor is abnormal because of the relatively low proportion of REM sleep.

An EEG appearance can be normal when occurring in association with one behavioral state and abnormal in association with another. This means that EEG records can be adequately assessed only if the animal is free to exhibit a range of behavior and the behavior is adequately observed and recorded. Early observers described a "dissociation" between the EEG and behavior in cats and dogs after the administration of atropine (Wikler, 1952; Bradley and Elkes, 1957). The animals appeared more alert than expected on the basis of the slow-wave activity in the EEG. This is explainable if spontaneous motor activity and apparent arousal are related to activity in subcortical arousal systems and atropine blocks only the last cortical stage of arousal. However, anticholinergics produce an acute toxic confusional state (termed the "central anticholinergic syndrome" by Longo, 1966) and perhaps the EEG changes are not inappropriate.

12.2. Nonepileptic Abnormal Rhythms

Some drug-induced EEG appearances are abnormal in that they are unlike anything occurring naturally. The enhanced fast activity seen after benzodiazepines is different from the low-voltage fast activity associated with the alert state because it has a more uniform frequency and amplitude. Delta activity induced by relatively high doses of sedative drugs is also more rhythmic and uniform than that in the EEG of slow-wave sleep. Even more distinctive are the bursts of mixed-frequency activity separated by relatively silent periods that are seen in deep barbiturate anesthesia. Toxic doses of several centrally acting drugs, including benzodiazepines, are associated with rhythmic sustained fast activity superimposed on equally rhythmic and sustained slow-wave activity.

12.3. Epileptic Features

Signs of epileptic activity take many forms and are one of the common-est findings during the investigation of newly synthesized centrally acting drugs. It is extremely important to make simultaneous records of the EEG and of motor signs of epileptic activity. Minor motor signs that may accompany epileptic discharges include masticatory movements (associated particularly with amygdaloid, hippocampal, or temporal lobe discharges), sudden vocalization, twitching of vibrissae, eyelids, or other facial muscula-ture, nystagmus, focal limb twitching, and brief generalized myoclonic jerks. Commonly, epileptic discharges in the cortex are accompanied by the absence of motor activity (akinetic epilepsy). All that is observed is a sudden loss of spontaneous motor activity, a postural change or loss of muscle tone, or a transient fixation of gaze. Drugs producing akinetic seizures are not uncommonly reported as having a sedative action and (because the threshold for motor seizures induced by electroshock or drugs such as pentylenetetrazol, picrotoxin, or thiosemicarbazide is usually raised) as being anticonvulsant. Skilled observation combined with adequate EEG recording is necessary to avoid this error. Another possibility also necessi-tates close observation of motor behavior. Animals may show either a running fit (rodents) or a tonic spasm and yet all that is seen on the conventional EEG as recorded at the scalp or over the neocortex is an activated pattern. Under these circumstances, very high frequency discharges may be recorded with an oscilloscope from the brain stem (Rodin et al., 1971).

Among the characteristic types of EEG changes associated with epilepsy are isolated spikes or sharp waves, which may be diffuse or focal, spikes and waves, bursts of spikes, and rhythmic spikes and waves. When the last are symmetrical and occurring regularly at about 3/s, they are often associated with absence of spontaneous motor activity as after Δ^9-tetrahydrocannabinol (Meldrum et al., 1974) or parachlorophenyl-GABA (Meldrum and Horton, 1974). Spikes and waves when irregular and more rapid are usually associated with myoclonic movements of the muscles of the face or limbs.

Convulsive seizures evolve according to rather rigid patterns characteristic of the species and the drug. A tonic seizure is often preceded by a running fit in rodents, and by isolated or rhythmic spikes and muscle jerks in cats and primates. The tonic seizure commonly progresses from an initial flexor phase into an extensor spasm and then into rhythmic generalized myoclonus. On the EEG, such a tonic seizure characteristically begins with low-voltage fast activity which becomes increasingly rhythmic and of higher amplitude until there is almost sinusoidal activity at 10–16 Hz of extremely high amplitude. During generalized myoclonus, this is replaced by repetitive polyspikes and waves. Rhythmic myoclonic activity can be extremely sustained, as after bicuculline in baboons (Meldrum and Horton, 1973). A sudden synchronous cessation of myoclonic activity (and the associated cortical polyspikes and waves) is usually followed by postictal depression of the EEG and of motor activity.

Most drug-induced seizure activity has an apparently symmetrical onset. However, this is not true of pyridoxal phosphate antagonists (see Section 13.4).

13. TRANSMITTERS AND EEG CHANGES

13.1. Acetylcholine

EEG activation following the intracarotid injection of acetylcholine in the cat cerveau isolé was described by Bonnet and Bremer (1937). Similar effects can be produced by anticholinesterases, such as physostigmine given systemically (Rinaldi and Himwich, 1955; Bradley and Elkes, 1957; Meldrum et al., 1970a). These and some other EEG-activating compounds can be antagonized by atropine and other muscarinic blocking agents (Bremer and Chatonnet, 1949; Domino et al., 1968).

Using histochemical stains specific for acetylcholinesterase in the rat, Shute and Lewis (1967) described an ascending reticular system which they presumed to be cholinergic and which may provide the anatomical basis for these pharmacological effects. Initial stages run in the dorsal and ventral tegmental pathways from the nucleus cuneiformis, ventral tegmental area, and substantia nigra to the thalamus, hypothalamus, and basal forebrain areas. A second system with cell bodies in the globus pallidus, entopeduncular nucleus, and lateral preoptic area projects diffusely to the neocortex. Stimulation of sensory nerves or electrical stimulation of deep structures forming part of this ascending system can produce EEG activation and enhance the release of acetylcholine from the pial surface of the cortex in rabbits and cats (Mitchell, 1963; Celesia and Jasper, 1966; Kanai and Szerb, 1965). The spontaneous efflux of acetylcholine is reduced during slow-wave sleep and is augmented during REM sleep (Jasper and Tessier, 1971). The release of acetylcholine is enhanced by atropine, suggesting that the system may be under a feedback control.

Microelectrode studies with iontophoretic application of acetylcholine to neurons is the deeper layer of the sensorimotor cortex have demonstrated a slow excitatory action of acetylcholine that can be blocked by atropine (Krnjević and Phillis, 1963b; Crawford and Curtis, 1966).

Pharmacological, physiological, and anatomical evidence supports the concept of a mesodiencephalic cholinergic EEG-activating system that is largely muscarinic. Its diffuse nature and the absence of a uniform inhibitory feedback probably explain the absence of the phasing that is seen during activity in the thalamic relay nuclei, and thus the EEG-desynchronizing or -activating effect.

The exact role of this system is far from defined in most pharmacological and physiological situations. In particular, it should not be assumed that antagonism of a particular activating effect by atropine establishes that the effect is mediated by this system.

13.2. Catecholamines

Evidence that dopamine acts as a neurotransmitter in the basal ganglia has been accumulating over the last decade (see York, Chap. 2, Vol. 6). More recently, neurons containing dopamine have been identified in the subcortical components of the limbic system in the rat and dopamine-containing terminals identified within the limbic cortex and the basal forebrain (Thierry et al., 1973; Hökfelt et al., 1974). Neuroleptic drugs such as the phenothiazines and butyrophenones are believed to block dopaminergic transmission postsynaptically (Carlsson and Lindqvist, 1963; see also York, Chap. 2, Vol. 6). In experimental and human studies, chlorpromazine and haloperidol produce a slowing of the EEG (the background rhythms become slower and more δ-activity and spindles appear) (Bradley and Hance, 1957; Longo and Florio, 1970; Borenstein et al., 1970). The EEG-activating effects of amphetamines are blocked by chlorpromazine and haloperidol, but the

EEG changes following atropine or eserine are not modified (Bradley and Hance, 1957; Consroe and White, 1972). There is some evidence that the EEG effects of chlorpromazine are produced by an action on dopaminergic rather than noradrenergic transmission. Chlorpromazine and butyrophenones block the EEG arousal induced by mesencephalic stimulation in the rabbit, and this effect is reversed by L-dopa (Florio and Longo, 1971). Apomorphine has an EEG-desynchronizing action which is potently and specifically blocked by chlorpromazine or haloperidol (Votava and Dyntarová, 1970). Destruction of the nigrostriatal dopaminergic system diminishes behavioral wakefulness but not EEG desynchronization (Jones et al., 1973).

Central neurons containing norepinephrine have been thoroughly mapped in the rat (Fuxe, 1965; Hillarp et al., 1966), but their functional role is not yet clear.

Epinephrine or norepinephrine given intravenously produces EEG alerting or desynchronization in the cat (Rothballer, 1956). However, this effect is secondary to peripheral cardiovascular changes (Baust et al., 1963; Baust and Niemczyk, 1964). Norepinephrine does not enter the brain from the blood except to a limited extent in the hypothalamus (Weil–Malherbe, 1960). In the newborn chick, which has an imperfectly developed blood–brain barrier, catecholamines given systemically induce behavioral sleep and a slow-wave EEG pattern (Key and Marley, 1962; Dewhurst and Marley, 1965c). Similarly, catecholamines given intracisternally or into ventricles or subarachnoid space produce sedation or anesthesia (Leimdorfer and Metzner, 1949; Feldberg and Sherwood, 1954; Feldberg, 1963; Marley and Stephenson, 1972).

When applied iontophoretically, norepinephrine depresses the activity of cortical neurons (Krnjević and Phillis, 1963a; Krnjević, 1974), but it can apparently act as an excitant in the hypothalamus (Moss et al., 1972).

However, evidence from lesion studies in which the ascending noradrenergic systems are partially destroyed and from pharmacological experiments in which the synthesis of norepinephrine is impaired suggests that the ascending systems contribute to the maintenance of wakefulness and of paradoxical sleep. Thus lesions induced by 6-hydroxydopamine injection in the dorsal bundle containing axons from cell bodies in the locus coeruleus produce a temporary reduction in EEG "wakefulness" (but no change in behavioral wakefulness) in the rat (Lidbrink, 1974). Similar effects are seen after electrolytic lesions of the mesencephalon in the cat (Jones, 1969; Jones et al., 1973). When norepinephrine synthesis is impaired with α-methyl-p-tyrosine or disulfiram, behavioral and EEG wakefulness are reduced and the proportion of REM sleep decreases (Jouvet, 1972). However, the role of these noradrenergic systems in functional states with a low-voltage fast EEG must be limited, as such states do still occur when the systems are partially or totally destroyed (Lindbrink, 1974; Jouvet, 1972).

13.3. 5-Hydroxytryptamine

The main ascending "serotoninergic" system as identified by his-tofluorescence has its cell bodies in the nuclei of the median raphe and its terminals scattered diffusely in the neocortex, striatum, lateral geniculate, hippocampus, and hypothalamus (Fuxe, 1965).

Both excitatory and inhibitory responses have been reported to follow the iontophoretic application of 5-hydroxytryptamine to neurons in the cortex, lateral geniculate, or brain stem (Hösli et al., 1971; Jordan et al., 1972; Johnson et al., 1969; Satinsky, 1967; Roberts and Straughan, 1967).

5-Hydroxytryptamine does not cross the blood–brain barrier, but given systemically in young chicks it induces behavioral and EEG (slow-wave) sleep (Spooner and Winters, 1967). Its immediate precursor, 5-hydroxytryptophan, given to rabbits, cats, or baboons enhances EEG slow-wave activity (Costa et al., 1960; Wada et al., 1972). Stereotaxic lesions involving bilateral destruction of a large part of the nuclei of the median raphe produce insomnia in the cat (Jouvet, 1969b), as does administration of p-chlorophenylalanine, which impairs the synthesis of 5-hydroxytryptamine by inhibiting the hydroxylation of tryptophan.

Lysergic acid diethylamide has a very powerful EEG-activating effect; low doses of hallucinogenic indolethylamines, such as psilocybin and di-methyltryptamine, also enhance fast activities on the EEG (Meldrum and Naquet, 1971), but higher doses of these compounds or of methysergide augment slow activities. At the lateral geniculate, these compounds, like 5-hydroxytryptamine, diminish postsynaptic responses (Curtis and Davis, 1962; Meldrum and Naquet, 1971), but they block the excitatory effects of 5-hydroxytryptamine on cortical neurons (Roberts and Straughan, 1967). The spontaneous firing of neurons in the midbrain raphe nuclei is reduced or abolished by lysergic acid diethylamide or dimethyltryptamine (Aghaja-nian et al., 1970). This is apparently due to a direct inhibitory action of lysergic acid diethylamide on raphe neurons (Haigler and Aghajanian, 1974).

The relationship between the EEG effects of drugs which block the action of 5-hydroxytryptamine on smooth muscle and their actions on serotoninergic neurons in the brain remains to be elucidated.

13.4. γ-Aminobutyric Acid

There is substantial evidence that GABA acts as a postsynaptic inhibitory transmitter at numerous sites within the central nervous system (see reviews by Krnjević, 1974, and Meldrum, 1975, and Krnjević, Chap. 4, Vol. 6), and GABA is probably also involved in presynaptic inhibition on primary afferent pathways. In the neocortex, thalamus, basal ganglia, hippocampus, and cerebellum, GABA appears, in general, to be released by small interneurons. Because GABA is involved in systems of recurrent inhibition, it probably plays a role in preventing sustained synchronous discharge of large groups of neurons.

Two alkaloids which block the postsynaptic (and presynaptic) inhibitory action of GABA, bicuculline and picrotoxin, both induce generalized seizures (Meldrum, 1975). These are of short latency of onset and tend to be exceptionally sustained (Meldrum and Horton, 1973). Their convulsant action may be more closely related to presynaptic inhibition than postsynaptic inhibition (Hill *et al.*, 1973).

Compounds which impair the synthesis of GABA by inhibiting glutamic acid decarboxylase also induce epileptic seizures. In the case of 3-mercaptopropionic acid, which inhibits glutamic acid decarboxylase by substrate competition, the seizures, in their timing and electrographic features, resemble those produced by picrotoxin (Horton and Meldrum, 1973). Drugs which are "pyridoxal phosphate antagonists" (interfering with either the synthesis or the coenzymic function of pyridoxal phosphate), such as isoniazid, thiosemicarbazide, and 4-deoxypyridoxine, inhibit many decarboxylases and transaminases, but usually show a major initial effect on glutamic acid decarboxylase. In primates, these compounds give rise to brief recurrent seizures with a characteristic unilateral onset (Meldrum *et al.*, 1970*b*; Meldrum and Horton, 1971). Focal spikes in the posterior parietal cortex of one side are associated with nystagmus and turning of the head to the opposite side.

One perplexing feature of the syndrome seen after just-convulsant doses of pyridoxal phosphate antagonists is the relative normality of the EEG record between seizures. However, the role of thalamic and neocortical GABA-containing neurons in the generation of normal EEG rhythms is largely a matter of speculation.

14. USES AND LIMITATIONS OF MACROELECTRODE RECORDINGS

In psychopharmacology, evidence from EEG studies is rarely, if ever, complete in itself. It has to be considered in relation to behavioral, neuroanatomical, biochemical, or pharmacological data obtained in the same or related experiments.

The EEG is an indispensable tool in two major areas—sleep and epilepsy. In both these topics, correlations among molecular biochemistry, neuroanatomy, and EEG changes have led to important hypotheses about (1) the physiological control systems and (2) the mode of action of drugs on behavior. As a tool for screening or classifying psychopharmacological agents, the EEG is empirically useful but lacks a coherent theoretical basis.

Macroelectrode recordings are also a vital ancillary procedure in many types of neuropharmacological experiments. This is particularly true for microelectrode studies, where the necessity for continuous monitoring of EEG background activity has only recently become widely appreciated. The significance of a change in the inhibitory effect of an iontophoretically applied compound is obviously different when generalized seizure activity is present but may also vary with less severe changes in the background EEG.

That EEG recording will continue to play a useful role in psychopharmacological research is evident. The extent of this future role will depend on the energy and intelligence with which EEG studies are combined with other approaches by currently active research workers.

15. REFERENCES

ADEY, W. R., DUNLOP, C. W., and HENDRIX, C. E., 1960, Hippocampal slow waves: Distribution and phase relationships in the course of approach learning, *Arch. Neurol.* **3:**74–90.

ADRIAN, E. D., 1935, Discharge frequencies in the cerebral and cerebellar cortex, *J. Physiol.* **83:**32–33.

ADRIAN, E. D., and MATTHEWS, B. H. C., 1934, The Berger rhythm: Potential changes from the occipital lobes of man, *Brain* **57:**355–385.

AGHAJANIAN, G. K., FOOTE, W. E., and SHEARD, M. H., 1970, Action of psychotogenic drugs on single midbrain raphe neurons, *J. Pharmacol. Exp. Ther.* **171:**178–187.

AKINDELE, M. O., EVANS, J. I., and OSWALD, I., 1970, Monoamine oxidase inhibitors, sleep and mood, *Electroenceph. Clin. Neurophysiol.* **29:**47–56.

ALBE-FESSARD, D., STUTINSKY, F., and LIBOUBAN, S., 1966, *Atlas Stéréotaxique du Diencephale du Rat Blanc*, Editions du Centre National de la Recherche Scientifique, Paris.

ALLISON, T., GOFF, W. R., ABRAHAMIAN, H. A., and ROSNER, B. S., 1963, The effects of barbiturate anaesthesia upon human somatosensory evoked responses, *Electroenceph. Clin. Neurophysiol. Suppl.* **24:**68–75.

ANDERSEN, P., and ANDERSSON, S. A., 1968, *The Physiological Basis of the Alpha Rhythm*, Appleton-Century-Crofts, New York.

ANDERSEN, P., and SEARS, T. A., 1964, The role of inhibition in the phasing of spontaneous thalamo-cortical discharge, *J. Physiol.* **173:**459–480.

ANDERSEN, P., ECCLES, J. C., and SEARS, T. A., 1964, The ventro-basal complex of the thalamus: Types of cells, their responses and their functional organization, *J. Physiol.* **173:**370–399.

BALDOCK, G., and WALTER, W. G., 1946, A new electronic analyzer, *Elec. Eng.* **18:**339–344.

BAUST, W., and NIEMCZYK, H., 1964, Further studies on the action of adrenergic drugs on cortical activity, *Electroenceph. Clin. Neurophysiol.* **17:**261–271.

BAUST, W., NIEMCZYK, H., and VIETH, J., The action of blood pressure on the ascending reticular activating system with special reference to adrenaline-induced EEG arousal, *Electroenceph. Clin. Neurophysiol.* **15:**63–72.

BELL, J. A., and ANDERSON, E. G., 1972, The influence of semicarbazide induced depletion of γ-aminobutyric acid on presynaptic inhibition, *Brain Res.* **43:**161–169.

BICKFORD, R. G., JACOBSON, J. L., and CODY, D. T. R., 1964, Nature of average evoked potentials to sound and other stimuli in man, *Ann. N.Y. Acad. Sci.* **112:**204–223.

BONNET, V., and BREMER, F., 1937, Action du potassium, du calcium, et de l'acétylcholine sur les activités électriques spontanés et provoquées de l'écorce cérébrale, *Compt. Rend. Soc. Biol.* **126:**1271–1275.

BORENSTEIN, P., CUJO, P., and CHILA, M., 1965, A propos de la classification des substances psychotropes suivant leurs effets sur l'électroencéphalogramme, *Ann. Med. Psychol.* **123**:429–452.

BORENSTEIN, P., DONGIER, M., FINK., M., FLORIO, V., ITIL, T., LONGO, V. G., MELLERIO, F., NAQUET, R., PAMPIGLIONE, G., TITERA, J., and VERDEAUX, G., 1970, Clinical and experimental electroencephalography, in: *The Neuroleptics* (D. P. Bobon, P. A. J. Janssen, and J. Bobon, eds.), pp. 109–125, Karger, Basel.

BRADLEY, P. B., and ELKES, J., 1957, The effect of some drugs on the electrical activity of the brain, *Brain* **80**:77–117.

BRADLEY, P. B., and HANCE, A. J., 1957, The effect of chlorpromazine and methopromazine on the electrical activity of the brain in the cat, *Electroenceph. Clin. Neurophysiol.* **9**:191–215.

BRADLEY, P. B., and KEY, B. J., 1958, The effects of drugs on arousal responses produced by electrical stimulation of the reticular formation of brain, *Electroenceph. Clin. Neurophysiol.* **10**:97–110.

BREMER, F., 1943. Etude oscillographique des résponses de l'aire acoustique corticale chez le chat, *Arch. Int. Physiol.* **53**:53–103.

BREMER, F., 1952, Analyse oscillographique des résponses sensorielles des écorces cérébrales et cérébelleuse., *Rev. Neurol.* **87**:65–92.

BREMER, F., and CHATONNET, J., 1949, Acetylcholine et cortex cérébral, *Arch. Int. Physiol.* **57**:106–109.

BROOKS, C. McL., GOODWIN, R. A., and WILLARD, H. N., 1941. The effects of various brain lesions on morphine induced hyperglycaemia and excitement in the cat, *Am. J. Physiol.* **133**:226–227.

BROUGHTON, R., REGIS, H., and GASTAUT, H., 1965, Modifications of somaesthetic evoked potentials during bursts of mu rhythm and during fist clenching, *Electroenceph. Clin. Neurophysiol.* **18**:720–726.

BROWN, B. B., 1969, Effect of LSD on visually evoked responses to color in visualizer and non-visualizer subjects, *Electroenceph. Clin. Neurophysiol.* **27**:356–363.

BYFORD, G. H., 1965, Signal variance and its application to continuous measurements of EEG activity, *Proc. Roy. Soc. Lond. Ser. B* **161**:421–427.

CALVET, J., CALVET, M. C., and SCHERRER, J., 1964, Etude stratigraphique corticale de l'activité EEG spontanée, *Electroenceph, Clin. Neurophysiol.* **17**:109–125.

CARLSSON, A., and LINDQVIST, M., 1963, Effect of chlorpromazine or haloperidol on formation of 3-methoxytyramine and normetanephrine in mouse brain, *Acta Pharmacol. Toxicol.* **20**:140–144.

CELESIA, G. G., and JASPER, H. H., 1966, Acetylcholine released from cerebral cortex in relation to state of excitation, *Neurology* **16**:1053–1064.

CONSROE, P. F., and WHITE, R. P., 1972, Effects of haloperidol and chlorpromazine on central adrenergic and cholinergic mechanisms in rabbits, *Arch. Int. Pharmacodyn.* **198**:67–75.

COSTA, E., PSCHEIDT, G. R., VAN METER, W. G., and HIMWICH, H. E., 1960, Brain concentrations of biogenic amines and EEG patterns of rabbits, *J. Pharmacol. Exp. Ther.* **130**:81–88.

CRAWFORD, J. M., and CURTIS, D. R., 1964, The excitation and depression of mammalian cortical neurones by amino acids, *Brit. J. Pharmacol. Chemother.* **23**:313–329.

CRAWFORD, J. M., and CURTIS, D. R., 1966, Pharmacological studies on feline Betz cells. *J. Physiol.* **186**:121–138.

CREUTZFELDT, O. D., WATANABE, S., and LUX, H. D., 1966a, Relations between EEG phenomena and potentials of single cortical cells. I. Evoked responses after thalamic and epicortical stimulation. *Electroenceph. Clin. Neurophysiol.* **20**:1–18.

CREUTZFELDT, O. D., WATANABE, S., and LUX, H. D., 1966b, Relations between EEG phenomena and potentials of single cortical cells. II. Spontaneous and convulsoid activity, *Electroenceph. Clin. Neurophysiol.* **20**:19–37.

CURTIS, D. R., and DAVIS, R., 1962, Pharmacological studies upon neurones of the lateral geniculate nucleus of the cat, *Brit. J. Pharmacol.* **18**:217–246.

DAVIS, H., MAST, T., YOSHI, N., and ZERLIN, S., 1966, The slow response of the human cortex to auditory stimuli recovery processes, *Electroenceph. Clin. Neurophysiol.* **21**:105–113.

DAVIS, R., and HUFFMAN, R. D., 1968, *A Stereotaxic Atlas of the Brain of the Baboon (Papio)*, University of Texas Press, Austin.

DAWSON, G. D., 1951, A summation technique for detecting small signals in a large irregular background, *J. Physiol.* **115**:2p–3p.

DEMENT, W., and KLEITMAN, N., 1957, Cyclic variations in EEG during sleep and their relation to eye movements, body motility and dreaming, *Electroenceph. Clin. Neurophysiol.* **9**:673–690.

DEWHURST, W. G., and MARLEY, E., 1965a, Methods for quantifying behaviour and cerebral electrical activity and the effect of drugs under controlled conditions, *Brit. J. Pharmacol.* **25**:671–681.

DEWHURST, W. G., and MARLEY, E., 1965b, The effects of α-methyl derivatives of noradrenaline, phenylethylamine and tryptamine on the central nervous system of the chicken, *Brit. J. Pharmacol.* **25**:682–704.

DEWHURST, W. G., and MARLEY, E., 1965c, Action of sympathomimetic and allied amines on the central nervous system of the chicken, *Brit. J. Pharmacol.* **25**:705–727.

DOMINO, E. F., YAMAMOTO, K., and DREN, A. T., 1968, Role of cholinergic mechanisms in states of wakefulness and sleep, in: *Anticholinergic Drugs and Brain Functions in Animals and Man*, pp. 113–133, Elsevier, Amsterdam.

DUNLEAVY, D. L. F., BREZINOVA, V., OSWALD, I., MACLEAN, A. W., and TINKER, M., 1972, Changes during weeks in effects of tricyclic drugs on the human sleeping brain, *Brit. J. Psychiat.* **120**:663–672.

DROHOCKI, Z., 1948a, Les bases physiques de l'électro-encéphalographie quantitative, *Rev. Neurol.* **80**:617–618.

DROHOCKI, Z., 1948b, L'integrateur de l'électroproduction cérébrale pour l'électroencephalographie quantitative, *Rev. Neurol.* **80**:619.

EBE, M., MEIER-EWERT, K.-H., and BROUGHTON, R., 1969, Effects of intravenous diazepam (Valium) upon evoked potentials of photosensitive epileptic and normal subjects, *Electroenceph, Clin. Neurophysiol.* **27**:429–435.

ECCLES, J. G., 1953, *The Neurophysiological Basis of Mind*, Clarendon Press, Oxford.

ECCLES, J. C., 1957, *The Physiology of Nerve Cells*, Johns Hopkins University Press, Baltimore.

ECCLES, J. C., 1964, *The Physiology of Synapses*, pp. 1–316, Springer, Berlin.

ELUL, R., 1972, The genesis of the EEG, *Int. Rev. Neurobiol.* **15**:227–272.

EMMERS, R., and AKERT, K., 1963, *A Stereotaxic Atlas of the Brain of the Squirrel Monkey* (Saimiri sciureus), University of Wisconsin Press, Madison.

FELDBERG, W., 1963, *A Pharmacological Approach to the Brain from Its Inner and Outer Surface*, Arnold, London.

FELDBERG, W., and SHERWOOD, S. L., 1954, Injections of drugs into the lateral ventricle of the cat, *J. Physiol.* **123**:148–167.

FINCKH, R., and KUGLER, J., 1961, Quantitative Bestimmung der cerebralen Elektrogenese unter dem Einfluss von Schafmitteln und Thymoleptica, *Med. Exp.* **5**:370–374.

FINK, M., 1964, A selected bibliography of electroencephalography in human psychopharmacology, 1951–1962, *Electroenceph. Clin. Neurophysiol. Suppl.* **23**, pp. 1–68.

FINK, M., 1969, EEG and human psychopharmacology, *Ann. Rev. Pharmacol.* **9**:241–258.

FLORIO, V., and LONGO, V. G., 1971, Neuroleptic drugs and the central dopaminergic system, *Neuropharmacology* **10**:45–54.

FROST, J. D., An automatic sleep analyzer, *Electroenceph. Clin. Neurophysiol.* **29**:88–92.

FUXE, K., 1965, The distribution of monoamine terminals in the central nervous system, *Acta Physiol. Scand.* **64**:37–85 (Suppl. 247).

GAILLARD, J. M., KRASSOÏEVITCH, M., and TISSOT, R., 1972, Analyse automatique du sommeil par un système hybride: Nouveaux resultats, *Electroenceph. Clin. Neurophysiol.* **33**:403–410.

GAILLARD, J.-M., SCHULZ, P., and TISSOT, R., 1973, Effect of three benzodiazepines (Nitrozepam, Fluritrazepam and bromazepam) on sleep of normal subjects, studied with an automatic sleep scoring system, *Pharmacopsychiatry* **6**:207–217.

GAY, P., and BINNIE, L. D., 1970, An improved write-out system for low frequency wave analysers, *Electroenceph. Clin. Neurophysiol.* **29**:313–315.

GOLDSTEIN, L., MURPHREE, H., SUGERMAN, A. A., PFEIFFER, C. C., and JENNEY, E. H., 1963*a*, Quantitative EEG analysis of naturally occurring and drug-induced psychotic states in human males, *Clin. Pharmacol. Ther.* **4**:10–21.

GOLDSTEIN, L., MURPHREE, H., and PFEIFFER, G. C., 1963*b*, Quantitative EEG in man as a measure of CNS stimulation, *Ann. N.Y. Acad. Sci.* **107**:1045–1056.

HAIGLER, H. J., and AGHAJANIAN, G. K., 1974, Lysergic acid diethylamide and serotonin. A comparison of effects on serotoninergic input, *J. Pharmacol. Exp. Ther.* **188**:688–699.

HILL., R. G., SIMMONDS, M. A., and STRAUGHAN, D. W., (1973), Presynaptic inhibition and the depressant actions of GABA and glycine in the feline cuneate nucleus: Changes related to electrographic seizure activity, *J. Physiol.* **234**:83p–84p.

HILLARP, N. A., FUXE, K., and DAHLSTRÖM, A., 1966, Demonstration and mapping of central neurons containing dopamine, noradrenaline and 5-hydroxytryptamine and their reactions to psychopharmaca, *Pharmacol. Rev.* **18**:727–741.

HOFFMAN, J. S., and DOMINO, E. F., 1969, Comparative effects of reserpine on the sleep cycle of man and cat, *J. Pharmacol. Exp. Ther.* **170**:190–198.

HÖKFELT, T., LUNGDAHL, Å., FUXE, K., and JOHANSSON, O., 1974, Dopamine nerve terminals in the rat limbic cortex; aspects of the dopamine hypothesis of schizophrenia, *Science* **184**:177–179.

HORTON, R. W., and MELDRUM, B. S., 1973, Seizures induced by allylglycine, 3-mercaptopropionic acid and 4-deoxypyridoxine in mice and photosensitive baboons, and different modes of inhibition of cerebral glutamic acid decarboxylase, *Brit. J. Pharmacol.* **49**:52–63.

HÖSLI, L., TEBÈCIS, A. K., and SCHÖNWETTER, H. P., 1971, A comparison of the effects of monoamines on neurones of the bulbar reticular formation, *Brain Res* **25**:357–370.

ITIL, T. M., 1973, Quantitative pharmaco-electroencephalography, in: *Psychotropic Drugs and the Human EEG* (T. M. Itil, ed.), Modern Problems of Pharmacopsychiatry Series, Karger, New York.

IZQUIERDO, I., and NASELLO, A. G., 1972, Pharmacology of the brain: The hippocampus, learning and seizures, *Prog. Drug Res.* **16**:211–228.

JASPER, H. H., 1958, Report of the committee on methods of clinical examination in electroencephalography, *Electroenceph. Clin. Neurophysiol.* **10**:370–375.

JASPER, H. H., and AJMONE-MARSAN, C., 1954, *A Stereotaxic Atlas of the Diencephalon of the Cat*, National Research Council of Canada, Ottawa, Canada.

JASPER, H. H., and DROOGLEEVER-FORTUYN, J., 1947, Experimental studies on the functional anatomy of petit mal epilepsy, *Res. Publ. Ass. Nerv. Ment. Dis.* **26**:272–298.

JASPER, H. H., and TESSIER, J., 1971, Acetylcholine liberation from cerebral cortex during paradoxical (REM) sleep. *Science* **172**:601–602.

JOHNSON, E. S., ROBERTS, M. H. T., and STRAUGHAN, D. W., 1969, The responses of cortical neurones to monoamines under differing anaesthetic conditions, *J. Physiol.* **203**:261–280.

JONES, B. E., 1969, *Catecholamine-Containing Neurons in the Brain Stem of the Cat and Their Role in Waking*, pp. 1–87, Imprimerie des Beaux Arts, Lyon.

JONES, B. E., BOBILLIER, P., PIN, C., and JOUVET, M., 1973, The effect of lesions of catecholamine-containing neurones upon monoamine content of the brain and EEG and behavioural waking in the cat, *Brain Res.* **58**:157–177.

JORDAN, L. M., FREDERICKSON, R. C. A., PHILLIS, J. W., and LAKE, N., 1972, Microelectrophoresis of 5-hydroxytryptamine: A clarification of its action on cerebral cortical neurones, *Brain Res.* **40**:552–558.

JOUVET, M., 1969a, Neurophysiological and biochemical mechanisms of sleep, in: *Sleep: Physiology and Pathology* (A. Kalès, ed.), Saunders, Philadelphia.

JOUVET, M., 1969b, Biogenic amines and the states of sleep, Science **163**:32–41.

JOUVET, M., 1972, The role of monoamines and acetylcholine-containing neurons in the regulation of the sleep-waking cycle, *Ergeb. Physiol.* **64**:166–307.

KALÈS, J., KALÈS, A., BIXLER, E., and SLYE, E. S., 1971, Effects of placebo and flurazepam on sleep patterns in insomniac subjects, *Clin. Pharmacol. Ther.* **12**:691–697.

KANAI, T., and SZERB, J. C., 1965, Mesencephalic reticular activating system and cortical acetylcholine output, *Nature* **205**:80–82.

KEY, B. J., and MARLEY, E. D., 1962, The effect of the sympathomimetic amines on the behaviour and electrocortical activity of the chicken, *Electroenceph. Clin. Neurophysiol.* **14**:90–105.

KILLAM, K. F., 1957, Pharmacological influences upon evoked electrical activity in the brain, in: *Psychotropic Drugs* (S. Garattini and V. Ghetti, eds), pp. 244–251, Elsevier, Amsterdam.

KÖNIG, J. F. R., and KLIPPEL, R. A., 1963, *The Rat Brain: A Stereotaxic Atlas of the Forebrain and Lower Parts of the Brain Stem*, pp. 1–162, Williams and Wilkins, Baltimore.

KOOI, K. A., and BAGCHI, B. K., 1964, Observations on early components of the visual evoked response and occipital rhythms, *Electroenceph. Clin. Neurophysiol.* **17**:638–643.

KRNJEVIĆ, K., 1974, Chemical nature of synaptic transmission in vertebrates, *Physiol. Rev.* **54**:418–540.

KRNJEVIĆ, K., and PHILLIS, J. W., 1963a, Actions of certain amines on cerebral cortical neurones, *Brit. J. Pharmacol. Chemother.* **20**:471–490.

KRNJEVIĆ, K., and PHILLIS, J. W., 1963b, Pharmacological properties of acetylcholine-sensitive cells in the cerebral cortex, *J. Physiol.* **166**:328–350.

KUFFLER, S. W., 1967, Neuroglial cells: Physiological properties and a potassium mediated effect of neuronal activity on the glial membrane potential, *Proc. Roy. Soc. Lond. Ser. B* **168**:1–21.

LEIMDORFER, A., and METZNÈR, W. R. T., 1949, Analgesia and anaesthesia induced by epinephrine, *Am. J. Physiol.* **157**:116–121.

LEVY, R. A., and ANDERSON, E. G., 1973, Bicuculline and picrotoxin blockade of positive dorsal root potentials, *Nature* **241**:156–157.

LEWIS, S. A., 1970, Comparative effects of some amphetamine derivatives on human sleep, in: *Amphetamines and Related Compounds* (E. Costa and S. Garattini, eds.), Raven Press, New York.

LIDBRINK, P., 1974, The effect of lesions of ascending noradrenaline pathways on sleep and waking in the rat, *Brain Res.* **74**:19–40.

LONGO, V. G., 1962, *Electroencephalographic Atlas for Pharmacological Research*, Elsevier, Amsterdam.

LONGO, V. G., 1966, Behavioral and electroencephalographic effects of atropine and related compounds, *Pharmacol Rev.* **18**:965–996.

LONGO, V. G., and FLORIO, V., 1970, Effects of neuroleptic drugs on the cerebral electrical activity of laboratory animals: Presentation of a model design for neuropharmacological experiments, *Acta Neuropsychiat. Belg.*

LUCAS, E. A., POWELL, E. W., and MURPHREE, O. D., 1974, Hippocampal theta in nervous pointer dogs, *Physiol. Behav.* **12**:609–613.

MARLEY, E., and STEPHENSON, J. D., 1972, Central actions of catecholamines, in: *Handbook of Experimental Pharmacology*, Vol. 33: *Catecholamines* (H. Blaschko and E. Muscholl eds.), pp. 463–537, Springer, Heidelberg.

MATOUŠEK, M., 1973, Frequency and correlation analysis in *Handbook of Electroencephalography and Clinical Neurophysiology*, Vol. 5A, editor A. Remand, pp. 1–108, Elsevier, Amsterdam.

MELDRUM, B. S., 1966, Drug-induced changes in EEG activity and the form of cortical potentials evoked by somatosensory stimulation, *Electroenceph. Clin. Neurophysiol.* **21**:309.

MELDRUM, B. S., 1975, Epilepsy and GABA-mediated inhibition, *Int. Rev. Neurobiol.* **17**:1–36.

MELDRUM, B. S., and HORTON, R. W., 1971, Convulsive effects of 4-deoxypyridoxine and of bicuculline in photosensitive baboons (*Papio papio*) and in rhesus monkeys (*Macaca mulatta*), *Brain Res.* **35**:419–436.

MELDRUM, B. S., and HORTON, R. W., 1973, Physiology of status epilepticus in primates, *Arch. Neurol.* **28**:1–9.

MELDRUM, B. S., and HORTON, R. W., 1974, Neuronal inhibition mediated by GABA and patterns of convulsions in photosensitive baboons with epilepsy (*Papio papio*), in: *The Natural History and Management of Epilepsy* (P. Harris and C. Maudsley, eds.), Churchill Livingstone, London.

MELDRUM, B. S., and NAQUET, R., 1971, Effects of psilocybin, dimethyltryptamine, mescaline and various lysergic acid derivatives on the EEG and on photically-induced epilepsy in the baboon (*Papio papio*), *Electroenceph. Clin. Neurophysiol.* **31**:563–572.

MELDRUM, B. S., NAQUET, R., and BALZANO, E., 1970a, Effects of atropine and eserine on the electroencephalogram, on behaviour and on light-induced epilepsy in the adolescent baboon (*Papio papio*), *Electroenceph. Clin. Neurophysiol.* **28**:449–458.

MELDRUM, B. S., BALZANO, E., GADEA, M., and NAQUET, R., 1970b, Photic and drug-induced epilepsy in the baboon (*Papio papio*): The effects of isoniazid, thiosemicarbazide, pyridoxine and amino-oxyacetic acid, *Electroenceph. Clin. Neurophysiol.* **29**:333–347.

MELDRUM, B. S., FARIELLO, R. G., PUIL, E. A., DEROUAUX, M., and NAQUET, R., 1974, Δ^9-Tetrahydrocannabinol and epilepsy in the photosensitive baboon, (*Papio papio*), *Epilepsia.* **15**:255–264.

MITCHELL, J. F., 1963, The spontaneous and evoked release of acetylcholine from the cerebral cortex, *J. Physiol.* **165**:98–116.

MONNIER, M., and GANGLOFF, H., 1961, *Atlas for Stereotaxic Brain Research on the Conscious Rabbit*, Elsevier, Amsterdam.

MORUZZI, G., and MAGOUN, H. W., 1949, Brain stem reticular formation and activation of the EEG, *Electroenceph. Clin. Neurophys.* **1**:455–473.

MOSS, R. L., URBAN, I., and CROSS, B. A., 1972, Microelectrophoresis of cholinergic and aminergic drugs on paraventricular neurons, *Am. J. Physiol.* **223**:310–318.

MURPHREE, H., GOLDSTEIN, L., PFEIFFER, C., SCHRAMM, L., and JENNEY, E., 1964, Computer analysis of drug effects on the EEG of normal and psychotic subjects, *Int. J. Neuropharmacol.* **3**:97–104.

OGUNREMI, O. O., ADAMSON, L., BŘEZINOVÁ, V., HUNTER, W. M., MACLEAN, A. W., OSWALD, I., and PERCY-ROBB, I. W., 1973, Two anti-anxiety drugs: A psychoneuroendocrine study, *Brit. Med. J.* **2**:202–205.

PAMPIGLIONE, G., 1963, *Development of Cerebral Function in the Dog*, pp. 1–68, Butterworths, London.

PARMEGGIANI, P. L., 1967, On the functional significance of the hippocampal ıW rhythm, in: *Progress in Brain Research: Structure and Function of the Limbic System.* (T. Tokizane, ed.), pp. 413–441, Elsevier, Amsterdam.

PELLEGRINO and CUCHMAN, 1967, *A Stereotaxic Atlas of the Rat Brain*, Century Psychology Series, Appleton-Century-Crofts, New York.

PHILLIPS, C. G., 1956, Intracellular records from Betz cells in the cat, *Quart. J. Exp. Physiol.* **41**:58–69.

RAY, C. D., BICKFORD, R. G., CLARK, L. C., JOHNSTON, R. E., RICHARDS, T. M., ROGERS, D., and RUSSERT, W. E., 1965a, A new multicontact, multipurpose, brain depth probe: Details of construction, *Mayo Clin. Proc.* **40**:771–780.

RAY, C. D., BICKFORD, R. G., CLARK, L. C., and RUSSERT, W. E., 1965b, A new multicontact, multipurpose, brain depth probe: First experimental results, *Mayo Clin. Proc.* **40**:781–790.

RECHTSHAFFEN, A., and KALÈS, A. (eds.), 1968, *A Manual of Standardized Terminology, Techniques and Scoring System for Sleep Stages of Human Subjects*, U.S. Public Health Service Publication No. 204, Government Printing Office, Washington, D.C.

REGAN, D., 1972, *Evoked Potentials in Psychology, Sensory Physiology and Clinical Medicine*, pp. 1–328, Chapman and Hall, London.

RICHE, D., CHRISTOLOMME, A., BERT, J., and NAQUET, R., 1968, *Atlas Stéréotaxique du Cerveau du Babouin, Papio papio*, Editions du Centre National de la Recherche Scientifique, Paris.

RINALDI, F., and HIMWICH, H. E., 1955, Alerting responses and actions of atropine and cholinergic drugs, *AMA Arch. Neurol. Psychiat.* **73**:387–395.

ROBERTS, M. H. T., and STRAUGHAN, D. W., 1967, Excitation and depression of cortical neurons by 5-hydroxytryptamine, *J. Physiol.* **193**:269–294.

RODIN, E., ONUMA, T., WASSON, S., PORZAK, J., and RODIN, M., 1971, Neurophysiological mechanisms involved in grand mal seizures induced by metrazol and megimide, *Electroenceph. Clin. Neurophysiol.* **30**:62–72.

ROSSI, G. F., and ZANCHETTI, A., 1957, The brain stem reticular formation: Anatomy and physiology, *Arch. Ital. Biol.* **95**:203–435.

ROTHBALLER, A. B., 1956, Studies on the adrenaline-sensitive component of the reticular activating system, *Electroenceph. Clin. Neurophysiol.* **8**:603–621.

SATINSKY, D., 1967, Pharmacological responsiveness of lateral geniculate nucleus neurons, *Int. J. Neuropharmacol.* **6**:387–397.

SATO, K., KITAJIMA, H., MIMURA, K., HIROTA, N., TAGAWA, Y., and OCHI, N., 1971, Cerebral visual evoked potentials in relation to EEG, *Electroenceph. Clin. Neurophysiol.* **30**:123–138.

SCHMIDT, R. F., 1971, Presynaptic inhibition in the vertebrate central nervous system. *Ergeb. Physiol.* **63**:20–101.

SHEER, D. E. (ed.), 1961, *Electrical Stimulation of the Brain*, University of Texas Press, Austin.

SHERWOOD, N. M., and TIMIRAS, P. S., 1970, *A Stereotaxic Atlas of the Developing Rat Brain*, University of California Press, Berkeley.

SHIPTON, H. W., 1961, Engineering considerations in the design of waveform analyser of the Walter type, *Electroenceph, Clin. Neurophysiol. Suppl.* **20**:25–30.

SHUTE, C. C. D., and LEWIS, P. R., 1967, The ascending cholinergic reticular system: Neocortical, olfactory and subcortical projections, *Brain* **90**:497–520.

SNIDER, R. S., and LEE, J. C., 1961, *A Stereotaxic Atlas of the Monkey Brain* (Macaca mulatta), University of Chicago Press, Chicago.

SNIDER, R. S., and NIEMER, W. T., 1961, *A Stereotaxic Atlas of the Cat Brain*, University of Chicago Press, Chicago.

SPOONER, C. E., and WINTERS, W. D., 1967, The influence of centrally active amine induced blood pressure changes on the electroencephalogram and behaviour, *Int. J. Neuropharmacol.* **6**:109–118.

STORM VAN LEEUWEN, W., BICKFORD, R., BRAZIER, M., COBB, W. A., DONDEY, M., GASTAUT, H., GLOOR, P., HENRY, C. E., HESS, R., KNOTT, J. R., KUGLER, J., LAIRY, G. C., LOEB, C., MAGNUS, O., OLLER-DAURELLA, L., PETSCHE, H., SCHWAB, R., WALTER, W. G., and WIDEN, L., 1966, Proposal for an EEG terminology, *Electroenceph. Clin. Neurophysiol.* **20**:306–310.

THIERRY, A. M., STINUS, L., BLANC, G., and GLOWINSKI, J., 1973, Some evidence for the existence of dopaminergic neurons in the rat cortex, *Brain Res.* **50**:230–234.

TOWE, A. L., 1966, On the nature of the primary evoked response, *Exp. Neurol.* **15**:113–139.

VERHAART, W. J. L., 1964, *A Stereotaxic Atlas of the Brain Stem of the Cat*, Van Gorcum, Assen.

VOTAVA, Z., and DYNTAROVÁ, H., 1970, in: *The Neuroleptics* (D. P. Bobon, P. A. J. Janssen, and J. Bobon, eds.), pp. 102–103, Karger, Basel.

VUILLON-CACCIUTTOLO, G., MELDRUM, B. S., and BALZAMO, E., 1973, Electrocorticogram and afferent visual transmission in the epileptic baboon (*Papio papio*), *Epilepsia* **14**:213–221.

WADA, J. A., BALZAMO, E., MELDRUM, B. S., and NAQUET, R., 1972, Behavioural and electrographic effects of L-5-hydroxytryptophan and D,L-parachlorophenylalanine on epileptic Senegalese baboon (*Papio papio*), *Electroenceph. Clin. Neurophysiol.* **33**:520–526.

WALTER, W. G., COOPER, R., ALDRIDGE, V. J., McCALLUM, W. C., and WINTER, A. L., 1964, Contingent negative variation: An electric sign of sensorimotor association and expectancy in the human brain, *Nature* **203**:380–384.

WEIL-MALHERBE, H., 1960, The passage of catecholamines through the blood–brain barrier, in: *Adrenergic Mechanisms* (J. R. Vane, G. E. W. Wolstenholme, and M. O'Connor, eds.), pp. 421–423, Churchill, London.

WIKLER, A., 1952, Pharmacologic dissociation of behaviour and EEG "sleep patterns" in dogs: Morphine, n-allylmorphine, and atropine, *Proc. Soc. Exp. Biol. Med.* **79:**261–265.

WHITE, R. P., and RUDOLPH, A. S., 1967, Neurophysiological comparison of subcortical actions of anticholinergic compounds, in: *Progress in Brain Research,* Vol. 28, (P. B. Bradley and M. Fink, eds.), Elsevier, Amsterdam, pp. 14–26.

WÜNSCHER, W., SCHOBER, W., and WERNER, L., 1965, *Architektonischer Atlas von Hirnstamm der Ratte,* pp. 1–61, Hirzel, Leipzig.

4

NEUROPHARMACOLOGICAL RESPONSES FROM NERVE CELLS IN TISSUE CULTURE

Bruce R. Ransom and Phillip G. Nelson

1. INTRODUCTION

It has been amply demonstrated over the past several years that nervous tissue can maintain and develop a high degree of differentiation in culture. Essentially every region of the neuraxis has been successfully grown in some form of culture, and neural tissue from bird, mouse, rat, and man as well as invertebrate material has proven suitable for *in vitro* work (Murray, 1971; Nelson, 1974). In this chapter, we will be particularly concerned with electrophysiological responses of nerve (and muscle) cells to iontophoretically applied neurohormones but will also deal with some biochemical effects of neuropharmacological agents.

The type of question that can be posed with respect to culture systems is strongly determined by the type of culture utilized. Explant cultures consist of small (approximately 1 mm³) fragments of tissue which, when maintained in an appropriate culture medium, exhibit a relatively high degree of functional and anatomical integrity and complexity and may rather faithfully reflect some organizational features of the intact nervous system. On the other hand, this complexity precludes morphological clarity so that experimental rigor is sacrificed to some degree. Preparation of dissociated cell

Bruce R. Ransom and *Phillip G. Nelson* ● Behavioral Biology Branch, National Institute of Child Health and Human Development, National Institutes of Health, Bethesda, Maryland

cultures involves the rigorous disruption of all intercellular contacts in fetal neural tissues by a combination of chemical and mechanical procedures (Paul, 1972). When a suspension of single cells produced in this way is inoculated into culture dishes and maintained for several days or a few weeks, functional neuronal networks may form. Such cultures allow considerable experimental control of the recording and stimulating conditions but undoubtedly fail to mimic many features of the normal neural organization. Continuous cell lines of neurobiological interest are transformed or neoplastic nervous system cells, which, while maintaining their capacity for cell division, are also capable of expressing a number of differentiated characteristics under appropriate culture conditions. These cell lines have a number of advantages as far as cell biological analysis is concerned but differ from the normal situation even more markedly than do cell cultures of normal material (Sato, 1973). The tradeoffs that must be made between analytical advantages and potential or actual sacrifice of normal biology can best be discussed with regard to specific experimental situations (Giller *et al.*, 1974).

2. MUSCLE

In vitro studies concerned with the responses of striated muscle cells to iontophoretically applied acetylcholine (ACh) and with synaptic potentials recorded at nerve–muscle junctions are excellent examples of how tissue culture model systems can be exploited for neuropharmacological research. A number of close parallels to *in vivo* nerve–muscle systems are found in culture, but some differences have also been noted which depend on the type of culture studied. In all cases, nerve–muscle synapses have been found to be cholinergic and transmitter release is quantal in nature and dependent on the external divalent cation concentrations. Calcium is necessary for release and Mg^{2+} reduces the quantum content of the evoked end-plate potential (EPP). Synaptic potentials have been found to reverse in size at a membrane potential of about -10 mV, as is the case in normal muscle synapses, and curare blocked the EPP completely (Fischbach, 1972). In explant cultures but not in cell cultures, anticholinesterases prolonged and augmented the EPPs. A histochemical correlate of this was the observation that cholinesterase stains demarcated the nerve–muscle region much more prominently in explant cultures than in cell cultures. Iontophoretically applied ACh evoked a membrane depolarization in cultured muscle cells, and this response was blocked by curare. A snake toxin, α-bungarotoxin, has been found to bind and inactivate the cholinergic receptor protein in a number of intact systems. α-Bungarotoxin also blocked the response of cultured muscle cells to applied ACh. The binding of α-bungarotoxin is irreversible, and the localization of radioactively labeled toxin can be determined by autoradiography. Some correlation between ACh sensitivity and density of bungarotoxin binding has been established (Hartzell and Fambrough, 1973) (Fig. 1). The synthesis and insertion of ACh receptor molecules into the membrane can thus be studied by both electrophysiological and autoradiographic means. In chick muscle, the receptor was distributed in an uneven manner, with occasional "hot spots" of high receptor density. This distribution was not markedly different in uninnervated and innervated fibers. Unlike the situation *in vivo*, innervation did not produce a major shift in receptor distribution (Fischbach and Cohen, 1973). The concentration of

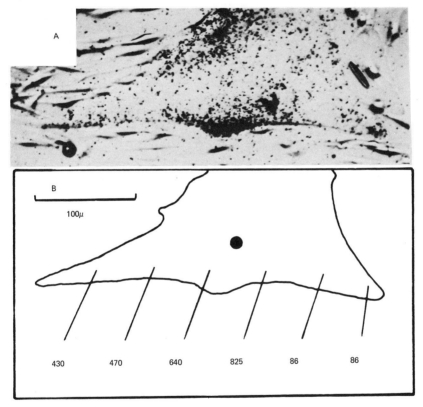

FIG. 1. Spatial distribution of acetylcholine sensitivity and α-bungarotoxin binding sites on cultured rat muscle. (B) The acetylcholine sensitivity at points along a large rat myotube in culture was measured electrophysiologically. Acetylcholine sensitivities are expressed as millivolts per nanocoulomb. The filled circle in the center of the cell outline indicates the position of the recording electrode. (A) After the acetylcholine sensitivities were measured, the culture was incubated in "saturating [^{125}I]α-bungarotoxin." It was then rinsed, and autoradiography was performed. Panel A is a phase contrast photomicrograph of the same cell shown in outline in B and illustrates the distribution of the α-bungarotoxin binding sites. From Hartzell and Fambrough (1973).

receptors was, however, substantially changed in noninnervated fibers by muscle activity. Suppression of muscle activity by tetrodotoxin (which eliminates spike and hence twitch activity) increased receptor density, and prolonged (more than 24 h) electrical stimulation produced a decrease in receptor density (Cohen and Fischbach, 1973; see also Purves and Sakmann, 1974) (Fig. 2). Development of the nerve–muscle synapse has been shown not to depend on functional cholinergic transmission. If nerve–muscle cultures from frog or rodent are grown in medium containing high concentrations of curare, synapses develop which can be shown to be functional when the curare is withdrawn (Cohen, 1972; Crain and Peterson, 1971). This system illustrates the sort of combined electrophysiological, biochemical, and morphological study of cultured material that can be used to explore mechanisms of drug and synaptic action and control mechanisms involved in receptor synthesis and disposition in the cell membrane.

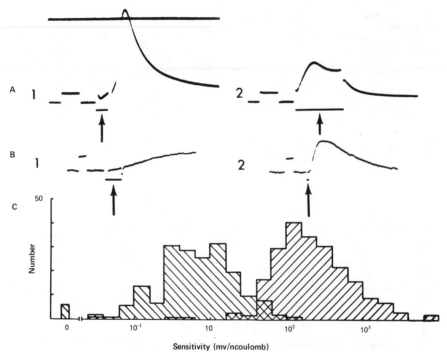

FIG. 2. Effects of muscle cell activity on acetylcholine sensitivity. (A₁) Action potential induced in muscle fiber by depolarizing current pulse (bar at arrow). (A₂) Failure to elicit action potential in muscle fiber bathed in 5.0×10^{-8} g/ml tetrodotoxin. Calibration pulse for A₁ and A₂ was 10 mV, 2 ms. (B₁) Acetylcholine response of a cell that had been electrically stimulated for 68 h. Bar indicates duration of drug application. Sensitivity to drug was 13.7 mV/nC. (B₂) Acetylcholine response of a cell exposed to tetrodotoxin for 137 h. Sensitivity to drug was 1943 mV/nC. (C) Histograms of all acetylcholine responses from 26 stimulated (\\\\) and 30 tetrodotoxin- or lidocaine-treated (///) fibers. The sensitivity is shown in millivolts per nanocoulomb on a log scale. From Cohen and Fischbach (1973).

3. CONTINUOUS CELL LINES

Continuous lines of neurons, especially the mouse neuroblastoma, and a number of glial tumor lines have been shown in a large number of biochemical studies to be capable of a number of biosynthetic activities related to nervous system function and to be responsive to psychopharmacological agents (Giller *et al.*, 1974). Neuroblastoma cells have been studied extensively by electrophysiological methods (Nelson *et al.*, 1969, 1971; Nelson, 1973; Peacock and Nelson, 1973; Peacock *et al.*, 1973*a*; Schubert *et al.*, 1973). These cells are responsive to iontophoretically applied acetylcholine, and both hyperpolarizing or inhibitory and depolarizing or excitatory membrane changes have been observed (Harris and Dennis, 1970; Peacock and Nelson, 1973). These opposite responses were sometimes seen in the same cell, with some spatial separation between the areas on the cell surface from which the depolarizing and hyperpolarizing responses could be elicited. The regional specificity is similar to the separation of excitatory and inhibitory synaptic contacts that is typical of central neurons *in vivo*. The ACh-induced potentials of opposite polarity also had differential sensitivities to blocking agents. Dopamine, norepinephrine, and serotonin were also tested on neuroblastoma cells. Dopamine caused a hyperpolarizing potential shift in about 30% of cells and the other drugs were ineffective (Peacock and Nelson, 1973).

4. GLIA

Neuroglia are also amenable to study *in vitro*. The major uncertainties which still remain concerning their role in the overall function of nervous tissue coupled with the attendant difficulties in selectively studying their behavior *in situ* (see Kuffler and Nicholls, 1966) makes the *in vitro* approach to the investigation of this cell type particularly inviting. Wardell (1966) used cultured glia from rabbit cerebellum to dispute the physiological significance of a previously described glial cell "response" to direct electrical stimulation (Tasaki and Chang, 1958). He concluded that this represented nothing more than a transient deterioration of the membrane caused by very large voltage gradients. He also surveyed this same preparation for pharmacological responsiveness to a wide range of putative neurotransmitters and found the glia to be completely insensitive. For the most part, *in vivo* studies on presumed glia have confirmed this finding (Krnjević and Schwartz, 1967). Where responses have been noted (Krnjević and Schwartz, 1967; Krnjević *et al.*, 1971), there is the possibility that these were the indirect result of stimulation of adjacent neurons with subsequent modulation of extracellular K^+ concentration. Electrophysiological experiments on dissociated cell cultures of embryonic mouse spinal cord and rat cerebrum have revealed the feasibility of intracellular recording from glial elements (Nelson and Ransom, unpublished observations) and should permit a reassessment of this issue. It has been frequently suggested that glia might serve to eliminate released transmitter substances from their sites of action in the extracellular space by an active uptake mechanism. A careful study of this possibility using neoplastic glial cell lines has been carried out (Schrier and Thompson, 1974), and the results are most intriguing. Not only did glioma cells exhibit uptake systems for various transmitter candidates—glutamate, aspartate, taurine, and γ-aminobutyric acid (GABA)— but they were also capable of synthesizing taurine and GABA and excreting these chemicals back into the extracellular milieu. These findings are consistent with autoradiographic observations made on more complicated and organotypic *in vitro* preparations of nervous tissue. Such studies have invariably implied glial involvement in the uptake of transmitter substances (Hösli *et al.*, 1973a; Lasher, 1974; Schon and Kelly, 1974). Studies showing that isoproterenol, a β-adrenergic agent, increases the intracellular level of cyclic adenosine monophosphate (cAMP) in glioma cultures suggests a possible further mechanism for neuron–glia interactions (Gilman and Nirenberg, 1971). Fascinating questions remain, however, regarding the actual physiological significance of these phenomena, and tissue culture methodology can be expected to remain an important experimental approach in this area.

5. EXPLANTS

Nervous system explants retain a high degree of structural and functional complexity. Development of complicated spontaneous bioelectrical activity and responses to electrical stimuli have been followed as the explants mature using extracellular recording techniques. The existence of prominent inhibitory components of the synaptic circuitry has been inferred from the effects of strychnine. Some mature cultures seemed to be dominated by inhibitory circuitry to the extent that electrical stimulation evoked only minimal activity unless inhibition was blocked by drugs or reversed by ionic manipulations of the extracellular milieu (Crain, 1972; see also Crain and Bornstein, 1974). As in the case of the neuromuscular synapse, blockade of all spike and synaptic activity in developing cultures did not prevent apparently normal synaptogenesis (Crain *et al.*, 1968). Calcium ions were necessary for normal functioning of the synaptically linked networks in the explants, and electrical activity was suppressed by low Ca^{2+} solutions. Very low concentrations of cAMP temporarily reversed this depression, suggesting that the cyclic nucleotide either mobilized some tissue stores of calcium or replaced Ca^{2+} by having its own immediate role in excitation–secretion coupling (Crain and Pollack, 1973). GABA and glycine in the culture medium rapidly and reversibly diminished spontaneous electrical activity in the explants, as might be expected from their possible role as inhibitory synaptic transmitters (Crain, 1973). The capability of explant and reaggregated CNS tissue to generate spontaneous and evoked repetitive electrical activity and the responsiveness of these cultures to a variety of neuropharmacological agents suggest that they may be valuable tools in assessing the activity of such agents. However, the complexity of explants makes the detailed analysis of drug action at the cell and membrane level difficult.

Hösli et al. (1973a,b) have used intracellular methods to study membrane effects of neurohormones in spinal cord and brain explants. Glutamate produced a sodium-dependent depolarization of morphologically identified neurons (electrophysiological identification, i.e., action and synaptic potentials, has not been presented), and glycine produced a chloride-dependent membrane hyperpolarization. These workers and Lasher (1974) have sought to identify specific cell types on histochemical grounds and on the basis of uptake of various putative neurotransmitters. Acetylcholinesterase activity has been demonstrated in the cytoplasm of the cell bodies, and sometimes the dendrites, of many of the neurons in explants of rat spinal cord and fetal human spinal cord (Hösli and Hösli, 1971; Hösli et al., 1973b). The presence of monoamines has also been established in cultured rat brain stem by histochemical techniques (Hösli et al., 1971). In these same preparations, autoradiography was used to determine the localization of transmitter substances taken up from the extracellular space. Although neuronal uptake was seen for glutamate, glycine, and GABA, no precise category of cell types could be distinguished which took up any one of these drugs selectively (Hösli and Hösli, 1972; Hösli et al., 1972, 1973a). In the cerebellum, glycine and glutamate did not appear to be taken up to any great extent, but GABA did appear to label a specific set of cells (Lasher, 1974). Autoradiographs frequently showed heavily labeled and unlabeled cells in close proximity. This is a potentially highly useful approach, but interpretation of these last results in terms of a specific set of GABA-transmitting cells still needs substantial corroboration.

Bunge et al. (1974) have employed two culture methodologies to develop a preparation consisting of dissociated cells from rat superior cervical ganglion and explants of rat thoracic spinal cord. An earlier study (Olson and Bunge, 1973) had established some degree of specificity regarding synaptogenesis in such preparations by demonstrating that when explants of cerebral cortex or spinal cord were given the opportunity to innervate sympathetic neurons only spinal cord was found to form morphologically defined synaptic contacts on these cells. Electron micrographs of sympathetic neurons grown in the presence of spinal cord revealed two types of synaptic terminals. One type, which was also present in the absence

of spinal cord, contained pleomorphic dense-core vesicles after KMnO₄
fixation and was presumably adrenergic, and the other contained uniform
round vesicles which were clear after KMnO₄ fixation and underwent
degeneration when the spinal cord explant was extirpated. It was possible to
obtain stable intracellular recordings from sympathetic neurons in these
cultures, and some evidence was obtained which suggested the presence of
spontaneous synaptic activity in those cells which were grown with spinal
cord (Bunge *et al.*, 1974). The specificity of this system makes it a favorable
one for analyzing the effects of synapse formation on a cell's pharmacological responsiveness.

6. DISSOCIATED PRIMARY CELL CULTURES

It is well documented that dissociated cell cultures of central nervous tissue
can express normal bioelectrical activity at the cellular level (Fischbach and
Dichter, 1974; Peacock *et al.*, 1973*b*). Action potentials and synaptic potentials, both inhibitory and excitatory, as well as complex patterned spontaneous activity are all present. The enormous reduction in the quantity of
interacting elements presumably eliminates some normal features of nervous function, but this reduction offers the opportunity to examine under
direct vision a discriminable number of nerve cells with their processes, laid
out in a two dimensional plane. We will discuss in some detail our recent
experiments on dissociated cell cultures of fetal murine brain and spinal
cord in which intracellular electrophysiological methods have been used to
assess the membrane effects of a number of neurotransmitter candidates.
These experiments illustrate the sort of resolution that cell culture allows in
terms of analyzing membrane mechanisms involved in neuropharmacological responses. In the discussion, we will explore some of the possible future
applications of this methodology to a wider spectrum of psychopharmacological problems.

Fetal mouse spinal cord was dissected free from surrounding tissues
and dissociated and plated in the manner described by Peacock *et al.* (1973*b*)
and modified by Giller *et al.* (1973). A few experiments utilized fetal rat
cerebrum prepared in a similar manner, but with mechanical dissociation.
Growth medium consisted of 90% Dulbecco modified Eagle's medium
(DMEM) and 10% horse serum.

Physiological experiments were done by placing culture dishes in a
special chamber on the stage of an inverted phase contrast microscope.
Temperature and pH of the culture medium were carefully controlled.
Standard electrophysiological techniques were utilized for intracellular
recording and iontophoretic drug application. These techniques are discussed elsewhere in this volume. A bridge circuit permitted current to be
injected through the recording pipette.

Iontophoretic pipettes were pulled from "theta tubing" (glass tubing constructed with a thin central partition dividing the lumen into two compartments) to a tip diameter of about 0.5 μm. The pipettes could be filled immediately before use since the capillary force caused by the central partition allowed solutions to enter the pipette tips almost immediately. Table 1 lists the various drugs which have been used.

Figure 3 shows some morphological features of the preparations. Mature spinal cord cultures were characterized by isolated cells and distributed cell clumps which varied from a few cells to aggregates too large to count. Favorable areas for electrophysiological analysis, as shown in Fig. 3A, consisted of large discrete cells whose multipolar branching patterns were easily discerned (see also Figs. 8 and 9). As described in an earlier publication (Peacock *et al.*, 1973*b*), dorsal root ganglion cells (DRG cells) were clearly distinguishable from spinal cord cells on the basis of distinctive electrophysiological properties and on the basis of their morphology (no DRG cells are seen in Fig. 3A). In comparison to multipolar spinal cord cells (SC

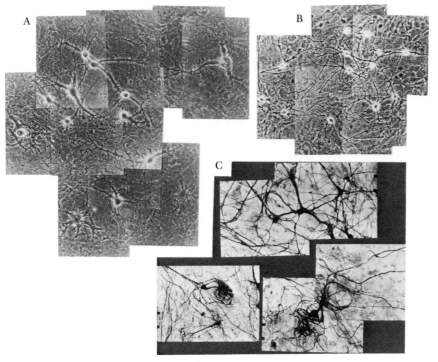

Fig. 3. (A) Montage of phase contrast photomicrographs from 10-wk-old spinal cord culture showing a group of large multipolar neurons. (B) Montage showing a field of neurons from a 5-wk-old culture of fetal rat cerebral cortex. Same phase optics as in A. (C) Selected examples of silver-stained neurons taken from mature mouse spinal cord cultures. Light field optics. The bar in B represents 50 μm for A–C.

TABLE 1

Drugs Used for Iontophoresis

Drug	Molarity (M)	pH
L-Glutamate	0.5	8.0
Aspartate	0.5	10.0
Glycine	1.5	3.5
β-Alanine	1.0	4.0
GABA	1.0	4.0
Acetylcholine chloride	1.0	—[a]

[a]Acetylcholine was passed as a cation.

cells), the DRG cells had fewer processes and their round cell bodies appeared brighter with phase contrast optics and had sharply defined nuclei and nucleoli. The large size of the spinal neurons is emphasized by comparing them to cultured cells from rat cerebral cortex (Fig. 3B). Figure 3C shows a group of silver-stained SC cells (see also Fig. 9). This histological technique reliably revealed a much more complex network of interconnecting processes than could be detected by phase contrast microscopy. It is possible to appreciate qualitative differences in morphology between the cells taken from these different areas, and a goal of future investigation is to develop morphological and physiological criteria for distinguishing specific cell types within the same preparation.

Large SC cells (Fig. 3A) were easily impaled and could be recorded from without difficulty for periods often greater than 1 h. In some instances, it was possible to reimpale a previously studied cell and obtain normal resting potential and spike electrogenesis. Furthermore, replacing the growth medium with a balanced salt solution of specified composition did not interfere with subsequent recording and provided a simple means of controlling the extracellular ionic environment.

A crucial problem in neurobiology is the identification of putative neurotransmitters within the mammalian central nervous system. One approach to this problem has been the iontophoretic application of various drugs to physiologically identified neurons buried within complex neural structures. An unavoidable shortcoming of this *in situ* methodology is the inability to know the exact location of the drug pipette in relation to the cell which is being recorded. In some instances, it is difficult to be certain that an elicited effect in the recorded cell is not secondary to the action of the applied drug on adjacent cells which synaptically interact with the monitored cell. Even when it can be assumed that the applied drug is acting on the recorded cell, it is impossible to determine the topographic distribution of sensitivity. Of particular interest is the sensitivity of synaptic regions on the cell surface.

Iontophoretic studies on neurons in dissociated cell culture circumvent some of these limitations of the *in vivo* situation.

The iontophoretic pipette was positioned as closely as possible to a cell's membrane using a phase contrast microscope at a magnification of about 190×. One could usually return repeatedly to a specific application site and each time elicit an essentially identical response to a constant test pulse of drug. A technical advantage of this recording situation is the ability to obtain large responses with iontophoretic currents which are an order of magnitude smaller than those typically employed *in situ*. This reduces stimulus artifacts and polarization potentials. Maximum current in these experiments rarely exceeded 30 nA, and significant responses could often be obtained with currents of only 1–5 nA and 20 ms duration. The large currents required *in situ* may be necessary for a number of reasons. Since the iontophoretic pipette cannot be carefully positioned close to the cell membrane, the applied drug must diffuse greater distances than *in vitro* in order to reach its site of action. This problem would be compounded by the complex glial investment often seen around neurons in the intact nervous system which could represent an anatomical barrier further increasing the diffusion distance. Finally, the *in vivo* nervous system may have much more efficient mechanisms for the uptake and/or inactivation of transmitter substances than is the case *in vitro*.

The majority of SC cells tested with L-glutamate responded with depolarizing potentials (Table 2), which often produced action potentials if enough drug was applied. The rise times of glutamate-induced depolarizations were variable but could be quite rapid, as shown in Fig. 4A. No evidence for membrane desensitization to glutamate was seen despite

TABLE 2

Drug Responses of Spinal Cord SC Cells[a]

	Glutamate		Acetyl-choline		Aspartate		Glycine		GABA		β-Alanine	
	GM[b]	BSS[c]	GM	BSS	GM	BSS	GM	BSS	GM	BSS	GM	BSS
Number tested	33	28	6	9	0	9	40	57	13	7	4	0
Percent responding	85	97	50	22	—	45	0	46	85	72	0	—

[a]All responses to glutamate, acetylcholine, and aspartate were depolarizations unassociated with large changes in conductance. Responses to glycine and GABA were often depolarizing at resting membrane potential but usually had reversal potentials of around −40 mV (Ransom, Giller, and Nelson, in preparation; *cf.* Figs. 12 and 13). These last responses were associated with marked increases in membrane conductance.

[b]Complete growth medium.

[c]Balanced salt solution.

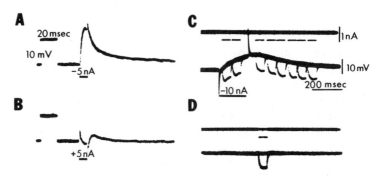

FIG. 4. Depolarizing responses elicited in spinal cord neurons by iontophoretic application of glutamate. (A) Intracellular record showing depolarizing
transient produced by a short pulse of glutamate applied to the cell soma. Bar
beneath trace indicates duration of ejection current; number and sign indicate
the amplitude and polarity of current. Negative indicates glutamate flowing
out of the pipette. Resting potential −64 mV. (B) Same cell as in A. Note the
lack of response when a current pulse of opposite polarity was passed through
the glutamate pipette. Pipette at same location as in A. (C) Depolarization
elicited in another SC cell by application of glutamate to the soma. During the
drug response, constant pulses of current (upper trace) were injected through
the intracellular pipette to measure the membrane resistance. Membrane
resistance during the action of glutamate was essentially the same as during the
control period (shown in D). Resting potential −60 mV. The records in C and
D were made by photographically superimposing several sweeps. In this and in
all subsequent figures, upward deflections are positive for intracellular records. The square-wave pulse on the initial segment of some intracellular traces
(e.g., A and B) is a calibration signal. Calibration pulses in A and B were 10 mV,
20 ms; calibration marks in C are for C and D.

large-amplitude, long-duration focal applications of this drug to a number
of cells. In contrast to SC cells, DRG cells never responded to glutamate. This
argues against glutamate being an entirely nonspecific neural excitant.

Glutamate-evoked depolarizations were not accompanied by large
changes in conductance (Fig. 4C,D), but small increases in conductance were
sometimes noted. This observation indicates that the density of glutamate
receptors and their associated ionophores is relatively low since the conductance was usually measured at the site of drug application, so significant
shunting would have been detected had it occurred. Another possibility
concerns the nature of the ionophores which are activated. Ionophores can
be pictured as shunt conductances added in parallel with the resting
membrane conductance. If the shunt conductances representing the individual ionophores are small enough, activating an area of high receptor
density (and ionophore density) would still result in only a small increase in
overall membrane conductance.

Aspartate could also cause SC cell depolarization (Table 2), and Fig. 5
compares the effects of this drug and glutamate on the same cell. When both

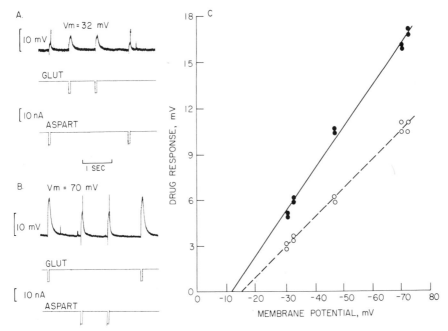

FIG. 5. Effects of membrane polarization on glutamate- and aspartate-induced depolarizing potentials. Constant amounts of glutamate and aspartate were applied to approximately the same site near the cell soma while the membrane potential was varied by intracellular injection of steady current. Sample penwriter recordings taken at two different membrane potentials (-32 and -70 mV) are shown on the left (A and B). The top trace in each group of records is the intracellular recording, and the bottom traces are appropriately labeled ejection current records for the two drugs (downward deflections indicate anodal current). The complete data obtained from this experiment are shown graphically in C. Note that the two drugs have approximately the same extrapolated equilibrium potential.

drugs were alternatively applied to approximately the same site on the cell membrane, depolarizations of similar time courses were elicited (Fig. 5A,B). Furthermore, the effects of membrane polarization on response amplitude were nearly identical, as indicated by the equilibrium potentials for the two drugs (Fig. 5C), suggesting similar ionic mechanisms. Most cells seemed more sensitive to glutamate than to aspartate, and in some cells which responded to glutamate no aspartate response could be obtained, raising the possibility of different receptors for these two amino acids.

Equilibrium potentials for glutamate were obtained in many cells and seemed to fall into two classes. One group of glutamate depolarizations was quite responsive to polarizing current and usually had equilibrium potentials of between 0 and -30 mV (e.g., Figs. 5 and 7). The other group, however, had much more positive equilibrium potentials, as shown in Fig. 6. One explanation of this would be the existence of two different ionic

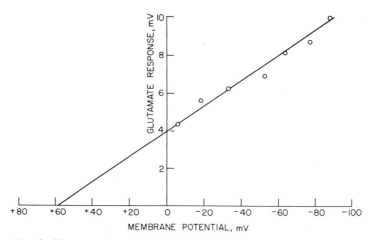

FIG. 6. Glutamate response with a highly positive equilibrium potential. An SC cell was tested with standardized pulses of glutamate (18 nA, 320 ms) applied to a sensitive site on a process about 125 μm from the soma while the membrane potential was varied by intracellular current injection. This cell had a constant input resistance over a membrane potential range of −33 to −87 mV. Resting potential −48 mV.

mechanisms which could be activated by glutamate receptors. The unique accessibility of the extracellular environment of cells in dissociated culture will permit careful investigation of this question by manipulation of ionic concentrations in the bath solution. Although drugs were sometimes applied to membrane sites up to 150 μm from the recording electrode in the soma, this did not cause large changes in the drug equilibrium potential (Ransom, Giller, and Nelson, in preparation).

Spontaneous excitatory postsynaptic potentials (EPSPs), sometimes of large amplitude, were commonly noted in SC cells, but were absent from DRG cells. EPSPs could be evoked in selected SC cells by impaling an appropriate presynaptic element, either another SC cell or a DRG cell. This provided an opportunity to compare the synaptic potential with drug-induced excitation in the same cell.

Figure 7 shows a pair of SC cells linked together by reciprocal excitatory synaptic connections (Fig. 7B,C). The equilibrium potential for the evoked EPSP in the bottom cell of Fig. 7A was determined and compared to the equilibrium potential of a glutamate response elicited at a distal site (shown by the arrow in Fig. 7A). There is a significant discrepancy between these two potentials, with the EPSP equilibrium potential being about 20 mV more positive. Two other similar experiments confirmed this observed discrepancy, with the EPSP equilibrium potential being more positive than the comparable value for glutamate by as much as 50 mV. These data suggest

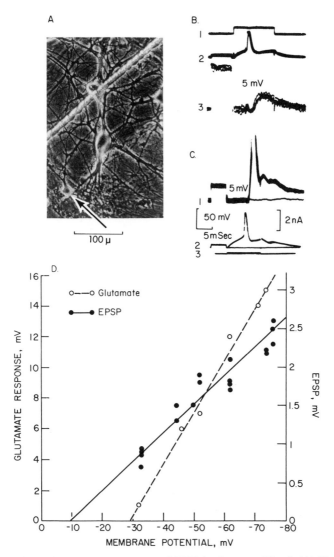

FIG. 7. Comparison of glutamate response and EPSP in the same SC cell. (A) Phase picture showing the cell pair from which records were taken. The top cell of the pair lies near a scratch in the bottom of the plastic culture dish. The arrow indicates the site at which glutamate was applied to the lower cell of the pair. (B) EPSP evoked in bottom cell (trace 3) by action potential in top cell (trace 2) elicited by injection of depolarizing current (trace 1). Calibration pulses 5 mV, 5 ms. (C) EPSP leading to an action potential evoked in the top cell (trace 1) by an action potential in the bottom cell (trace 2). Calibration pulse 5 mV, 5 ms on trace 1. The 50-mV, 5-ms calibration bars are for trace 2 only; the 2-nA calibration bar is for current traces in B and C. (D) Effect of membrane polarization on amplitude of EPSP and glutamate response elicited in bottom cell. Glutamate was applied to the site shown in A (arrow) by a standardized current pulse (−30 nA, 30 ms). Note the discrepancy between the extrapolated equilibrium potentials. Resting potentials: bottom cell −55 mV, top cell −47 mV.

that for some excitatory connections between pairs of SC cells glutamate is unlikely to be the excitatory transmitter (see Krnjević, 1974, for review). One might argue that the driving force for the synaptic potentials would not have been as affected by membrane polarization as was the glutamate response if the synapses were located distally from the cell body. This issue could be resolved by a more detailed analysis of EPSP time course and the neuronal anatomical and passive electrical properties (see Rall *et al.*, 1967, for methodology). In addition, it seems feasible in cell culture to develop techniques for precise localization of synaptic connections which will permit an unambiguous comparison between the equilibrium potentials of drug responses and synaptic potentials.

It is important to recall that glutamate responses in some cells had much more positive equilibrium potentials than those discussed immediately above (compare Fig. 6 with Fig. 7D). The ionic mechanism of such glutamate responses would seem to correspond more closely to that of the EPSP shown in Fig. 7. It will be necessary, however, to obtain evoked EPSPs in those same cells in which glutamate responses have very positive equilibrium potentials in order to have a valid comparison. An interesting and specific excitatory synapse to study in this regard is the one seen between DRG and SC cells, since some neurochemical evidence indicates that the proximal projections of DRG cells contain increased amounts of glutamate (Johnson, 1972).

Focal applications of glutamate to different areas of SC cells were usually not equipotent in eliciting depolarization. The majority of these cells exhibited areas on their processes where the membrane was particularly sensitive to glutamate as judged by the response magnitude and rise time. It should be noted, however, that a differential topography of glutamate receptors is probably best assessed by variance in rise times as opposed to absolute response magnitudes (Harris *et al.*, 1971). Figures 8 and 9 show both uniform and nonuniform receptor densities, respectively, based on maps of glutamate responsiveness. All cells which had "hot spots" to glutamate had excitatory synaptic input, either spontaneous or evoked. As mentioned above, it seems feasible to identify sites of synaptic contact in spinal cord cultures by physiological methods, and it will be important to learn whether such sites coincide with areas of increased drug sensitivity as is the case for some synaptic junctions. This approach could prove a powerful one in helping to evaluate various putative transmitters with regard to their role in physiological transmission. Another issue raised by the finding of "hot spots" on innervated nerve cells is the possible trophic influence which the development of synaptic contacts might exert on the aggregation of receptors.

Figure 9 also demonstrates that cells which are physiologically studied can be readily recovered for subsequent histological examination. This fact is significant in that it permits reliable correlation between function and structure, even at the electron microscopic level.

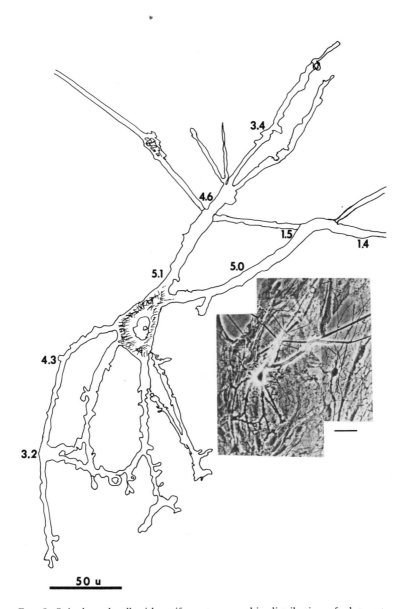

FIG. 8. Spinal cord cell with uniform topographic distribution of glutamate sensitivity. The inset shows a phase photomicrograph of the sketched cell. The response to a standard pulse of glutamate (−20 nA, 300 ms) in millivolts is indicated at each site tested. The bar below the phase picture represents 50 μm. Resting potential −38 mV.

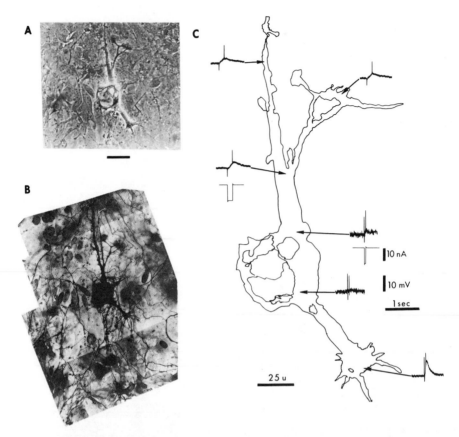

FIG. 9. Spinal cord cell demonstrating local area of increased sensitivity to glutamate. (A) Phase optics photomicrograph of cell. The bar indicates 50 μm for A and B. (B) Silver stain of cell seen in A. (C) Sketch of same cell showing the glutamate responses obtained at various sites of application. The bottom three responses were obtained using a short pulse (shown adjacent to current calibration bar). The top three responses were obtained using a longer pulse (shown under the bottom response on the left side). Note the faster rise time at the "hot spot." Resting potential −53 mV. Calibrations as shown.

A large number of cells in spinal cord culture were tested with the putative inhibitory transmitters GABA and glycine. In general, SC cells which responded to both of these drugs did not exhibit any striking preferential sensitivity to either of the drugs. A few cells were spatially mapped with regard to their sensitivity to glycine or GABA, and in all cases the sensitivity was highest on the soma and gradually decreased as one tested farther out on the processes. Some evidence of desensitization was noted for both drugs, but the phenomenon was much more strongly established for glycine (see below).

Unlike glutamate, the inhibitory drugs glycine and GABA caused very large conductance increases in the cells which responded (Fig. 10); in fact, this was the most characteristic aspect of the response, since the direction of the induced potential fluctuation was often in the depolarizing direction at resting potential (see below). The conductance increase was proportional to the amount of drug applied, as shown in Fig. 10A–C where the largest dose of GABA (Fig. 10C) caused approximately a 600% increase in conductance.

On the basis of experimental results from a number of neuronal preparations, it seems probable that an increase in membrane permeability to Cl⁻ was involved in the GABA and glycine responses. A variable leakage of Cl⁻ from the extracellular fluid into the neuron interior probably accompanies penetration of the cell by the recording electrode. An increase in intracellular Cl⁻ would tend to shift a chloride-dependent GABA or glycine response in the depolarizing direction. This set of circumstances may well

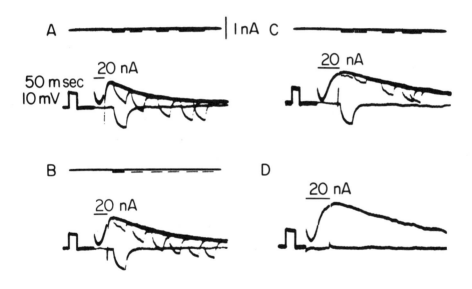

FIG. 10. Membrane conductance during GABA application. (A–C) A 20-nA pulse of GABA was applied for various lengths of time as indicated by the bars. At various times after the drug was applied, constant-current pulses were injected through the intracellular electrode to test membrane resistance. Note the decrease in the size of the potentials produced by the test pulses during the response to GABA. The response to a test pulse in the absence of GABA is shown in each case as a control. These records were made by superimposing many sweeps. The magnitude of the conductance change appears dependent on the length of the GABA pulse. (D) Record from same cell illustrating the lack of any response when the current pulse used to eject GABA was reversed in polarity (flat line). A response to the same magnitude current pulse of the usual polarity is shown for comparison. Resting potential −43 mV. Calibration pulses 10 mV, 50 ms.

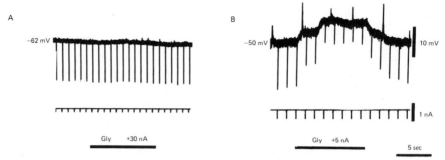

FIG. 11. Development of glycine responsiveness in an SC cell after switching from complete growth medium to a balanced salt solution. (A) Glycine applied to an SC cell bathed in complete growth medium including DMEM, which contains 0.4 mM glycine. Constant-current pulses (bottom trace) were injected through the intracellular electrode to monitor the cell's conductance. Note the lack of voltage fluctuation or change in membrane conductance when glycine was applied. (B) Same cell as in A after switching to a balanced salt solution containing no amino acids. Note the voltage fluctuation and increased conductance which accompanied the glycine application. The bars in A and B indicate the duration of drug application and the number signifies the average current strength. Some variation in current strength was present during a given application, which accounts for the variation in response amplitude seen in B.

explain the observation of depolarizing responses to the drugs at resting membrane potential.

When the glycine and GABA were tested on spinal cord cells which were bathed in growth medium (containing 0.4 mM glycine), no glycine responses were ever seen (Fig. 11A), but GABA responses were common (Figs. 10 and 12C; Table 2). When the growth medium was exchanged for a defined salt solution containing no amino acids, cells which were previously unresponsive to glycine now responded (Fig. 11B; the decrease in the cells' resting potential between Fig. 11A and 11B was probably due to the fact that this was the second impalement). Since such cells were unresponsive to glycine in DMEM, which contains glycine, and since there was no obvious difference between the resting potentials or input resistances of cells in DMEM as compared to those in a balanced salt solution (suggesting the absence of chronic stimulation of glycine receptors in DMEM), it is concluded that chronic application of high concentrations of glycine causes complete desensitization to this drug. Furthermore, the fact that SC cells do respond to GABA in cultures desensitized to glycine suggests that the GABA receptor is distinct from the glycine receptor.

Glycine and GABA equilibrium potentials were highly variable (about −30 to −80 mV) and could change with time during the same impalement (Ransom, Giller, and Nelson, in preparation). Equilibrium potentials were sometimes determined, as shown in Fig. 12B,C where long intracellular current pulses polarized the membrane while a drug response was elicited. Note the enormous increase of the GABA response with membrane

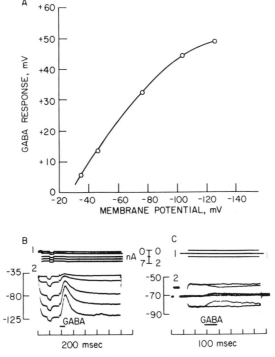

FIG. 12. Effects of membrane polarization on GABA responses. (B) GABA responses were obtained at various hyperpolarized membrane potentials (trace 2). A short pulse of hyperpolarizing current was also injected at each membrane potential to detect changes in the cell's input resistance (note that the size of the elicited IR drop first increased and then decreased with increasing hyperpolarization, indicating the presence of both delayed and anomalous rectification). (A) Graph of the data from panel B. (C) Similar data taken from a different cell, clearly illustrating a reversal of the response polarity with membrane depolarization. The current trace is labeled 1 in B and C.

hyperpolarization in Fig. 12B and also the clear-cut reversal of the response in Fig. 12C. The data in Fig. 12B have been graphed in Fig. 12A. The small current pulse in Fig. 12B elicits a voltage change at each resting potential and demonstrates the presence of both anomalous and delayed rectification. Both of these latter processes can be expected to affect the relationship between the magnitude of the drug response and the membrane potential. This effect is obvious in the high membrane potential range shown in Fig. 12A. Figure 13 shows how measurement of a cell's voltage-dependent changes in input resistance can be used to correct for such distortion. The main point of Fig. 13, however, is to illustrate the similarity between the equilibrium potentials for glycine and GABA when these were measured in the same cell. This is true for all the cells which have been tested, suggesting that a common ionic mechanism subserves both responses.

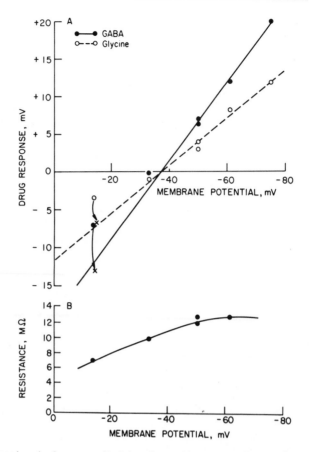

FIG. 13. Comparison in the same cell of the effects of membrane polarization on glycine- and GABA-induced potential fluctuations. Constant-sized pulses of GABA (13 nA, 320 ms) and glycine (25 nA, 320 ms) were applied to approximately the same location near the cell soma while membrane potential was varied. (A) Response amplitude graphed as a function of membrane potential. (B) Variation of input resistance of the cell with membrane potential. The drug responses obtained at the most depolarized membrane potentials were corrected for rectification (crosses in A). Note that both drugs had approximately the same equilibrium potential. Resting potential −50 mV.

Unlike SC cells, DRG cells never responded to glycine in glycine-free medium. In preliminary experiments, some DRG cells were found to respond with small depolarizing potentials to the application of GABA, but in all cases they were much less sensitive than SC cells which responded to this drug. Since GABA has been implicated in the genesis of the dorsal root potential associated with presynaptic inhibition in the spinal cord (see Krnjević, 1974, for review), it is possible that the DRG response to GABA may prove a helpful model for further analysis of the ionic mechanisms involved.

Brain cell cultures are suitable for neuropharmacological studies similar to those described above (Godfrey *et al.*, 1975). Morphologically differentiated neurons exhibit a wide range of ongoing action potential and synaptic activity. Excitatory and inhibitory synaptic activity can be elicited by stimulating neurons in the vicinity of recorded cells. Both GABA and glycine, when iontophoretically applied, elicit a large membrane conductance change with an equilibrium potential of about -50 mV. The glycine response can be obtained in DMEM, in contrast to the situation in spinal cord cultures. It is clear from preliminary experiments that the various cells in the culture respond in a selective manner to a number of neuropharmacological agents such as glutamate, acetylcholine, and norepinephrine.

7. DISCUSSION

The preceding presentation has examined the utility of various culture methods for studying some pharmacological responses of nervous tissue. Observations from dissociated cell cultures were emphasized, and some advantages of these systems have already been mentioned, but a more complete consideration of their assets and liabilities is needed.

A high degree of resolution of cellular detail is provided in dissociated cell cultures, and the size of neurons is quite adequate for careful intracellular studies of drug action. These features permit assessment of topographic drug sensitivity (e.g., Figs. 8 and 9) and biophysical experiments to determine the influence that the site of drug application has on the characteristics of the elicited response. Relating these neuropharmacological data to the problem of identification of neural transmitters is a difficult task, as has been discussed in detail elsewhere (Werman, 1966). Positive identification of the precise locus of synaptic contact in the cell cultures would be helpful in this regard and should be feasible. The sensitivity to the putative transmitters can then be determined at the synaptic regions and interactions between iontophoretically and naturally applied transmitter studied and the action of antagonists compared. Since an identified cell's morphology can be described by both light and electron microscopic studies (Giller *et al.*, 1974) and is readily correlated with its physiological and pharmacological properties, it is reasonable to expect that specific cell types will eventually become recognizable in these cultures. Some preliminary investigations suggest that measurements of enzyme and macromolecular biosynthetic activity may also be possible on single cells of a specific type (e.g., DRG cells), thus establishing their biochemical identity. Since the extracellular environment of cell cultures is easily manipulated, studies can be conducted on the ionic mechanisms of various drug responses or on the interaction between different drugs. Finally, it should be mentioned that other regions of the nervous system besides cerebrum and spinal cord can be grown in cell culture. Interactions between different areas of the brain can be studied by growing various combinations of two or more specific regions in the same culture.

It is appropriate to discuss some of the significant limitations associated with cell cultures. Many intact neural structures, despite their enormous quantitative complexity, have the simplifying feature that homogeneous cell populations are aggregated into specific areas which can be reliably located (e.g., granule cells of cerebellar cortex). This is naturally lost in cell culture and specific criteria for cell typing will need to be developed before this deficit can be circumvented. A tacit assumption of the cell culture method which deserves explicit consideration is that normal nerve cell differentiation is occurring in the disturbed microenvironment of the culture dish. The differences between the *in vivo* and *in vitro* situations during development are not only enormous, but are also at present undefined. As demonstrated in the case of glycine (Fig. 11), the manipulation of various aspects of the external chemical milieu can have powerful effects on drug actions and conceivably on the normal physiological function of nervous tissue. Some degree of neuronal cell death is seen in developing cultures, and it is not known whether this represents a random process or the selective elimination of a specific cell type. Finally, the vagaries of growing cells in dissociated cultures must be mentioned. The exact formula necessary to consistently obtain mature cultures which are optimal for electrophysiological study has not been developed. Unknown factors in the animal sera used to supplement the growth medium seem very important in this regard, and only by trial and error can particularly suitable lots of serum be determined. It is reasonable to speculate that certain aspects of differentiation, morphogenesis, and synaptogenesis might be influenced by such variables, but these questions remain unanswered.

The results presented here indicate that detailed study of the membrane mechanisms involved in neuronal responses to pharmacological agents is feasible using dissociated cell cultures. In addition to those described, many other agents which have actions on the nervous system including anesthetics, narcotics, catecholamines, the cyclic nucleotides, and epileptogenic agents such as penicillin could be easily examined using cell cultures in order to assess their mechanisms of action. Do these agents produce specific changes in membrane conductance, do they affect synaptic inputs, are the effects on synaptic action presynaptic or postsynaptic, are divalent cations (especially Ca^{2+}) involved in any of the effects? These are some of the questions readily approached in this system.

To fully explore these questions, it is essential to develop a full range of identified cell types in culture so that the varieties of cell responses that characterize the nervous system will be available for study. At present, we have worked with cells prepared from whole brain, cerebral cortex, the remainder of the cerebrum after removal of cortical tissue, cerebellum, midbrain, spinal cord, and dorsal root ganglion. The yield of viable, relatively mature neurons from these different regions is variable; cerebellum, for example, is rather difficult to maintain in our experience. Useful morphological and electrophysiological studies can be done, however, on cultures in which the overall survival rate is low.

A general question may be raised as to the relevance of the cellular neurobiology which we have described to the field of psychopharmacology, which has some behavioral connotations. The cell culture methodology totally disrupts all of the organization that is so crucial to the function of the nervous system *in vivo*. Moderately complex synaptic networks develop in culture, but the degree to which the specific patterns of innervation that characterize the intact nervous system are maintained *in vitro* is unknown at present. The assumption underlying the application of the culture system to psychopharmacological questions is that the fundamental membrane mechanisms and mode of action of pharmacological agents are operative *in vitro*. Furthermore, information about these basic mechanisms is important for the understanding of their action in more complex, behaviorally relevant systems, and the efficient development and application of new agents may be furthered by their study *in vitro*.

8. REFERENCES

BUNGE, R. P., REES, R., WOOD, P., BURTON, H., and KO, C.-P., 1974, Anatomical and physiological observations on synapses formed on isolated autonomic neurons in tissue culture, *Brain Res.* **66**:401–412.

COHEN, M. W., 1972, The development of neuromuscular connexions in the presence of D-tubocurarine, *Brain Res.* **41**:457–463.

COHEN, S. A., and FISCHBACH, G., 1973, Regulation of muscle acetylcholine sensitivity by muscle activity in cell culture, *Science* **181**:76–78.

CRAIN, S. M., 1972, Tissue culture model of epileptiform activity, in: *Experimental Models of Epilepsy—A Manual for the Laboratory Worker* (D. P. Purpura, J. K. Penry, D. Tower, C. W. Woodbury, and R. Walter, eds.), pp. 291–316, Raven Press, New York.

CRAIN, S. M., 1973, Tissue culture studies of central nervous system maturation, in: Early Development, *Res. Publ. Assoc. Res. Nerv. Ment. Dis.* **51**:113–131.

CRAIN, S. M., and BORNSTEIN, M. B., 1974, Early onset in inhibitory transactions during synaptogenesis in fetal mouse brain cultures, *Brain Res.* **68**:351–357.

CRAIN, S. M., and PETERSON, E. R., 1971, Development of paired explants of fetal spinal cord and adult skeletal muscle during chronic exposure to curare and hemicholinium, *In Vitro* **6**:373.

CRAIN, S. M., and POLLACK, 1973, Restorative effects of cyclic AMP on complex bioelectric activities of cultured fetal rodent CNS tissues after acute Ca^{++} deprivation, *J. Neurobiol.* **4**:321–342.

CRAIN, S. M., BORNSTEIN, M. B., and PETERSON, E. R., 1968, Maturation of cultured embryonic CNS tissue during chronic exposure to agents which prevent bioelectric activity, *Brain Res.* **8**:363–372.

FISCHBACH, G. D., 1972, Synapse formation between dissociated nerve and muscle cells in low density cell cultures, *Develop. Biol.* **28:**407–429.

FISCHBACH, G. D., and COHEN, S. A., 1973, The distribution of acetylcholine sensitivity over uninnervated and innervated muscle fibers grown in cell culture, *Develop. Biol.* **31:**147–162.

FISCHBACH, G. D., and DICHTER, M. A., 1974, Electrophysiologic and morphologic properties of neurons in dissociated chick spinal cord cell cultures, *Develop. Neurol.* **37:**100–116.

GILLER, E. L., SCHRIER, B. K., SHAINBERG, A., FISK, H. R., and NELSON, P. G., 1973, Choline acetyltransferase activity is increased in combined cultures of spinal cord and muscle cells from the mouse, *Science* **182:**588–589.

GILLER, E. L., BREAKEFIELD, X. O., CHRISTIAN, C. N., NEALE, E. A., and NELSON, P. G., 1974, Expression of neuronal characteristics in culture: Some pros and cons of primary cultures and continuous cell lines, in: *Proceedings of the Golgi Centennial Symposium* (M. Santini, ed.), Raven Press, New York, in press.

GILMAN, A., and NIRENBERG, M., 1971, Effect of catecholamines on adenosine 3':5'-cyclic monophosphate concentration of clonal satellite cells of neurons, *Proc. Natl. Acad. Sci.* **68:**2165–2168.

GODFREY, E. W., NELSON, P. G., SCHRIER, B. K., BREUER, A. C., and RANSOM, B. R., 1975, *Brain Res.* (in press).

HARRIS, A. J., and DENNIS, M. J., 1970, Acetylcholine sensitivity and distribution on mouse neuroblastoma cells, *Science* **67:**1253–1255.

HARRIS, A. J., KUFFLER, S. W., and DENNIS, M. J., 1971, Differential chemosensitivity of synaptic and extrasynaptic areas on the neuronal surface membrane in parasympathetic neurons of the frog tested by micro-application of acetylcholine, *Proc. Roy. Soc. Lond. Ser. B* **177:**541–553.

HARTZELL, H. C., and FAMBROUGH, D. M., 1973, Acetylcholine receptor production and incorporation into membranes of developing muscle fibers, *Develop. Biol.* **30:**153–165.

HÖSLI, E., and HÖSLI, L., 1971, Acetylcholinesterase in cultured rat spinal cord, *Brain Res.* **30:**193–197.

HÖSLI, E., MEIER-RUGE, W., and HÖSLI, L., 1971, Monoamine-containing neurones in cultures of rat brain stem, *Experientia* **27:**310.

HÖSLI, E., LJUNGDAHL, A., HÖKFELT, T., and HÖSLI, L., 1972, Spinal cord tissue cultures—A model for autoradiographic studies on uptake of putative neurotransmitters such as glycine and GABA, *Experientia* **28:**1342–1344.

HÖSLI, L., and HÖSLI, E., 1972, Autoradiographic localization of the uptake of glycine in cultures of rat medulla oblongata, *Brain Res.* **45:**612–616.

HÖSLI, L., HÖSLI, E., and ANDRES, P. G., 1973a, Nervous tissue culture: A model to study action and uptake of putative neurotransmitters such as amino acids, *Brain Res.* **62:**597–602.

HÖSLI, L., HÖSLI, E., and ANDRES, P. F., 1973b, Electrophysiological and histochemical properties of fetal human spinal cord, in: *Dynamics of Degeneration and Growth in Neurones*, Wenner-Gren Center International Symposium, Stockholm.

JOHNSON, J. L., 1972, Glutamic acid as a synaptic transmitter in the nervous system: A review, *Brain Res.* **37:**1–19.

KRNJEVIĆ, K., 1974, Chemical nature of synaptic transmission in vertebrates, *Physiol. Rev.* **54:**418–540.

KRNJEVIĆ, K., and SCHWARTZ, S., 1967, Some properties of unresponsive cells in the cerebral cortex, *Exp. Brain Res.* **3:**206–219.

KRNJEVIĆ, K., PUMAIN, R., and RENAUD, L., 1971, The mechanism of excitation by acetylcholine in the cerebral cortex, *J. Physiol.* **215:**247–268.

KUFFLER, ST. W., and NICHOLLS, J. G., 1966, The physiology of neuroglial cells, *Ergeb. Physiol. Biol. Chem. Exp. Pharmakol.* **57:**1–90.

LASHER, R. S., 1974, The uptake of [^{3}H]GABA and differentiation of stellate neurons in cultures of dissociated postnatal rat cerebellum, *Brain Res.* **69:**235–254.

MURRAY, M. R., 1971, Nervous tissues isolated in culture, in: *Handbook of Neurochemistry*, Vol. 5A (A. Lajtha, ed.), pp. 373–438, Plenum, New York.

NELSON, P. G., 1973, Electrophysiological studies of normal and neoplastic cells in tissue culture, in: *Tissue Culture of the Nervous System* (G. Sato, ed.), pp. 135–160, Plenum, New York.

NELSON, P. G., 1975, Nerve and muscle cells in culture, *Physiol. Rev.* **55**:1–6.

NELSON, P. G., and PEACOCK, J. H., 1973, Electrical activity in dissociated cell cultures from fetal mouse cerebellum, *Brain Res.* **61**:163–174.

NELSON, P., RUFFNER, W., and NIRENBERG, M., 1969, Neuronal tumor cells with excitable membranes grown *in vitro*, *Proc. Natl. Acad. Sci.* **64**:1004–1010.

NELSON, P. G., PEACOCK, J. H., and AMANO, T., 1971, Responses of neuroblastoma cells to iontophoretically applied acetylcholine, *J. Cell Physiol.* **77**:353–362.

OLSON, M. I., and BUNGE, R. P., 1973, Anatomical observations on the specificity of synapse formation in tissue culture, *Brain Res.* **59**:19–33.

PAUL, J., 1972, *Cell and Tissue Culture*, Williams and Wilkins, Baltimore.

PEACOCK, J. H., and NELSON, P. G., 1973, Chemosensitivity of mouse neuroblastoma cells *in vitro*, *J. Neurobiol.* **4**:363–374.

PEACOCK, J. H., McMORRIS, F. A., and NELSON, P. G., 1973a, Electrical excitability and chemosensitivity of mouse neuroblastoma × mouse or human fibroblast hybrids, *Exp. Cell Res.* **79**:199–212.

PEACOCK, J. H., NELSON, P. G., and GOLDSTONE, M. W., 1973b, Electrophysiologic study of cultured neurons dissociated from spinal cords and dorsal root ganglia of fetal mice, *Develop. Biol.* **30**:137–152.

PURVES, D., and SAKMANN, B., 1974, The effect of contractile activity on fibrillation and extrajunctional acetylcholine-sensitivity in rat muscle maintained in organ culture, *J. Physiol.* **237**:157–182.

RALL, W., BURKE, R. E., SMITH, T. G., NELSON, P. G., and FRANK, K., 1967, Dendritic location of synapses and possible mechanisms for the monosynaptic EPSP in motoneurons, *J. Neurophysiol.* **30**:1169–1193.

SATO, G. (ed.), 1973, *Tissue Culture of the Nervous System*, Vol. 1 of *Current Topics in Neurobiology*, Plenum, New York.

SCHON, F., and KELLY, J. S., 1974, Autoradiographic localization of [^{3}H]GABA and [H^3]glutamate over satellite glial cells, *Brain Res.* **66**:275–288.

SCHRIER, B. K., and THOMPSON, E. J., 1974, On the role of glial cells in the mammalian nervous system, *J. Biol. Chem.* **219**:1769–1780.

SCHUBERT, D., HARRIS, A. J., HEINEMANN, S., KIDOKORO, Y., PATRICK, J., and STEINBACH, J. H., 1973, Differentiation and interaction of clonal cell lines of nerve and muscle, in: *Tissue Culture of the Nervous System* (G. Sato, ed.), pp. 55–86, Plenum, New York.

TASAKI, I., and CHANG, J. J., 1958, Electric response of glia cells in cat brain, *Science* **128**:1209–1210.

WARDELL, W. M., 1966, Electrical and pharmacological properties of mammalian neuroglial cells in tissue culture, *Proc. Roy. Soc. Lond. Ser. B* **165**:326–361.

WERMAN, R., 1966, Criteria for identification of a central nervous system transmitter, *Comp. Biochem. Physiol.* **18**:745–766.

5

BIOCHEMICAL IDENTIFICATION OF MEMBRANE RECEPTORS: PRINCIPLES AND TECHNIQUES

M. D. Hollenberg and P. Cuatrecasas

1. INTRODUCTION

Since the earliest pharmacological studies, the cell membrane has been considered a likely site of drug interaction (Clark, 1933). Yet only within the past decade has considerable progress been made in the identification and purification of a variety of membrane-localized hormone receptors. This chapter will not attempt a comprehensive summary of all such studies completed to date; rather, an attempt will be made to elaborate on a few specific studies which, it is felt, will not only illustrate the general approaches that can be used to study ligand–membrane interactions but will also reveal some of the successes and pitfalls of these approaches. Examples will be drawn largely from work done in this laboratory, primarily because of our familiarity with the intimate details of these studies, both published and unpublished. Furthermore, examples will deal only with several of the polypeptide hormones and with catecholamines and will thus omit a large body of work on cholinergic receptors and on membrane receptors for an enlarging number of polypeptide hormones and other compounds. Studies

M. D. Hollenberg and *P. Cuatrecasas* ● Department of Pharmacology and Experimental Therapeutics and Department of Medicine, The Johns Hopkins University School of Medicine, Baltimore, Maryland

on cytoplasmic receptors for steroids are considered beyond the scope of this discussion. For details of these studies, the reader is referred to review articles elsewhere (Hall, 1972; Cuatrecasas, 1973a, 1974; Lis and Sharon. 1973; Hollenberg and Cuatrecasas, 1975a).

In general, the approach has been to study the physiochemical interaction between a radioactively labeled ligand and the plasma membrane, either in the intact cell or in an isolated membrane preparation. For receptors of endogenous hormones, the ligands used will generally require labeling to very high specific activity (e.g., ^{125}I or ^{131}I, at about 2 Ci/μmol) because of the scarcity of receptor structures in the target cells. Many methods are available for measuring the binding interaction (to be described in a later section). In such studies, it is essential to satisfy a number of criteria in order to establish that the binding measurements obtained truly reflect a hormone–receptor interaction in a pharmacological sense: (1) The labeled ligand used as a membrane probe must be fully active biologically so as to mimic the activity of the parent compound; it is presumed that such an analogue will be interchangeable with the parent compound at the receptor site. (2) The binding must exhibit absolute structural and steric specificity *pari passu* with the known biological activity of the parent ligand, its structural analogues, and its antagonists. (3) The binding should demonstrate saturability within a concentration range that can be meaningfully related to that of agonists which elicit the known biological response in intact biological systems. (4) The binding interaction should reflect high affinity, in harmony with the sensitivity of the tissue to the physiologically active concentration range of the ligand. (5) The presence of this binding should be restricted to tissues (or species) known to be physiologically sensitive to the agonist. (6) The binding should in most if not all cases be reversible, in accord with the rapidity of several of the known biological responses upon removal of the agonist from the medium in the given system. In the case of hormones, the affinity and number of binding sites must be consistent with the physiological concentration of the hormone. The essential meaning of these criteria is that considerable care and caution must be exercised in correlating the properties of the binding interaction with the biological properties of the *in vivo* or intact system to ascertain the true identity of the receptor interaction.

Since the binding data (specificity, affinity, number of sites) must be evaluated by careful and detailed comparisons with the biological activity of the ligand, it is desirable that the initial preparation used for binding studies be a simple, intact system (e.g., isolated, homogeneous, and viable cells) so that the binding and biological responses can be measured in the same system, before disruptive procedures are performed. With the use of an appropriate system, it is possible to avoid many complications (e.g., heterogeneous cell populations, presence of connective tissues and basement membrane, or diffusion barriers presented by thick multicellular matrices such as tissue slices) which may seriously compromise the interpretation of the binding data (rates of association and dissociation, saturability, role of nonspecific binding, etc.). When the binding–activity relationships are ascertained, a proper setting is established in which to evaluate studies in isolated, particulate (plasma membrane), and solubilized preparations. In many cases, a ligand-responsive biological activity (e.g., adenylate cyclase activity) can also be determined in isolated membrane preparations. With the proviso that very important differences may exist between the hormonal modulation of an enzyme system in the intact cell and the modulation by regulators in membrane preparations, it is also profitable to study binding–activity relationships in such subcellular isolates.

For studies on receptors in the central nervous system, it is difficult to obtain an intact preparation whereby ligand binding can be compared directly with a biological response. Rather, studies of binding to membrane preparations can be performed, as have been done for [^{3}H]opiate analogues (Goldstein *et al.*, 1971; Pert and Snyder, 1973*a,b*; Simon *et al.*, 1973; Snyder, Chap. 6, Vol. 5). While absolute comparisons of ligand affinities with biological activities cannot be made directly in the same membrane preparations, it is still possible to study accurately the steric and structural properties of the ligand interaction and to compare the relative potencies of known agonists and antagonists with the measured membrane affinities. Most of criteria outlined above can thus be met. It is likely that propagable cell lines, e.g., those derived from mouse neuroblastoma, or other cultured cell systems such as those discussed by Richelson (Chap. 6, Vol. 1), will find increasing use as biologically responsive systems in which to study ligand–membrane interactions. It has been possible, for instance, to compare the affinity of ^{125}I-labeled β-nerve growth factor for membrane receptors in ganglia with the biological action of β-NGF in chick sensory ganglia (Banerjee *et al.*, 1973*b*).

It should not be overlooked that a biologically responsive membrane activity, e.g., adenylate cyclase, may be used to complement studies on ligand binding. Specific responsive membrane-localized enzyme activities derived from central nervous system structures would prove most useful in further work on ligand binding, e.g., in connection with studies on opiate receptors, or on bungarotoxin binding sites in the brain.

2. PROPERTIES OF RECEPTOR INTERACTIONS AND TECHNICAL CONSIDERATIONS

2.1. Number and Affinity of Membrane Receptors

It is possible to generalize somewhat on the properties of hormone–receptor interactions. The affinities involved are remarkably high, with dissociation constants usually less than 10^{-8} M—e.g., 10^{-10} M for insulin in fat cells (Cuatrecasas, 1971a) and 5×10^{-10} M for epidermal growth factor (EGF) in fibroblasts (Hollenberg and Cuatrecasas, 1973a). In addition, the receptors found on any given cell are present in vanishingly small numbers—e.g., 10^4 insulin receptors per fat cell (Cuatrecasas, 1971a), 8×10^4 EGF receptors per fibroblast (Hollenberg and Cuatrecasas, 1973a), and 1.6×10^5 atropine receptors per smooth muscle cell (Paton and Rang, 1965). These figures are in excellent agreement with early estimates of the numbers of specific drug receptors present on responsive cells (Clark, 1926a,b).

Because of the small number of receptors generally present, it is desirable to use radioactively labeled compounds of very high specific activity (e.g., 1000–3000 Ci/mmol). For example, with the fat cell (approximately 10^6 cells) the use of a compound possessing only 10–20 Ci/mmol (the value usually attainable for ^{3}H-labeled compounds) would restrict measurements to a maximum of a few hundred cpm above background. Since experiments with enormous quantities of cells or membranes are both impractical and subject to special kinds of complications, most studies, e.g., with peptides, have employed compounds substituted with ^{125}I or ^{131}I (less than one atom per molecule) to attain the desired specific activity.

2.2. Preparation of Radioactive Ligand Derivatives

2.2.1. Iodination (^{125}I, ^{131}I)

Most frequently, peptides are iodinated by procedures originally developed by Greenwood and Hunter (1963) with minor modifications (Cuatrecasas, 1971a). In a typical experiment with insulin, 5 μl of a solution of peptide (1 mg/ml) is gently mixed into 100 μl of 0.25 M sodium phosphate buffer, pH 7.4, containing 1–3 MCi of freshly made carrier-free Na^{125}I (usually added in 5 or 10 μl). Immediately, 20 μl of chloramine T (2.5 mg/ml) is added with agitation of the solution, and the reaction is allowed to proceed for 20 s. Sodium metabisulfite (20 μl of 5 mg/ml) is then added, and the reaction is allowed to proceed for a further 10 s. The mixture is then diluted with 2–3 ml of 0.1 M sodium phosphate buffer, pH 7.4, containing 0.1% (w/v) crystalline bovine albumin (PBA) and rapidly transferred to a centrifuge tube containing a crushed pellet of talc (25 mg) for adsorption of the iodinated peptide. The small amount of solution remaining in the reaction vessel is taken up in approximately 0.5 ml of PBA and saved for the measurement of the percent incorporation of ^{125}I into peptide.

The talc-adsorbed insulin is washed with five successive 12-ml portions of PBA, and the final pellet is suspended in 2–3 ml of a solution of 1 N HCl–H$_2$O–20% crystalline albumin in Krebs–Ringer bicarbonate buffer, pH

7.4 (3:2:1, v/v). The suspension is clarified by centrifugation (2500 rpm for 40 min) and the insulin eluted into the supernatant is decanted with a pasteur pipette. The solution is adjusted to pH 4–6 (indicator paper) by the dropwise addition of 1 N NaOH and then frozen in aliquots for further use.

The incorporation of ^{125}I is estimated in the following manner. An aliquot, e.g., 50 μl of the final diluted reaction mixture, is mixed into 1 ml of sodium phosphate buffer, pH 7.4, containing 1% albumin. An equal aliquot (50 μl) is then withdrawn for crystal scintillation counting. Trichloroacetic acid (0.5 ml of 10% w/v in H_2O) is then added, and the resulting precipitate is sedimented in a clinical centrifuge. An aliquot of the supernatant (50 μl) is withdrawn and the radioactivity is measured. It is assumed that the radioactivity remaining in the supernatant represents nonincorporated ^{125}I. The percent incorporation of iodine is thus given by the formula

$$\frac{\text{R.A. initial} - 1.5 \text{ R.A. supernatant}}{\text{R.A. initial}}$$

where "R.A. initial" and "R.A. supernatant" refer, respectively, to the radioactivity in aliquots before and after the addition of trichloroacetic acid. It can be demonstrated by this procedure that more than 97% of the [^{125}I]insulin prepared is precipitable in the presence of trichloroacetic acid.

When [^{125}I]insulin is synthesized by the technique outlined above, on average less than one atom of iodine is incorporated per molecule of insulin. Such derivatives of insulin retain their biological activity.

However, it should be emphasized that while applicable in general for the substitution of ^{125}I into peptides the above technique must be specifically tailored for each particular peptide. For example, the talc purification step does not work well for the isolation of [^{125}I]cholera toxin or plant lectins; Sephadex G75 chromatography or affinity chromatography is a suitable alternative.

The chemical procedures used in the iodination reaction may be harmful to the integrity of the particular protein being modified. For example, sodium metabisulfite may destroy or alter the biological activity of a given peptide by reducing disulfide bonds, and alternative methods to stop the iodination reaction must be employed. Thus for preparing biologically active derivatives of ^{125}I-labeled nerve growth factor, the reduction step is omitted; the reaction is rapidly "quenched" by dilution with 0.5 ml of 0.1 M sodium phosphate buffer, adsorption for 1 min on 25 mg crushed talc, and repeated washing of the [^{125}I]NGF adsorbed to talc with PBA as outlined above (Banerjee et al., 1973b). The oxidizing agent used, chloramine T, may destroy peptide activity by oxidizing susceptible methionine, tryptophan, or sulfhydryl residues. In such cases, the concentration of the oxidizing agent and the time of exposure to this chemical must be decreased to the minimal values compatible with effective iodination. Alternatively, the iodide may be oxidized to iodine immediately before addition of the protein. The use of the lactoperoxidase technique (Thorell and Johansson, 1971) can yield biologically active ^{125}I-substituted peptides of sufficient specific activity to permit binding studies. However, it must be remembered that this technique uses H_2O_2 and thus does not avoid exposure to a strong oxidizing agent. The enzyme simply acts to generate free, activated iodine molecules from iodide, which subsequently iodinate the protein spontaneously. Thus it does not offer a fundamentally distinct chemical iodination procedure. Although the iodination procedures described above generally result in the substitution of tyrosyl residues, it must be remembered that histidine and sulfhydryl groups can also react. In fact, sulfhydryl groups are much more reactive than phenolic groups. Lactoperoxidase does not introduce iodine into specific peptide residues since the acceptor for the iodine produced is not a substrate for the enzyme.

The biological potency of iodinated insulin derivatives can be correlated with several physicochemical criteria. Fully active iodoinsulin is precipitated more than 97% in the presence of 20% trichloroacetic acid, 97% is adsorbed to talc, and 98% is adsorbed to microfine silica QUSO G32 (Philadelphia Quartz Co.) (Yalow and Berson, 1966; Cuatrecasas, 1968a). For peptides other than insulin, it may be possible to use similar criteria to test the quality of a particular preparation.

Compounds lacking substituents capable of accepting iodine (e.g., phenolic, sulfhydryl, or imidazole groups) may be difficult to modify with ^{125}I by the procedure outlined above. This is especially true of very small peptides or nonpeptide chemical substances which are to be used as receptor ligands. However, it is feasible to synthesize appropriate biologically active analogues, e.g., peptides substituted at noncritical positions with tyrosine or histidine, which can be subsequently iodinated for binding studies.

2.2.2. Other Methods of Labeling Ligands

Other methods of preparing radioactively labeled ligands exist, although none of these achieves the very high specific activities (e.g., 2 Ci/μmol) obtained with carrier-free ^{125}I or ^{131}I. Among the more useful alternatives are tritium exchange, especially with the use of microwave discharge activation of tritium gas (Hembree et al., 1973); chemical modification of sulfhydryl groups with radioactive organomercurials or analogous metals; substitution of free amino groups with [^{3}H]acetyl moieties by using [^{3}H]acetic anhydride (available commercially at 8 Ci/mmol) (Cuatrecasas, 1969b; Cuatrecasas et al., 1971b); reaction of primary amino groups with tritiated methyl ester of acetamide to give acetamidino derivatives (Zull and Repke, 1972); oxidation (reversible) of terminal galactose residues followed by reduction with NaB^3H_4; dehalogenation of an iodinated derivative by substitution of tritium for iodine (Meunier et al., 1972) and by the specific substitution of tritiated pyridoxal groups (Cooper and Reich, 1972). In the past, the incorporation of [^{35}S]sulfate into insulin has also been used (Stadie *et al.*, 1952, 1953).

2.3. Rates of Association and Dissociation

While most measurements of ligand–receptor interactions are done under equilibrium (or steady-state) conditions, it is useful to consider the rates of association (k_1) and dissociation (k_{-1}) of ligand. Not only do such measurements provide an independent estimate of the affinity ($K_D = k_{-1}/k_1$) but the rates determined may also reveal serious limitations in the techniques whereby it is desired to measure ligand binding. For example, most measurements require efficient and complete separation of membrane-bound from free ligand. How rapidly must such separations be achieved? It has been observed for insulin (at 24°C) that $k_1 = 1.5 \times 10^7\,M^{-1}s^{-1}$ and that $k_{-1} = 7.4 \times 10^{-4}s^{-1}$. Since the half-life (at 24°C), $t_{1/2} = 0.693/k_{-1}$, can be calculated to be 16 min, a variety of methods can be used to isolate the membrane-bound insulin, especially if the procedures are performed at 4°C. However, should the affinity of a ligand for the membrane be less than that of insulin (e.g., $K_D = 10^{-9}\,M$) and the rate of association similar to that of insulin, the half-life of the receptor–ligand complex could be as short as 46 s. In practice, it is likely that both k_1 and k_{-1} will alter to yield the quotient of K_D of $10^{-9}\,M$. However, even with a ligand–receptor association limited solely by diffusion, i.e., $k_1 = 10^{10}\,M^{-1}\,s^{-1}$, it can be calculated that, given a K_D of $10^{-8}\,M$, half-life for the ligand–receptor complex would be about 7 ms. From such calculations, it is evident that in many instances it may be necessary to use very rapid techniques, e.g., centrifugation (El-Allawy and Gliemann, 1972) or filtration (Cuatrecasas, 1971a), to separate the free from the membrane-bound ligand for further analysis. Techniques employing columns or the washing of centrifugally pelleted material may not suffice. Since the rate of dissociation will in general be highly dependent on temperature, it is advisable to perform the separation procedures at 4°C.

2.4. Competitive Antagonists as Tools for Binding Studies

Because of considerations of rates and affinities of ligands as outlined above, it may be impractical if not impossible to perform binding studies with compounds which have low receptor affinities, e.g., $\leqslant 10^{-8}\,M$, or which dissociate rapidly. It is often the case, however, that well-characterized competitive antagonists of a particular ligand agonist have a greater affinity for the membrane binding site than the agonist itself. The binding of the antagonist may thus be amenable to examination, and such studies may *pari passu* yield information about the agonist and similar analogues. For example, studies of the binding of [³H]atropine (Paton and Rang, 1965) and [¹²⁵I]neurotoxins (Cooper and Reich, 1972) have yielded much information about cholinergic receptors (Hall, 1972), and competitive binding studies of opiates employing [³H]naloxone and other opiate antagonists have yielded a great deal of information about opiate receptors in the central nervous system (Snyder, Chap. 6, Vol. 5). Similarly, studies with [³H]strychnine have been useful in elucidating the distribution of glycine receptors of the central nervous system (Young and Snyder, 1973). Studies on the binding of pharmacological antagonists can thus play an important role in the detailed analysis of agonist action at the receptor site.

2.5. The Problem of Specific vs. Nonspecific Binding

In studies of the binding of ligands at very low concentrations, it is often a problem to determine the quantity of total binding which relates specifically to the biological process in question. For practical purposes, it is assumed that the amount of radioactive ligand not "displaced" (when added before or together with the tracer) from the membrane by "reasonably high" concentrations of the parent ligand is bound in a "nonspecific manner" (e.g., to glass, filters, connective tissue, or nonreceptor membrane structures, radioisotope exchange). Such "nonspecific" binding may be of very high affinity (e.g., comparable to or higher than that of the specific receptor), and it may thus constitute a substantial amount of the total binding even when very low concentrations of the ligand are used. Nonspecific binding, however, will nearly always exhibit such a high capacity that it is difficult if not impossible to demonstrate saturation of the binding. For this reason, reasonably low concentrations of the unlabeled compound will not cause displacement of binding. The criteria outlined above are therefore usually sufficient to determine the proportion of binding which is "specific." For example, the "reasonable" concentration of unlabeled insulin (approximately 10^{-7} M) used to displace [¹²⁵I]insulin and to determine the nonspecific binding is chosen with the knowledge that this concentration of insulin is several orders of magnitude above that at which insulin ceases to have a biological effect in fat cells and above that concentration which obtains in serum.

It is important, however, to determine experimentally for each system that the concentrations being used are indeed below those which may cause saturation of nonspecific adsorption. Since the latter can be considered to exhibit an "infinite" number of binding sites only within reasonable limits, the possibility always exists that extremely small quantities of materials may be present which possess special nonspecific adsorptive properties for the ligand. For example, it should be noted that in certain experiments

(Cuatrecasas and Hollenberg, 1975) apparently specific (high-affinity, saturable, and displaceable) binding of insulin has been detected in the absence of any cellular material. This binding is possibly due to a small amount of an unknown substance (silica dust?) eluted from a particular batch of glass—but not plastic tubes. In other experiments, stereospecific displacement of [³H]naloxone from glass filters has been observed (Snyder, 1973) in the absence of cellular constituents. Thus even when the criteria of saturability and stereospecificity of binding are satisfied, caution should be exercised in interpreting binding data.

2.6. Methods of Obtaining Binding Data

One of the simplest techniques of measuring ligand binding to an insoluble matrix (whole cell or membrane) employs centrifugation as a means of separating bound from free ligand. The operation is performed at 4°C, the pellet obtained from a cell or membrane suspension is rapidly washed, and the bound radioactivity is measured. Because of the problem of the rate of dissociation outlined above, it may be impractical to employ this technique in its simplest form because of the relatively long periods of time involved in the washing step.

With the use of suitable water-immiscible oils (Gliemann *et al.*, 1972; Livingston *et al.*, 1974; Chang and Cuatrecasas, 1974) of the desired density (e.g., mixtures of dinonyl- and dibutylphthalate), it is possible to separate, efficiently and free from contaminating aqueous medium, membrane or cell components which either float (e.g., fat cells) or sink (e.g., liver membranes) in the aqueous phase under the influence of a centrifugal field. With small, high-velocity centrifuges (e.g., Beckman 152 microfuge), the separation of free from bound ligand by this oil flotation technique is achieved extremely rapidly, permitting measurements of systems with $t_{1/2}$ of dissociation the order of 60 s.

Filtration on microporous glass or synthetic polymer filters provides a second method whereby membrane-bound ligand is separated from free ligand in the suspension. In practice, the filter is usually immobilized in a multiple manifold apparatus and the suspension filtered under reduced pressure. The collected material is rapidly (less than 10–15 s) washed with an aliquot of ligand-free buffer, and the radioactivity trapped on the filter is measured. The proper design of this filtration machine is quite important, since the fitting around the periphery of the filter must be tight and free of dead space which can act to trap the radioactive medium. For such studies, it is often a problem to select a filter which itself does not interfere with binding measurements. For example, glass filters are a particularly poor choice for studies on peptide binding, since peptides at low concentrations bind avidly to glass. For this reason, filters composed of cellulose acetate are most often used. Studies on the binding of concanavalin A require the use of teflon filters to reduce the "background" binding to an acceptable level (Cuatrecasas, 1973h). Since, in general, adsorption is related to the available surface area of the filter, it is preferable to use filters of the largest acceptable pore size, so as to minimize the effective filter surface area. For the unwary, artifacts of "filter binding" can seriously compromise studies of ligand–membrane affinities.

Although not widely used, it is possible with particulate preparations to employ the method of Hummel and Dreyer (1962), originally developed for soluble enzymes, so as to obtain equilibrium estimates of ligand–membrane affinities (Cuatrecasas et al., 1967). Other column techniques designed to separate free from bound ligand may not achieve separation rapidly enough to obtain meaningful data. In all column methods, care must be given to prevent the trapping or adsorption of the membrane particles on the gel bed.

2.7. Measurements on Solubilized Receptors

Receptors for a number of hormones such as insulin (Cuatrecasas, 1972b), glucagon (Giorgio et al., 1974), and acetylcholine (Changeux et al., 1970, 1971; Meunier et al., 1972) can be obtained in soluble form from appropriate tissues with the use of nonionic detergents. In the presence of modest amounts (0.2% w/v) of the detergent Triton X100, the receptor for insulin retains its peptide affinity and behaves as a large protein with a molecular weight of approximately 300,000, a frictional ratio of 1.5, and an axial ratio (prolate ellipsoid) of about 9 (Cuatrecasas, 1972a). It is remarkable that the receptor specificity and affinity for insulin are unaltered in the presence of detergent, and it is of utmost importance that the receptor properties can be compared directly with observations in the whole cell (fat cell) or intact membrane preparations (liver). Similar results have been obtained with detergent-solubilized acetylcholine receptors from electric tissues of fish (Changeux et al., 1970; Miledi et al., 1971; Eldefrawi and O'Brien, 1971; Raftery et al., 1972). Since the data for the solubilized insulin receptor do agree well with data obtained in intact systems, it becomes possible to compare the physicochemical properties of the receptor solubilized both from different tissues and from different species. It is essential that studies on solubilized membrane receptors be compared directly with parallel measurements on an intact system, for only by such comparisons can one have confidence that the measurement on the soluble receptor truly reflects the properties of the physiologically active ligand–receptor combination.

The techniques used to measure ligand binding in soluble receptor systems differ somewhat from the methods used for particulate systems. A convenient and frequently used method employs polyethylene glycol to precipitate the soluble ligand–receptor complex from solution, leaving the free ligand in the supernatant (Desbuquois and Aurbach, 1971; Cuatrecasas, 1972d). The precipitate is rapidly collected and washed on an appropriate filter, e.g., cellulose acetate, millipore (EHWP or EAWP), and the amount of bound radioactively labeled ligand is determined. It is of interest that the identical technique proves extremely useful for particulate membrane preparations which cannot be efficiently trapped by small-pore membrane filters. The addition of polyethylene glycol agglutinates the particulate membrane, permitting the use of relatively large-pore filters for efficient collection and washing of the filtrate. The column technique of Hummel and Dreyer (1962), described earlier, has been used to study solubilized glucagon receptors (Giorgio et al., 1974).

2.8. Membrane Receptors and Proteolytic Agents

While many studies on ligand–membrane interactions focus attention on the stability of the ligand in the presence of membranes, it is often overlooked that the membrane receptor itself can be exquisitely sensitive to proteolytic agents. The specific insulin binding of isolated fat cells is reduced more than 70% by trypsin at concentrations as low as 10 μg/ml acting at 37°C for 15 min in the presence of 1% bovine albumin (Cuatrecasas, 1971b). It is pertinent that low amounts of trypsin (10 μg/ml) do not abolish the action of insulin. Rather, the apparent K_D of both the measured membrane affinity and the biological activity of insulin is raised from about 10^{-10} M to approximately 10^{-9} M. Higher concentrations of trypsin lower the receptor affinity further and reduce the insulin-mediated response (conversion of [U^{14}C]glucose to ^{14}CO$_2$). Other membrane receptors (e.g., for glucagon, opiates, and epidermal growth factor) are also sensitive to proteolytic agents. It may be impossible to completely prevent the exposure of membrane preparations to tissue cathepsins. However, when the measured affinity or activity of a particular ligand in a membrane or whole cell preparation does not agree with other data derived from in vivo measurements or from serum levels, the problem of receptor degradation in the in vitro system should be explored.

2.9. Comparative Studies of Ligand–Membrane Interactions

Once an interaction between a particular ligand and a membrane receptor has been characterized, it is often of interest to compare such interaction either for different tissues in the same animal or for the same tissue in different species. It also may be of interest to map receptor distribution, as has been done for opiate receptors in the brain (Kuhar *et al.*, 1973). Qualitative differences between tissues, e.g., presence or absence of a specific membrane–ligand interaction, are relatively easy to determine. However, quantitative comparisons may prove difficult because of lack of an appropriate denominator to serve as reference for the amount of receptor present. A meaningful and direct comparison is possible between whole cells of a clearly defined and homogeneous type, e.g., dissociated fat cells. It has, for instance, been possible to demonstrate equivalent numbers of insulin receptors in large and small fat cells derived from obese and "normal" rats, respectively; despite equivalent numbers of insulin-binding sites, the large fat cells are resistant to the biological action of insulin (Bennett and Cuatrecasas, 1972). With other cells, e.g., lymphocytes, or with membrane preparations derived from a heterogeneous tissue such as liver, animal-to-animal comparisons are not clear-cut. For example, it is known that the lymphocyte population is heterogeneous, comprised of two major classes of cells (thymus derived vs. bone marrow derived). Further, the proportions of such cells present in the peripheral circulation can vary. Thus, even if a relatively homogeneous population of lymphocytes is obtained with respect to morphology, it is difficult, because of their functional heterogeneity, to quantitatively compare receptors on lymphocytes obtained either at different times from the same animal or at the same time from different animals. Clearly, refined techniques are necessary to define the exact nature of the cell studied so as to permit a quantitative comparison.

A quantitative comparison of receptors in different membrane preparations presents other difficulties. Simply applying the same differential or gradient centrifugation technique to a particular tissue does not ensure recovery of the same membrane fraction, e.g., from fatty vs. normal liver. It is pertinent, however, that techniques are available to isolate specifically the plasma membrane fraction by prelabeling intact cells with essentially irreversibly bound membrane markers before disruptive procedures are employed (Chang *et al.*, 1975). Once the plasma membrane fraction is isolated, quantitative comparison of the numbers of receptors per milligram of membrane may be possible. The detailed comparison of membrane receptors derived from different areas of the central nervous system may require the use of similar specialized techniques for characterization of the membrane preparation before the ligand–receptor interaction is determined.

2.10. Other Methods for the Study of Ligand–Receptor Interactions

This chapter deals mainly with techniques for the use of soluble, highly radioactive ligands to characterize ligand–receptor interactions. Other methods of study which have met with limited success will be dealt with only briefly. It is, for example, possible to use spectroscopic techniques to detect changes in the state of the membrane. Growth hormone, at extremely low concentrations (10^{-15} M), perturbs the fluorescence polarization of human erythrocyte membrane preparations (Sonenberg, 1971). However, it is difficult with this technique to obtain exact quantitative data for the rate and affinity of this hormone–membrane interaction. Alternatively, autoradiographic techniques can localize the site of interaction, as has been observed for [^{125}I]α-bungarotoxin in rat diaphragm (Barnard et al., 1971), in muscle (Porter et al., 1973), or in cultured muscle cells (Cohen and Fishbach, 1973; Giacobini et al., 1973; Sytkowski et al., 1973). With this method, it is difficult to determine either the extent of "nonspecific" binding of the ligand or the affinities and rate constants of binding. Immunofluorescence techniques may also be of use for the study of membrane–ligand interactions. However, the scarcity of receptors (fewer than 10^5 per cell) for homones and other active compounds outlined earlier renders the immunofluorescence techniques of limited value. Nonetheless, with specialized immunological techniques it is possible to detect about 10^5 antibody combining sites on the surface of lymphocytes, and further refinements of such methods might permit the detection of as few as 10^4 sites per cell.

For each of the techniques outlined above, it should be possible to satisfy, at least in part, most of the criteria outlined earlier regarding the structural and steric specificity of the ligand–membrane interaction, the saturability of binding, and the correlation of binding with the biological activity of the ligand and its analogues in membranes from sensitive tissues.

2.11. Mathematical Analysis of Binding Data

Binding data are often interpreted either according to the method of Scatchard (1949) or using double-reciprocal plots to estimate the affinities and numbers of receptors of a given class. It should be pointed out that analysis by these methods was originally developed for systems where soluble ligands interact with one or more independent binding sites on a soluble macromolecule. It may be naive to assume that such a mathematical model will hold for the case of particulate membrane receptors with extremely high affinity. In some cases, as much as 30–40% of a ligand, e.g., [^{125}I]cholera toxin (Cuatrecasas, 1973c,d,e,f), can be bound at concentrations well below the apparent K_D for this compound. Under such conditions, the frequently employed mathematical analysis does not apply (Henderson, 1973). The difficulty in applying Scatchard plots in systems of very high affinity can be illustrated by the fact that in such systems the binding is directly proportional to the concentration of ligand over the low range of concentration provided that the receptor (or second binding component) is in large excess relative to the number of complexes formed. This is usually the case in studies of ligand–membrane receptor interactions. Such data give a horizontal line (parallel to the y axis) on a Scatchard plot, which by definition implies an infinite number of binding sites. Furthermore, since, as the concentration of ligand is increased, the direct proportionality will no longer hold, curvatures (downward) will be obtained which indicate that the affinity estimated from the original horizontal line is grossly underestimated. In addition, since in almost all instances some nonspecific binding sites exist which have not been completely excluded experimentally, the data will almost always contain other curvatures at the highest concentrations of ligand; these may be mistakenly interpreted as indicating "another" binding site of low affinity and high capacity. It is perhaps preferable to use analysis based on a Langmuir-type isotherm such as has been used for the binding of [^{3}H]atropine to guinea pig ileum (Paton and Rang, 1965). In cases where a single saturable binding site is observed, a simple binding isotherm (e.g., Fig. 1) may be sufficient to estimate the maximum possible binding so as to calculate the number of binding sites per cell or per milligram of protein.

3. EXAMPLES OF STUDIES ON HORMONE–MEMBRANE RECEPTOR INTERACTIONS

3.1. Insulin–Receptor Interaction in Fat and Liver Cells

The measurements of the binding and biological activity of [^{125}I]insulin in the fat cell provide an example of a 1:1 correspondence between the physicochemical measurements and the biological response (Cuatrecasas, 1971a). The biological activity of [^{125}I]insulin containing less than one atom of iodine per insulin molecule (Fig. 1, lower) is indistinguishable from the action of native insulin in enhancing the conversion of [U-^{14}C]glucose to $^{14}CO_2$ (Garrat, 1964; Izzo et al., 1964; Massaglia et al., 1969; Cuatrecasas, 1971a). The concomitant specific binding of [^{125}I]insulin to the fat cells is a saturable process with respect to insulin concentration within the physiological range of hormone concentration (Fig. 1, upper), and there is an excellent correlation between the binding curve and the dose–response curve for glucose oxidation (Fig. 1, lower). [^{125}I]Insulin bound in small amounts in fat cells is displaced by increasing amounts of native insulin in a manner predicted by the near identity of these two molecules (Fig. 2). The plateau of the displacement curve (80–150 μunits/ml) agrees well with the corresponding plateau of the binding curve (Fig. 1, upper). It is of interest that very high concentrations of native insulin will displace further substantial amounts of [^{125}I]insulin, perhaps suggesting the presence on the fat cell of a second "non-specific" binding site for insulin which is unrelated to the known

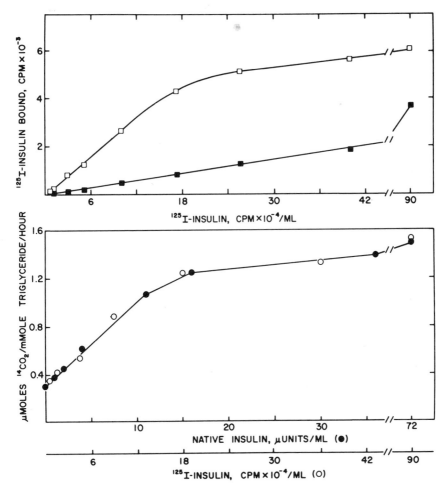

FIG. 1. Ability of native (●) and [^{125}I]insulin (○) to enhance the rate of glucose oxidation by isolated fat cells (lower), correlated with the specific binding of [^{125}I]insulin (□) to fat cells (upper). For each concentration of [^{125}I]insulin studied, control incubations were done in the presence of a displacing amount of native insulin. The nonspecific binding, not represented in the curve for specific binding, is plotted in the upper graph (■). From Cuatrecasas (1971a).

actions of insulin on this cell. Unrelated peptides and biologically inactive derivatives do not displace [^{125}I]insulin even at high concentration (Table 1). However, proinsulin, desoctapeptide insulin, and des-ala-insulin, all of which possess biological activity, are observed to displace insulin, approximately in step with their measured biological potencies (Cuatrecasas *et al.*, 1971a, Cuatrecasas 1972c; Freychet *et al.*, 1971a,b, 1972). The rate data of binding and dissociation of insulin (Fig. 3, top and bottom) indicate that the

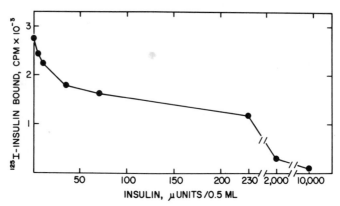

FIG. 2. Displacement by native insulin of [^{125}I]insulin bound to isolated fat cells. Fat cells were incubated at 24°C for 30 min with 1.9×10^{-11} M [^{125}I]insulin and increasing amounts of native insulin. From Cuatrecasas (1971a).

TABLE 1

Displacement of [^{125}I]Insulin Binding by Peptide Hormones[a]

Tissue	Peptide	Concentration (μg/ml)	Specific binding [^{125}I]insulin ($10^6 \times$ nmol)
Fat cells	None		2.4
	Insulin	0.002	1.4
	Insulin	0.012	0.7
	Adrenocorticotropin	40	2.4
	Growth hormone	40	2.4
	Prolactin	40	2.5
	Vasopressin	40	2.4
	Oxytocin	40	2.4
	Glucagon	40	2.5
	Carboxymethyl chains of insulin	0.2	2.3
	Oxidized chains of insulin	0.2	2.2
	Reduced insulin[b]	0.3	2.2
Liver membranes	None		4.2
	Insulin	0.002	3.0
	Insulin	0.008	2.1
	Insulin	0.4	0.1
	Proinsulin	0.2	3.4
	Proinsulin	10	0.9
	Desoctapeptide insulin	5	4.0
	Glucagon	50	4.3
	Growth hormone	50	4.2

[a]The ability of each peptide to affect the specific binding of [^{125}I]insulin (2.8×10^{-11} M for fat cells, 2×10^5 cells in 0.5 ml; 1.7×10^{-11} M for liver membranes, 71 μg protein in 0.2 ml) was determined at 24°C by filtration methods. Data for fat cells from Cuatrecasas (1972c); data for liver membrane from Cuatrecasas et al. (1971a).
[b]Treated for 90 min at 24°C with 20 mM dithiothreitol in 0.1 M NaCHO$_3$ buffer, pH 8.1.

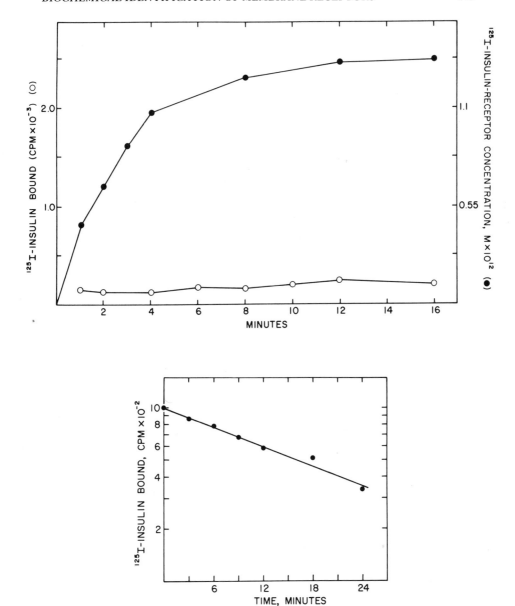

FIG. 3. Top: Rate of binding of [^{125}I]insulin to isolated fat cells at 24°C. Fat cells were incubated with 6.8×10^{-11} M [^{125}I]insulin in the presence (○) and absence (●) of native insulin. The left ordinate describes the uptake of radioactivity, the right ordinate the corresponding concentration of the complex used to calculate the kinetic constants. Bottom: Semilog plot of the dissociation of [^{125}I]insulin bound to fat cells as a function of time at 24°C. Fat cells were equilibrated at 24°C with [^{125}I]insulin (4.6×10^{-11} M), collected, and washed at 4°C on millipore filters, and the dissociation at 24°C of the bound insulin was then measured. From Cuatrecasas (1971a).

TABLE 2

Equilibrium and Kinetic Constants for the Specific Interaction of Insulin with Fat Cell Membranes, Liver Cell Membranes and Isolated Fat Cells

	Membranes		
Constant	Fat[a]	Liver[b]	Fat cells[c]
Association rate (k_1, mol^{-1} s^{-1})	8.5×10^6	3.5×10^6	1.5×10^7
Dissociation rate (k_{-1}, s^{-1})	4.2×10^{-4}	2.7×10^{-4}	7.4×10^{-4}
Dissociation constant			
From k_{-1}/k_1	$5 \ \times 10^{-11}$ M	7.7×10^{-11} M	$5 \ \times 10^{-11}$ M
From equilibrium data	7.5×10^{-11} M	6.7×10^{-11} M	$8 \ \times 10^{-11}$ M

[a]From Cuatrecasas (1971c).
[b]From Cuatrecasas *et al.* (1971a).
[c]From Cuatrecasas (1971a).

hormone–receptor interaction is freely reversible. Both from the binding curve (Fig. 1, upper) and from the rate data (Fig. 3), a dissociation constant of approximately 10^{-10} M can be calculated (Table 2).

The nonspecific binding of insulin is not saturable (Fig. 1, upper). It also differs markedly from the specific binding in that the rate of nonspecific binding is extremely rapid (equilibrium obtained in less than 1 min), and the rate is not appreciably temperature dependent. In contrast, the rate of dissociation of specific binding is decreased at least tenfold by lowering the temperature from 24 to 4°C.

The dissociable nature of the insulin–receptor interaction has been confirmed, and the insulin which dissociates (spontaneously or with acid) is chemically and biologically intact (Cuatrecasas, 1971a, Cuatrecasas *et al.*, 1971a). Binding *per se* thus does not cause degradation of the hormone.

It is possible to obtain similar data for the binding of insulin in liver membrane preparations (Fig. 4). It has also been possible to solubilize the insulin receptor from rat liver membranes, to purify it by affinity chromatography techniques (Cuatrecasas, 1972a,b), and to demonstrate that the purified receptor complex retains insulin-binding properties which are similar, if not identical, to those observed in the intact fat cell. From the studies on insulin binding, it is seen that the hormone–receptor interaction is a highly specific, temperature-sensitive, dissociable process endowed with high affinity.

3.2. Insulin Receptors in Human Lymphocytes and Fibroblasts

It has been observed that human peripheral white blood cells possess specific binding sites for insulin (Gavin *et al.*, 1972, 1973; Krug *et al.*, 1972).

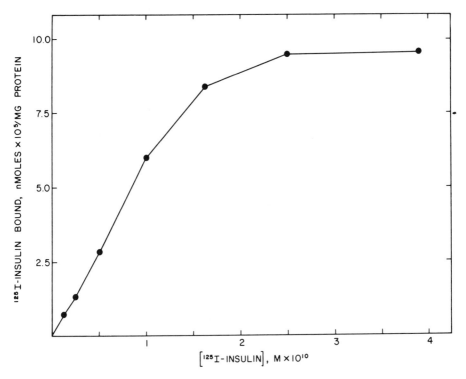

FIG. 4. Binding of [^{125}I]insulin to rat liver membranes. Membranes (50 µg of protein) were incubated with increasing amounts of [^{125}I]insulin, and binding was measured by filtration methods. Values are corrected for nonspecific adsorption of insulin. From Cuatrecasas *et al.* (1971*a*).

However, the studies of Krug *et al.* (1972) reveal that whereas some leukocytes (e.g., macrophages) can bind considerable amounts of insulin, nylon column–purified lymphocytes free from macrophages, polymorphs, and platelets possess less than one insulin-binding site per cell, whether binding is measured in whole cells, broken cell preparation, detergent-solubilized membrane preparation, or phospholipase C–treated cells. The last treatment is observed to unmask insulin receptors in fat cells, liver cell membranes, permanent cell line lymphocytes (RPMI 6237), and lectin-stimulated lymphocytes (Cuatrecasas, 1971*b*; Krug *et al.*, 1972; Krug and Cuatrecasas, 1973).

When nylon column–purified lymphocytes are stimulated with a phytomitogen such as concanavalin A (Con A), there is a dramatic appearance of insulin binding sites in step with the onset of DNA synthesis (Figs. 5 and 6). Cell division *per se* is not a prerequisite for the appearance of the insulin binding sites since cytochalasin B–treated cells, when stimulated with Con A, possess increased numbers of receptors in proportion to their

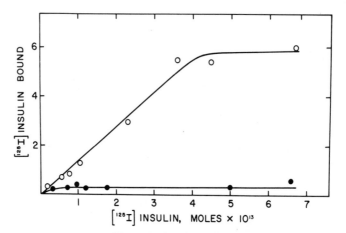

FIG. 5. Binding of [^{125}I]insulin to lectin-transformed (○) and un-transformed (●) lymphocytes as a function of [^{125}I]insulin concentration. Binding, in $10^{16} \times$ mol per 10^6 cells, is corrected for nonspecific adsorption of insulin. Measurements were made on aliquots of cells (3–4 × 10^6) in 0.2 ml of Hanks buffer at 24°C. From Krug *et al.* (1972).

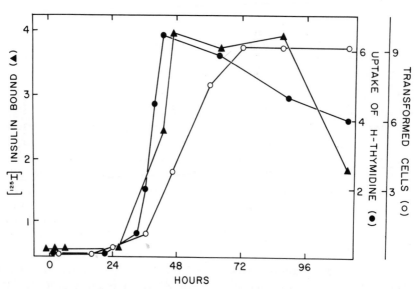

FIG. 6. Binding of insulin to lymphocytes during transformation. Measurements were made at intervals after the addition of concanavalin A to the culture medium. Specific binding of [^{125}I]insulin ($10^{16} \times$ mol) (▲), incorporation of [^{3}H]thymidine into DNA (●), and the number of morphologically transformed cells (×10^{-5}) (○) are expressed per 10^6 cells. From Krug *et al.* (1972).

increased surface area compared with untreated Con A–stimulated cells. It is presumed either that the emergent insulin binding sites are synthesized *de novo* or that before transformation they are present in a cryptic form not detectable by present techniques.

The emergence of the insulin binding sites is not dependent on the nature of the mitogenic stimulus; either phytohemagglutinin or periodate induces the appearance of insulin binding sites in step with cell transformation (Hollenberg and Cuatrecasas, 1974*a*) (Fig. 7). Insulin binding sites are not the only "new" binding sites to appear during the process of mitogenesis. Specific binding sites for nerve growth factor (Banerjee *et al.*, 1973*a*; Hollenberg and Cuatrecasas, 1974*a*) and for growth hormone (Bockman and Sonenberg, 1973) can also be detected on lectin-transformed lymphocytes. However, no binding sites either for glucagon or for epidermal growth factor can be detected in either transformed or untransformed lymphocytes (Hollenberg *et al.*, 1973). Data from studies (Krug *et al.*, 1973) of the binding of Con A and wheat germ agglutinin (WGA) to lymphocytes indicate that during transformation there is a disproportionate change in the density of binding sites for these two lectins (Fig. 8). As the cells enlarge with transformation, the number of Con A binding sites increases, leaving the density of such sites unchanged. The number of sites for WGA is unchanged, and the density of such sites must therefore fall as the cell

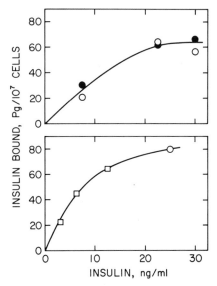

FIG. 7. Insulin binding by transformed human peripheral lymphocytes. Above: Cells transformed by Con A (○) and by PHA (●). Below: Cells transformed by periodate (□) and by Con A (○). Data from Hollenberg and Cuatrecasas (1974*a*).

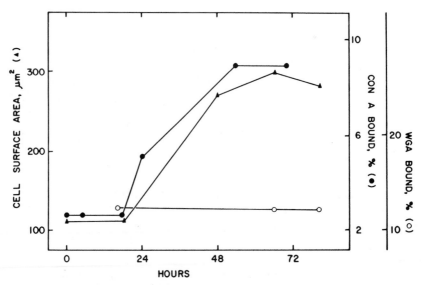

FIG. 8. Binding of Con A and WGA during *in vitro* transformation by Con A. The proportion of lectin added to the medium (0–1 μg/ml) which is specifically bound is described. The mean cell surface area was calculated from microscopic measurement of the average cell diameter. From Krug *et al.* (1973).

enlarges. Thus during transformation there may be a coordinated appearance of a number of specific ligand receptors. In this respect, it may be of considerable importance that acute lymphocytic lymphoblasts possess insulin binding sites equivalent in number to those found in normal cells transformed *in vitro* with Con A (Krug *et al.*, 1972) (Table 3). In contrast, insulin receptors are not detected in human chronic lymphocytic leukemia cells (Krug and Cuatrecasas, 1973). It is unknown whether T-cells, B-cells, or

TABLE 3

Density of Insulin Binding Sites on the Cell Surface

	Mean cell surface area (μm^2)	Insulin binding sites	
		Per cell	Per μm^2
Untransformed lymphocytes	130	<6	<0.05
Transformed lymphocytes (and leukemic lymphoblasts)	1400	350	0.3
Polynucleated, transformed lymphocytes (cytochalasin B)	12700	3500	0.3
Isolated fat cells, rat	5000	11000	2.2

Data from Cuatrecasas (1971a) and Krug *et al.* (1972).

perhaps both have the capacity when stimulated to develop insulin binding sites.

As yet, it has not been possible to demonstrate reproducibly biological responses to physiological concentrations of insulin with either the lectin-transformed cells or the RPMI 6237 permanent cell line lymphocytes (glucose transport, enhanced conversion of [U-^{14}C]glucose to CO_2, protein and glycogen synthesis, RNA or DNA synthesis) (Krug and Cuatrecasas, 1973). Effects of insulin on α-aminoisobutyric acid transport in suckling rat thymocytes have been observed (Goldfine et al., 1972). However, insulin is active in these cells only at concentrations from 1 to 4 orders of magnitude above those found in serum (approximately 10^{-10} M). Thus no physiological function can yet be ascribed to the emergent hormone receptors. It has been suggested (Hollenberg and Cuatrecasas, 1974a) that the emergent receptors may be required either for completion of the transformation process itself or for some new function of the activated lymphocyte.

It is possible to measure simultaneously the biological activity and the binding of insulin in explanted human fibroblast monolayers (Hollenberg and Cuatrecasas, 1975b). While it has been known for some time that insulin can act as a serum substitute to support the growth of cells in culture (Gey and Thalhimer, 1924; Temin et al., 1972), it is recognized that insulin does so only at concentrations far above those which occur in vivo. Insulin at low concentrations is indeed a poor mitogen for human fibroblasts (Fig. 9).

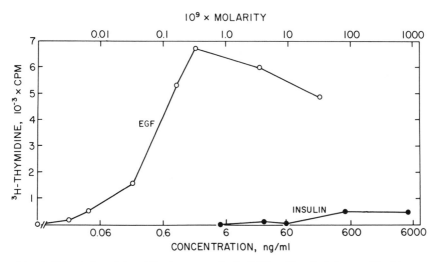

FIG. 9. Stimulation of thymidine incorporation by EGF and insulin in human fibroblasts. Confluent cells were refed with serum-free growth medium containing 0.1% (w/v) bovine albumin and either EGF or insulin. [^{3}H]Thymidine incorporation, measured at 23 h, is expressed as cpm/100 μg protein and is corrected for the amount incorporated in the absence of stimulant (390 ± 100 cpm for insulin; 900 ± 180 cpm for EGF). From Hollenberg and Cuatrecasas (1973a).

However, if cells are first "primed" with a fibroblast mitogen such as epidermal growth factor (EGF), at a dose insufficient to cause significant DNA synthesis, insulin becomes effective at low concentrations in stimulating appreciable DNA synthesis (Fig. 10). The binding of [^{125}I]insulin to the same fibroblasts is saturable and appears to correspond to the pharmacological action of insulin in stimulating DNA synthesis in these cells (Fig. 10).

It is pertinent that the affinity of insulin for receptors on fibroblasts and on lectin-stimulated lymphocytes differs significantly from that measured in the fat and liver cell: the K_D is approximately 10^{-9} M in lymphocytes and fibroblasts vs. 10^{-10} M in fat and liver cells. What can be the significance of receptor sites which at physiological concentrations of insulin ($\leqslant 150$ μ units/ml) would be virtually inoperative? It is possible that the fibroblast and lymphocyte binding sites interact with a noninsulin impurity present in small amounts even in the best available preparation. For example, contamination of 1% by an unrelated peptide having an actual $K_D \simeq 10^{-11}$ M could account for such a result. Nonetheless, experiments with highly purified

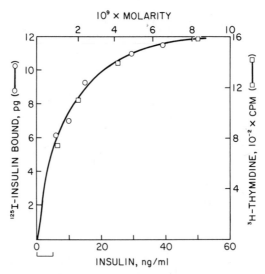

Fig. 10. Insulin-mediated thymidine incorporation and insulin binding in human fibroblasts. Stimulation of [^{3}H]thymidine incorporation was measured 23 h after the addition of insulin to cells which had attained confluency in a growth medium of 5% fetal calf serum in minimal essential medium. EGF (50 pg/ml), present as a "primer," did not stimulate thymidine incorporation significantly above the baseline value (2500 cpm). Incorporation, corrected for the baseline, is in cpm/100 μg protein ($\square$). The binding of [^{125}I]insulin corrected for nonspecific adsorption, was measured in intact monolayers and is in pg bound per monolayer (approximately 3×10^5 cells) ($\bigcirc$). The horizontal bar indicates the physiological range of insulin concentrations. From Hollenberg and Cuatrecasas (1975b).

"single-component" insulin indicate a dose–response curve in fibroblasts identical to that obtained with other preparations. Alternatively, it is possible that insulin receptors exist in these cells in a very large excess of those required for biological activation, such that maximal effects would occur with occupancy of only a small portion of receptors. It should be noted that receptor studies performed in recent years indicate that one should rigorously question previous data suggesting that some systems have a large portion of "spare" receptors (Cuatrecasas, 1974). It is perhaps more likely that the lymphocyte and fibroblast binding sites do indeed interact specifically with insulin, but that the receptors are intended for another as yet unidentified peptide.

Other peptides (somatomedin, multiplication stimulating activity, Con A, and WGA) are thought to interact with insulin receptor structures (Hintz et al., 1972; Pierson and Temin, 1972; Dulak and Temin, 1973a,b; Cuatrecasas and Tell, 1973). Is it not also possible that insulin will be found to cross-react with the physiological receptors for other, perhaps similar or related anabolic peptides? For instance, it is known that oxytocin can at high concentrations elicit an antidiuretic response, presumably interacting with vasopressin receptors; the action of vasopressin on the uterus at pharmacological concentrations is also well documented. Other examples of cross-reactivity of peptides at receptor sites are becoming apparent. Vasoactive intestinal polypeptide (VIP) and secretin can interact at a common receptor site in liver membranes (Desbuquois et al., 1973; Desbuquois, 1974). This is an especially instructive example since the binding sites which were originally discovered using ^{125}I-labeled secretin were assumed to be specific receptors for this hormone despite a relatively low apparent affinity for secretin. Actually, liver membrane receptors demonstrate a much greater affinity for VIP and are therefore likely to be the true receptors for this hormone. Human growth hormone and prolactin are thought to compete for receptor sites in pregnant rabbit breast and liver tissue (Shiu et al., 1973; Tsushima and Friesen, 1973). The meticulous analysis of the interaction of membrane binding sites with peptide hormones of known structure may thus unexpectedly yield evidence for the existence of other as yet unidentified but physiologically important hormones and receptors.

3.3. Insulin-like Activity and Binding of Plant Lectins

The plant lectins Con A and wheat germ agglutinin (WGA) exhibit insulin-like activity in both liver and fat cells (Cuatrecasas and Tell, 1973) (Figs. 11 and 12). In the fat cell, these lectins both enhance the production of $^{14}CO_2$ from [U-^{14}C]glucose and inhibit epinephrine-stimulated lipolysis (Fig.

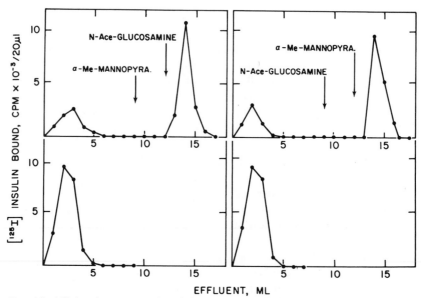

FIG. 11. Affinity chromatography of detergent-solubilized insulin receptor from rat
liver membranes on columns containing wheat germ agglutinin–agarose (left) and
concanavalin A–agarose (right). After application of the sample, columns were eluted
with buffers containing either 0.3 M α-methyl-D-mannopyranside or 0.3 M N-acetyl-D-
glucosamine. In control columns (lower graphs), the lectin-specific sugar was added to
the crude sample before chromatography. Data from Cuatrecasas and Tell (1973).

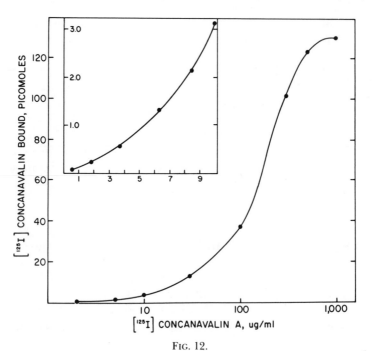

FIG. 12.

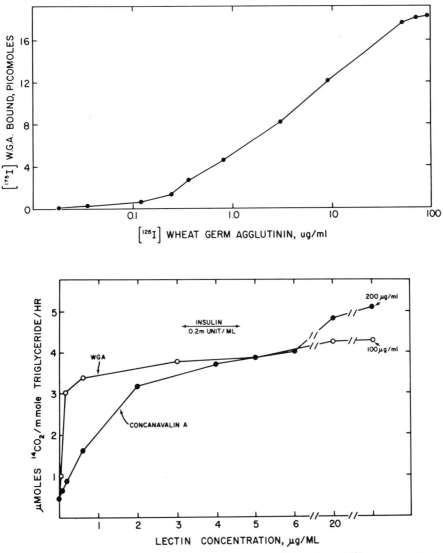

FIG. 12. Lectin binding and action in isolated fat cells. Specific binding of [^{125}I]concanavalin A (at left) and [^{125}I]wheat germ agglutinin (top) was determined at 24°C in isolated rat fat cell suspensions (2.2×10^5 cells in 0.2 ml for Con A; 3.4×10^4 in 0.2 ml for WGA). The effect of Con A and WGA on the conversion of [^{14}C]glucose to $^{14}CO_2$ by isolated rat fat cells (bottom) was measured at 37°C for 2 h. The horizontal arrow indicates the maximum response to insulin (200 μunits/ml). From Cuatrecasas (1973*h*) and Cuatrecasas and Tell (1973).

12 and Table 4). In liver cell membranes, these lectins inhibit both baseline and epinephrine-stimulated adenylate cyclase activity. These lectins can directly inhibit the binding of [^{125}I]insulin to membrane-bound or detergent-solubilized receptors (Table 5). Furthermore, lectin–agarose columns can be

TABLE 4

Suppression by Wheat Germ Agglutinin and Concanavalin A of Epinephrine-Stimulated Lipolysis in Fat Cells[a]

Additions	Glycerol released[b]
None	6.8 ± 0.5
Epinephrine, 0.16 μg/ml	24.0 ± 1.1
Epinephrine, 0.16 μg/ml +	
Wheat germ agglutinin, 0.11 μg/ml	20.5 ± 0.8
Wheat germ agglutinin, 0.33 μg/ml	14.0 ± 0.6
Wheat germ agglutinin, 1.0 μg/ml	10.3 ± 0.7
Wheat germ agglutinin, 5.0 μg/ml	6.4 ± 0.5
Concanavalin A, 2 μg/ml	25.7 ± 1.4
Concanavalin A, 6 μg/ml	20.1 ± 0.8
Concanavalin A, 30 μg/ml	10.9 ± 0.7
Concanavalin A, 100 μg/ml	8.8 ± 0.9
Insulin, 20 μunits/ml	6.3 ± 0.5
Insulin, 5 μunits/ml	12.9 ± 0.6

[a]Fat cells (3×10^4 cells/ml) were incubated for 2 h at 37°C in Krebs–Ringer bicarbonate buffer containing 3% (w/v) albumin. Data from Cuatrecasas and Tell (1973).
[b]Micromoles of glycerol released per millimole of triglyceride; average value ±SEM of three replications.

used to isolate solubilized insulin receptor structures by affinity chromatography (Cuatrecasas and Tell, 1973) (Fig. 11).

It is of interest to compare the binding of WGA and Con A to fat cells (Cuatrecasas, 1973b) with the biological dose–response curve (Fig. 12). It is evident that for both lectins saturation of binding is achieved only at very high concentrations relative to those which elicit a maximum biological response. It is difficult to discern even at low lectin concentrations a discrete binding site responsible for the insulin-like effect on the cell. Clearly, the membrane binding sites for these lectins in the fat cell are heterogeneous, as they are in the human lymphocyte (Krug et al., 1973). The binding of lectins to the much larger number of membrane sites unrelated to insulin-like activity (10^6–10^7 for the former; 10^4 for the latter) by far overshadows the binding to the "receptor" structures. While the lectins may represent an extreme case of binding to physiologically nonspecific membrane sites, it is possible that similar difficulties may be encountered in studies of hormone binding where the presence in disparate quantities of two or more sites (e.g., one related to hormone action, the other to degradation) with different affinities may make interpretation of binding data difficult if not impossible.

TABLE 5

Effect of Wheat Germ Agglutinin and Concanavalin A on the Specific Binding of Insulin to Isolated Fat Cells and Liver Membranes[a]

	Specific [^{125}I]insulin bound[b]	
Addition	Fat cells	Liver membranes
None	$6,500 \pm 300$	$16,200 \pm 900$
Wheat germ agglutinin		
1 μg/ml	$16,100 \pm 650$	
4 μg/ml		$30,700 \pm 1050$
16 μg/ml	$3,100 \pm 270$	
40 μg/ml		$19,300 \pm 700$
Concanavalin A		
5 μg/ml	$2,900 \pm 210$	
40 μg/ml	$1,200 \pm 80$	$13,100 \pm 400$
500 μg/ml		$5,700 \pm 200$

[a]Fat cell (10^6 cells/ml) and liver membrane (0.6 mg protein/ml) suspensions (0.2 ml) were incubated in Krebs–Ringer bicarbonate–0.1% *w/v* albumin for 60 min at 24°C with the plant lectins. [^{125}I]Insulin (1.8×10^5 cpm for fat cells and 1.2×10^5 cpm for membranes) was added to each sample, and the specific binding of insulin was determined after incubation for 50 min at 24°C. All of the effects of wheat germ agglutinin and concanavalin A are completely reversible if 80 mM *N*-acetyl-D-glucosamine or α-methyl-D-mannopyranoside, respectively, is included in the incubation medium. From Cuatrecasas and Tell (1973).
[b]Cpm bound, average value ±SEM of three replicates.

3.4. Glucagon Binding and Action in Liver Membranes

There have been extensive studies on the binding of glucagon to liver membranes (Tomasi *et al.*, 1970; Rodbell *et al.*, 1971*a,b,c*; Pohl *et al.*, 1971, 1972; Desbuquois and Cuatrecasas, 1972; Bataille *et al.*, 1973; Rubalcava and Rodbell, 1973; Desbuquois *et al.*, 1974; Livingston *et al.*, 1974). Radioiodinated glucagon retains its biological activity and binds to liver membranes with properties expected for a specific receptor interaction. The binding of [^{125}I]glucagon is saturable, indicating a finite number of membrane sites, and is reduced as expected by native glucagon but not by other polypeptides or by biologically inactive glucagon fragments. The apparent affinity for binding ($K_D \simeq 4 \times 10^{-9}$ M) corresponds to the apparent affinity for glucagon activation of liver membrane adenylate cyclase (Rodbell *et al.*, 1971*a,b*). In addition, certain treatments of the membranes (phospholipase A, digitonin, and urea) depress binding and biological responsiveness in parallel. The concentrations at which the binding to membranes saturates,

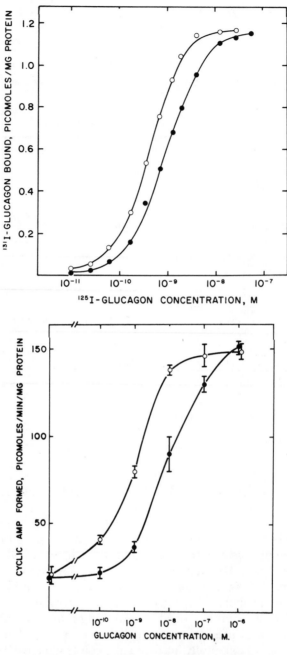

FIG. 13. Binding and action of glucagon in liver microsomal membranes in the presence and the absence of bacitracin. Top: Binding of [^{131}I]glucagon (10^{-11} to 8×10^{-8} M) was determined by filtration procedures with ($\bigcirc$) and without ($\bullet$) bacitracin (1 mg/ml). Bottom: Glucagon-stimulated activity of adenylate cyclase was measured at 30°C with 3 mM [α-^{32}P]ATP and increasing concentrations of native glucagon with ($\bigcirc$) and without ($\bullet$) bacitracin (0.5 mg/ml). From Desbuquois *et al.* (1974).

and at which adenylate cyclase is activated, do not, however, correspond to the known serum levels of glucagon.

The studies with glucagon are complicated by the fact that glucagon is very rapidly degraded by isolated liver membranes. Since membrane-bound glucagon which is eluted with acid or by protein denaturants or which dissociates spontaneously can bind again to fresh membranes, while inactivated glucagon cannot, it is likely that receptor binding and inactivation are separate and independent processes. Furthermore, certain small polypeptides such as bacitracin as well as other reagents can protect glucagon from degradation without modifying binding (Desbuquois and Cuatrecasas, 1972; Desbuquois et al., 1974). When inactivation is blocked by bacitracin, the dose–response curves for binding and for adenylate cyclase activation are both shifted to lower concentrations, which more closely approximate physiological levels (Fig. 13). That the binding and enzyme activation dose–response curves shift in concert reinforces the view that binding is occurring with specific receptors. It is unknown whether the potent glucagon-inactivating system in these membrane preparations is physiologically relevant in the normal process by which this hormone is inactivated.

Undoubtedly, certain other ligands are rapidly inactivated in the same system in which it is desired to obtain receptor binding data. Besides peptide hormones, acetylcholine and other cholinergic esteratic analogues are rapidly hydrolyzed by acetylcholinesterases or by nonspecific nucleophils; catecholamines can be oxidized spontaneously (this can be catalyzed by divalent cations) or metabolized by specific membrane-bound enzymes. The experiments with glucagon illustrate such a problem and suggest an approach which can partially overcome the complication in studies of peptide hormones.

Some data suggest that not all of the glucagon binding may be related to receptors. For instance, there is complete activation of glucagon-stimulated adenylate cyclase with occupation of only 10–20% of the binding sites (Birnbaumer and Pohl, 1973). Moreover, the complete inhibition of this activity by des-his-glucagon is observed when only 10–20% of the membrane-bound [^{125}I]glucagon is displaced by this hormone analogue.

It is possible that a certain proportion of binding sites are related to inactivation mechanisms, or to receptor structures for other peptides (perhaps for glucagon-like immunoreactivity) with which glucagon can cross-react. It is probable, nonetheless, that despite the apparent discrepancies described above, the majority of glucagon binding is related to specific receptors. It will be important in future work to obtain binding and dose–response relationships for glucagon in a convenient glucagon-responsive whole cell system, and to obtain more detailed and precise simultaneous kinetic relationships between binding and activation of adenylate cyclase in membrane fractions.

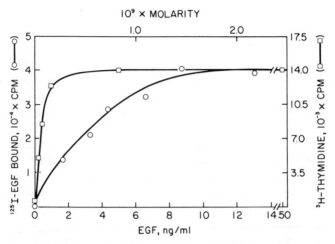

FIG. 14. Binding and action of EGF on fibroblast monolayers. Specific binding of [^{125}I]EGF (○) and EGF-mediated [^{3}H]thymidine incorporation (□) were measured in replicate intact monolayers (approximately 3×10^5 cells). From Hollenberg and Cuatrecasas (1975*b*).

3.5. Epidermal Growth Factor Receptors in Human Fibroblasts

Epidermal growth factor, a 6000 mol w single-chain polypeptide possessing three disulfide bridges which is derived from the submaxillary gland of the adult male mouse (Cohen, 1962, 1972), is a potent mitogen for human fibroblasts (Hollenberg and Cuatrecasas, 1973*a*) (Fig. 9). It is possible to demonstrate specific membrane receptors for this peptide in a variety of tissues (Covelli *et al.*, 1972; Frati *et al.*, 1972; Hollenberg and Cuatrecasas, 1973*a*; O'Keefe *et al.*, 1974). In the fibroblast system, it is possible to compare the binding data directly with the dose–response curve for EGF-stimulated DNA synthesis (Fig. 14). In contrast to the data obtained with insulin either in fat cells or in fibroblasts (Figs. 1 and 10), with EGF the maximum response (DNA synthesis) is attained at only 20% occupancy of the membrane binding sites for EGF. The lack of 1:1 correspondence between the binding curve and the biological dose–response curve may indicate significant differences in the manner whereby the EGF– and insulin–membrane interactions are coupled to the measured biological response (sugar transport vs. DNA synthesis).

The lack of correspondence between the binding isotherm and DNA synthesis may reflect the fact that a metabolic step is being measured (some

20 h later) which is probably very distant from the original site of interaction of the hormone with the cell membrane. Perhaps if the initial rate of production of the primary mediator (presently unknown) responsible for this effect could be measured, or if an early, primary metabolic effect could be measured, a closer correspondence would be found. It is possible, for example, that although occupancy of only 20% of the receptors is sufficient to lead to maximal effects on DNA synthesis, the full expression of other metabolic events requires activation of all the receptors. In systems which try to correlate binding with enzyme activation in isolated membrane preparations, discrepancies may possibly be attributed to differential effects of the isolation procedure itself on the binding site and on the activation coupling mechanism. However, the experiments with EGF in the whole cell system suggest that the noncorrespondence, *within a relatively narrow concentration range*, of the biological dose–response curve and the binding curve may, in the membrane systems, not be attributable simply to artifacts of the isolation procedure.

3.6. Catecholamine Binding and β-Adrenergic Receptors

Radioactively labeled catecholamines have been used successfully for many years in the elucidation of important transport, storage, and reuptake functions of adrenergic neurons (Kirshner, 1962; Stjarne, 1964; Iversen, 1967; Molinoff and Axelrod, 1971; Shore, 1972). However, only recently have such labeled compounds (primarily [³H]norepinephrine $\simeq 12$ Ci/mmol) been used to demonstrate specific binding to isolated liver (Marinetti *et al.*, 1969; Tomasi *et al.*, 1970; Dunnick and Marinetti, 1971) and heart (Lefkowitz and Haber, 1971; Lefkowitz *et al.*, 1972, 1973*b*; Lefkowitz and Levey, 1972) microsomal preparations, spleen capsule (DePlazas and DeRobertis, 1972), cultured myocardial cells (Lefkowitz *et al.*, 1973*a*), and turkey erythrocyte ghosts (Schramm *et al.*, 1972; Bilezikian and Aurbach, 1973*a,b*). The binding (Fig. 15) is observed to be saturable, with two apparent binding sites. The high-affinity site ($K_D \simeq 10^{-6}$ to 10^{-7} M) is thought to reflect reasonably closely the apparent affinity calculated from measurements of biological activity. It is pertinent, however, that most estimates of "biological activity" have been obtained from measurements of catecholamine-stimulated adenylate cyclase activity in particulate membrane preparations; it is well recognized that in many situations stimulation of this particulate enzyme *in vitro* requires much higher concentrations of hormone than are required *in vivo*. In contrast, in the isolated fat cell, the half-maximal concentration for (−)-norepinephrine-mediated lipolysis (Fig. 16) is about 6×10^{-8} M (when catechol oxidation is prevented), while the binding of (−)-[³H]norepinephrine indicates an apparent K_D of about 10^{-6} M. Similarly, in intact turkey erythrocytes, D,L-isoproterenol

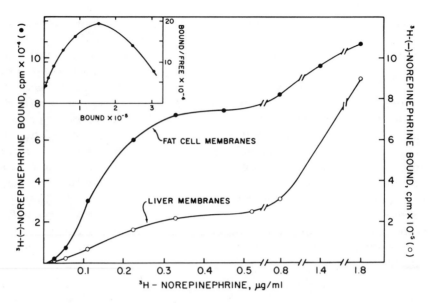

FIG. 15. Specific binding curve of [³H](−)-norepinephrine (6.4 Ci/mmol) to liver and fat cell membranes of rats. Binding in $10^{-4} \times$ cpm (●, fat cell membranes; ○, liver membranes) is corrected for the amount of radioactivity adsorbed in the presence of an excess of unlabeled (−)-norepinephrine (50 μg/ml). From Cuatrecasas *et al.* (1974).

stimulates sodium transport maximally at 10^{-7} M, with a half-maximal response observed at about 10^{-8} M (Gardner *et al.*, 1973); the binding measurements of D,L-[³H]isoproterenol to turkey erythrocyte ghosts yield a K_D of 4×10^{-6} M (Bilezikian and Aurbach, 1973a).

Even in early work on catecholamine binding, it was recognized that (+)-norepinephrine was as effective as (−)-norepinephrine in displacing [³H]norepinephrine from membranes (Fig. 17). However, many recognized β-adrenergic agonists are effective in displacing [³H]norepinephrine, and it has been proposed that the binding, despite the lack of stereospecificity, is related to the β-adrenergic receptor (Lefkowitz *et al.*, 1972). More recently (Cuatrecasas *et al.*, 1974), it has been observed that the specificity of binding is restricted solely to the catechol moiety of the catecholamine (Fig. 18).

Compounds lacking the ethanolamine portion and without any β-adrenergic activity, such as pyrocatechol and 3,4-dihydroxymandelic acid, compete as effectively for binding as does (−)-norepinephrine. It is of particular significance that the catechol compounds, so effective in blocking (−)-[³H]norepinephrine binding (e.g., dopamine, pyrocatechol, 3,4-dihydroxymandelic acid), which themselves are devoid of biological activity, have virtually no effect in altering the β-adrenergic potency of active compounds (Table 6). In particular, (+)-norepinephrine does not alter the

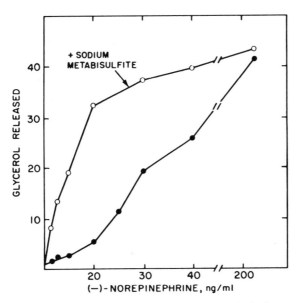

FIG. 16. (−)-Norepinephrine-mediated lipolysis in isolated fat cells. The lipolytic response (glycerol release in μmol glycerol per mmol of cell triglyceride) to increasing amounts of (−)-norepinephrine was determined at 37°C (for 90 min) in isolated fat cell suspensions with (○) and without (●) sodium metabisulfite (10 μg/ml). For experimental details, see Cuatrecasas *et al.* (1974).

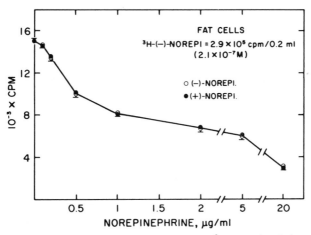

FIG. 17. Competition with binding of (−)-[³H]norepinephrine by unlabeled (+)- and (−)-norepinephrine in isolated fat cells. The unlabeled compound was added 3 min before (−)-[³H]norepinephrine. From Cuatrecasas *et al.* (1974).

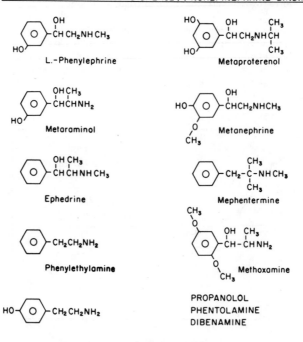

FIG. 18. Structures of compounds that have been tested for competition with [³H]norepinephrine for binding to membranes. For experimental details, see Cuatrecasas *et al.* (1974).

TABLE 6

Lipolytic Activity of Catechol Substances and Their Effect on the
Lipolytic Activity of (−)-Norepinephrine in Isolated Fat Cells[a]

Addition	Concentration (ng/ml)	Glycerol released[b]
None		13.6
(−)-Norepinephrine	10	48.7
	50	71.0
(−)-Isoproterenol	0.5	27.4
(+)-Norepinephrine	500	14.4
Pyrocatechol	2000	14.5
Dopamine	500	16.2
3,4-Dihydroxymandelic acid	500	15.1
(+)-Norepinephrine +	500	
(−)-Norepinephrine	10	51.4
(−)-Isoproterenol	0.5	28.2
Pyrocatechol +	2000	
(−)-Norepinephrine	10	49.8
Dopamine +	500	
(−)-Norepinephrine	10	52.9
3,4-Dihydroxymandelic acid +	500	
(−)-Norepinephrine	10	50.1

[a]The lipolytic potency of (−)-phenylephrine, pronetholol, phentolamine, and
6-hydroxydopamine was at least 100 times lower than that of (−)-
norepinephrine, while the potency of (−)-isoproterenol was 5–10 times
greater. Data from Cuatrecasas et al. (1974).
[b]Micromoles of glycerol per millimole of cell triglyceride.

dose–response curve of (−)-norepinephrine either for lipolysis in fat cells
(Fig. 19) or for norepinephrine-stimulated adenylate cyclase activity in liver
and fat cell membranes (Fig. 20) (Tell and Cuatrecasas, 1974).

A variety of catechol substances lacking β-adrenergic activity as well as
the (+)-isomers of norepinephrine and isoproterenol do not inhibit (−)-
norepinephrine-stimulated adenylate cyclase activity in fat, liver, or heart
cell membranes or in turkey or rat erythrocyte ghosts unless the concentrations of these catechols exceed 10^{-3} M (Cuatrecasas et al., 1974; Tell and
Cuatrecasas, 1974) (Fig. 21). Such high concentrations of these catechols
have been found to inhibit profoundly the unstimulated cyclase activity as
well as NaF- and glucagon-stimulated activity. Furthermore, such high
concentrations of the (−)-isomers of epinephrine and isoproterenol cause a
marked paradoxical inhibition of enzyme activity. The inhibitory effect is
thus due to a nonspecific (nonreceptor) suppression of activity. The apparent residual activity (about 0.1–1%) of (+)-norepinephrine (Figs. 19 and 20)
most probably results from contamination with the (−)-isomer (Tell and

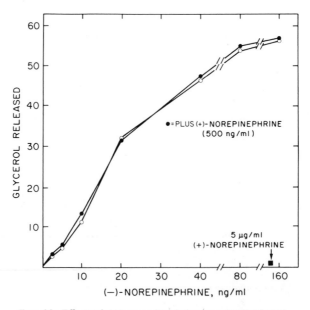

FIG. 19. Effect of (+)-norepinephrine on the lipolytic response of fat cells to (−)-norepinephrine. The lipolytic response after 80 min at 37°C is expressed as μmol of glycerol
released in the medium per mmol of cell triglyceride. From
Cuatrecasas *et al.* (1974).

Cuatrecasas, 1974). D,L-Dopa, dopamine, vanilmandelic acid, and 3,4-
dihydroxyphenylacetic acid, all potent blockers of [³H]norepinephrine
binding, fail to inhibit the ability of D,L-isoproterenol (10^{-8} M) to stimulate
sodium transport in intact erythrocytes, even when these compounds are
present at concentrations 1000 times greater than that of isoproterenol
(Gardner *et al.*, 1973). Finally, the noncatechol, *m*-methanesulfonamide
derivative of D,L-isoproterenol, soterenol (compound 49) (Uloth *et al.*, 1966),
which is as potent as (−)-norepinephrine in stimulating lipolysis and which is
inhibited by propranolol, fails to compete for the binding of
[³H]norepinephrine to fat cell membranes.

On the basis of the data above, it is evident that the measured membrane
binding of [³H]norepinephrine cannot represent a direct interaction with
the β-adrenergic receptor (Cuatrecasas *et al.*, 1974; Maguire *et al.*, 1974;
Wolfe *et al.*, 1974). The binding is thus "nonspecific" in the pharmacological
sense, in that it appears to be related to a moiety which is separate from the
adrenergic receptor. These binding sites are, however, specific in the sense
that they are present in a restricted, finite number and in that they have a
nearly absolute specificity for the 3,4-dihydroxyphenolic moiety. The
importance of the catechol function suggests a possible relationship with the

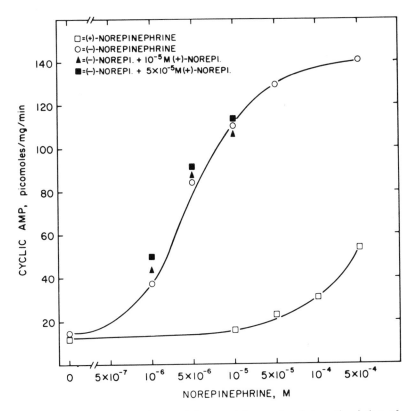

Fig. 20. Effect of (+)-norepinephrine on (−)-norepinephrine stimulation of adenylate cyclase activity in isolated fat cell microsomes. Dose–response data were obtained at 37°C after a 5-min incubation period. From Cuatrecasas *et al.* (1974).

enzyme catechol-*O*-methyltransferase (COMT). Indeed, recognized inhibitors of COMT (tropolone, pyrogallol, quercitin, and U-0521) as well as other specific compounds (3-mercaptotyramine, *S*-adenosylmethionine, and *S*-adenosylethionine) all modify [³H]norepinephrine binding (Cuatrecasas *et al.*, 1974). It has been suggested that the binding of catecholamines to microsomes may reflect binding to an altered form of COMT (Cuatrecasas *et al.*, 1974).

3.7. Macromolecular Hormone Derivatives and Plasma Membrane Receptors

Part of the evidence to indicate that polypeptide hormone receptors are localized on the cell surface has been obtained using insoluble hormone

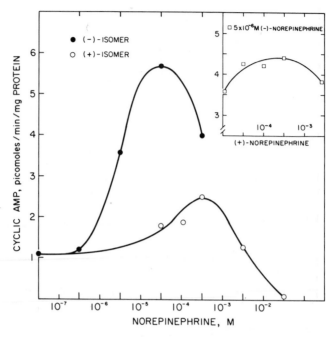

FIG. 21. Effect of (−)- and (+)-norepinephrine on adenylate cyclase activity of turkey erythrocyte ghosts. From Tell and Cuatrecasas (1974).

derivatives such as insulin–agarose (Cuatrecasas, 1969*a*). In properly controlled experiments, where the problem of the leakage of soluble ligand from the inert support is eliminated, the biological activities of such derivatives can be demonstrated in isolated cell systems. For instance, insulin–agarose can enhance the conversion of [U-^{14}C]glucose to CO_2 (Cuatrecasas, 1969*a*) in fat cells, and soluble insulin–dextran derivatives are active *in vivo* in reducing blood sugar levels and inducing hepatic enzymes (Suzuki *et al.*, 1972; Armstrong *et al.*, 1972).

It is of considerable interest that while the macromolecular derivatives exhibit biological activities on the whole similar to those of the parent active ligand, in some cases qualitative and quantitative differences can be observed. For instance, insulin–agarose, which in fat cells mimics the action of insulin, may act via fewer contacts at the fat cell surface than does soluble insulin and may thus in some respects be more potent than insulin itself. Similarly, insulin–dextran derivatives administered intravenously in alloxan-diabetic rats appear more potent than soluble insulin in their ability to lower blood glucose and induce hepatic enzyme synthesis (Suzuki *et al.*,

1972). In the virgin mouse, mammary cells which do not respond (α-aminoisobutyric acid uptake) to soluble insulin do respond to insulin–agarose in the way that insulin-sensitive mammary cells from pregnant mice respond. It is striking that the effect of insulin–sepharose on mammary cells from virgin mice can be blocked by soluble insulin (Oka and Topper, 1971). Similar kinds of results have been obtained with derivatives of phytohemagglutinin (PHA). Mouse B-lymphocytes, which ordinarily do not respond (DNA synthesis) well to soluble PHA, do respond to agarose–PHA derivatives (Greaves and Bauminger, 1972). Additionally, it has been observed that a multiplication factor from chick embryo, which stimulates DNA synthesis in embryonic rat pancreas fragments, appears to be more active as an insoluble agarose derivative than it is in its native form; the total amount of multiplication factor which when bound to agarose stimulated DNA synthesis was insufficient when in solution to effect stimulation (Ronzio and Rutter, 1973; Levine *et al.*, 1973). Such studies not only emphasize the plasma membrane location of the receptors but also suggest that the traditionally accepted response of such receptors may be amenable to manipulation by pharmacological agents which act outside the cell.

With the aid of ligand–agarose derivatives, it is possible to infer the presence of receptors in whole cells by direct microscopic observation. Fat cells, which normally float on aqueous buffers, can be seen to stick to insulin–sepharose beads so that the cells sink with the beads or the cells cause the beads to float with the cells, depending on the degree of derivatization of beads with insulin (Soderman *et al.*, 1973). The addition of soluble insulin reverses the binding of cells to insulin–agarose. Similarly, elegant studies with insoluble agarose–ligand derivatives have suggested the presence of histamine and norepinephrine receptors on the surface of selected leukocytes (Melmon *et al.*, 1972; Weinstein *et al.*, 1973). The binding of leukocytes to histamine–rabbit serum albumin–sepharose is prevented by high concentrations of histamine and histamine antagonists, but not by catecholamines or their pharmacological antagonists. The binding of cells to a similar norepinephrine derivative is blocked by some catecholamines and propranolol but not by histamine or antihistamines. Results of other work suggest that catecholamines immobilized on a glass support are also biologically active (Venter *et al.*, 1972, 1973).

The interaction of insoluble ligand derivatives with cell receptors may differ substantially from that of the soluble ligand. For instance, a striking redistribution of surface receptors is observed when lymphocytes adhere to Con A–derivatized nylon fibers; the receptors migrate to cluster at the region of cell–fiber contact (Edelman, 1973). It may be difficult therefore to interpret some of the data obtained with macromolecular hormone derivatives in terms of the known biological activity relationships for the soluble ligands. Nonetheless, given this restriction, these derivatives can be extremely useful in studying plasma membrane receptors.

4. CONCLUSIONS

It is felt that the examples of ligand–receptor interaction cited above provide a perspective for much work of a similar nature accomplished in this and other laboratories. Studies on insulin binding in fat and liver cells undoubtedly do reflect a true hormone–receptor interaction; there is a clear correlation between the biological and physicochemical data. On the other hand, studies on the interaction of insulin with fibroblasts and stimulated lymphocytes reveal significant quantitative discrepancies between the K_D in these cells and both the K_D observed in fat and liver cells and the known serum levels of insulin. These observations suggest interesting possibilities which can be elucidated by further work. The studies on the biological activity and binding of plant lectins illustrate difficulties which can be met when a ligand binds in large amounts to structures in addition to those responsible for a biological response. Studies with glucagon demonstrate the problem encountered when substantial amounts of ligand are degraded during binding measurements; similar difficulties are present in studies on catecholamine binding, where a rapid destruction of the catechol function is observed even in the absence of cell membrane constituents (Cuatrecasas, 1973g). In this context, it should be mentioned that degradation of the receptor structure as well (e.g., insulin receptors are remarkably sensitive to low concentrations of trypsin) can substantially compromise studies on ligand–membrane interactions. The data comparing EGF binding with its biological activity exemplify a case of noncoincidence of the biological and physicochemical data. While the shift in the two dose–response curves is small (approximately fivefold), it may be of importance in terms of the mode of action of this and other active peptides. In the case of catecholamine binding, it can be seen how careful simultaneous studies on binding and biological activity can be used to test the relation between binding and a putative pharmacological receptor. The significance of highly specific catechol binding in microsomes, which appears to be related to the enzyme catechol–O-methyltransferase, remains to be elucidated. Finally, it is seen that while macromolecular hormone derivatives can be used to answer certain questions, e.g., localization of receptors, these compounds may have modes of action which differ from those of the parent compounds and may thus provide special tools for examining the mechanism of action of those hormones. On the whole, the application of the general approaches outlined in this chapter has yielded some answers, as well as many interesting questions, concerning the interaction of hormones with plasma membrane receptors.

5. REFERENCES

ARMSTRONG, K. J., NOALL, M. W., and STOUFFER, J. E., 1972, Dextran-linked insulin: A soluble high molecular weight derivative with biological activity *in vivo* and *in vitro*, *Biochem. Biophys. Res. Commun.* **47**:354–360.

BANERJEE, S. P., HOLLENBERG, M. D., and CUATRECASAS, P., 1973*a*, unpublished observations.

BANERJEE, S. P., SNYDER, S. H., CUATRECASAS, P., and GREENE, L. A., 1973*b*, Binding of nerve growth factor in sympathetic ganglia, *Proc. Natl. Acad. Sci.* **70:**2519–2523.

BARNARD, E. A., WIECKOWSKI, J., and CHIU, T. H., 1971, Cholinergic receptor molecules and cholinesterase molecules at mouse skeletal muscle junctions, *Nature* **234:**207–209.

BATAILLE, D. P., FREYCHET, P., KITABGI, P. E., and ROSSELIN, G. E., 1973, Gut glucagon: A common receptor site with pancreatic glucagon in liver cell plasma membranes, *FEBS Letters* **30:**215–218.

BENNETT, G. V., and CUATRECASAS, P., 1972, Insulin receptor of fat cells in insulin resistant metabolic states, *Science* **176:**805–806.

BILEZIKIAN, J. P., and AURBACH, G. D., 1973*a*, A β-adrenergic receptor of the turkey erythrocyte. I. Binding of catecholamines and relationship to adenylate cyclase activity, *J. Biol. Chem.* **248:**5577–5583.

BILEZIKIAN, J. P., and AURBACH, G. D., 1973*b*, A β-adrenergic receptor of the turkey erythrocyte. II. Characterization and solubilization of the receptor, *J. Biol. Chem.* **248:**5584–5589.

BIRNBAUMER, L., and POHL, S. L., 1973, Relation of glucagon-specific binding sites to glucagon-dependent stimulation of adenylyl cyclase activity in plasma membranes of rat liver, *J. Biol. Chem.* **248:**2056–2061.

BOCKMAN, R. S., and SONENBERG, M., 1973, personal communication.

CHANG, K.-J., and CUATRECASAS, P., 1974, ATP-dependent inhibition of insulin-stimulated glucose transport in fat cells—Possible role of membrane phosphorylation, *J. Biol. Chem.*, **249:**3170–3180.

CHANG, K.-J., BENNETT, V., and CUATRECASAS, P., (1975) Membrane receptors as general markers for plasma membrane isolation procedures—The use of [^{125}I]-labelled wheat germ agglutinin, insulin, and cholera toxin, *J. Biol. Chem.* **250:**488–500.

CHANGEUX, J.-P., KASAI, M., HUCHET, M., and MEUNIER, J.-C., 1970, Extraction à partir du tissu électrique de gymnote d'une proteine presentant plusieurs propriétés characteristiques du recepteur physiologique de l'acetylcholine, *Compt. Rend. Acad. Sci. Paris* **270:**2864–2867.

CHANGEUX, J.-P., MEUNIER, J.-C., and HUCHET, M., 1971, Studies on the cholinergic receptor protein of *Electrophorus electricus*. 1. An assay *in vitro* for the cholinergic receptor site and solubilization of receptor protein from electric tissue, *Mol. Pharmacol* **7:**538–553.

CLARK, A. J., 1926*a*, The reaction between acetylcholine and muscle cell, *J. Physiol.* **61:**530–546.

CLARK, A. J., 1926*b*, The antagonism of acetylcholine by atropine, *J. Physiol.* **61:**547–556.

CLARK, A. J., 1933, *Mode of Action of Drugs on Cells*, Edward Arnold, London.

COHEN, S., 1962, Isolation of a mouse submaxillary gland protein accelerating incisor eruption and eyelid opening in the new-born animal, *J. Biol. Chem.* **237:**1555–1562.

COHEN, S., 1972, Epidermal growth factor, *J. Invest. Dermatol.* **59:**13–16.

COHEN, S. A., and FISHBACH, G. D., 1973, Regulation of muscle acetylcholine sensitivity by muscle activity in cell culture, *Science* **181:**76–78.

COOPER, D., and REICH, E., 1972, Neurotoxin from venom of the cobra, *Naja naja siamensis:* Purification and radioactive labelling, *J. Biol. Chem.* **247:**3008–3013.

COVELLI, I., MOZZI, R., ROSSI, R., and FRATI, L., 1972, The mechanism of action of the epidermal growth factor, *Hormones* **3:**183–191.

CUATRECASAS, P., 1969*a*, Interaction of insulin with the cell membrane, the primary action of insulin, *Proc. Natl. Acad. Sci.* **63:**450–457.

CUATRECASAS, P., 1969*b*, Insulin-sepharose: Immunoreactivity and use in the purification of antibody, *Biochem. Biophys. Res. Commun.* **35:**531–537.

CUATRECASAS, P., 1971*a*, Insulin–receptor interaction in adipose tissue cells: Direct measurement and properties, *Proc. Natl. Acad. Sci.* **68:**1264–1268.

CUATRECASAS, P., 1971*b*, Unmasking of insulin reception in fat cells and fat cell membranes, *J. Biol. Chem.* **246:**6532–6542.

CUATRECASAS, P., 1971*c*, Properties of the insulin receptor of isolated fat cell membranes, *J. Biol. Chem.* **246:**7265–7274.

CUATRECASAS, P., 1972a, Properties of the insulin receptor isolated from liver and fat cell membranes, *J. Biol. Chem.* **247:**1980–1991.

CUATRECASAS, P., 1972b, Affinity chromatography and purification of the insulin receptor of liver cell membranes, *Proc. Natl. Acad. Sci.* **69:**1277–1281.

CUATRECASAS, P., 1972c, The insulin receptor, *Diabetes* **21:**396–402 (Suppl. 2).

CUATRECASAS, P., 1972d, Isolation of the insulin receptor of liver and fat cell membranes, *Proc. Natl. Acad. Sci.* **69:**318–322.

CUATRECASAS, P., 1973a, Insulin receptor of liver and fat cell membranes, *Fed. Proc.* **32:**1838–1846.

CUATRECASAS, P., 1973b, Interaction of concanavalin A and wheat germ agglutinin with the insulin receptor of fat cells and liver, *J. Biol. Chem.* **248:**3528–3534.

CUATRECASAS, P., 1973c, The interaction of *Vibrio cholerae* enterotoxin with cell membranes, *Biochemistry* **12:**3547–3557.

CUATRECASAS, P., 1973d, Gangliosides and membrane receptors for cholera toxin, *Biochemistry* **12:**3558–3566.

CUATRECASAS, P., 1973e, Cholera toxin–fat cell interaction and the mechanism of activation of the lipolytic response, *Biochemistry* **12:**3567–3576.

CUATRECASAS, P., 1973f, *Vibrio cholerae* choleragenoid—Mechanism of inhibition of cholera toxin action, *Biochemistry* **12:**3577–3581.

CUATRECASAS, P., 1973g, unpublished observations.

CUATRECASAS, P., 1973h, Interaction of wheat germ agglutinin and concanavalin A with isolated fat cells, *Biochemistry* **12:**1312–1323.

CUATRECASAS, P., 1974, Membrane receptors, *Ann. Rev. Biochem.* **43:**169–214.

CUATRECASAS, P., and HOLLENBERG, M. D., 1975, Binding of insulin and other hormones to non-receptor materials: saturability, specificity and apparent "negative cooperativity", *Biochem. Biophys. Res. Commun.* **62:**31–41.

CUATRECASAS, P., and TELL, G. P. E., 1973, Insulin-like activity of concanavalin A and wheat germ agglutinin—Direct interactions with insulin receptors, *Proc. Natl. Acad. Sci.* **70:**485–489.

CUATRECASAS, P., FUCHS, S., and ANFINSEN, C. B., 1967, Catalytic properties and specificity of the extracellular nuclease of *Staphylococcus aureus*, *J. Biol. Chem.* **242:**3063–3067.

CUATRECASAS, P., DESBUQUOIS, B., and KRUG, F., 1971a, Insulin receptor interactions in liver cell membranes, *Biochem. Biophys. Res. Commun.* **44:**333–339.

CUATRECASAS, P., ILLIANO, G., and GREEN, I., 1971b, Production of anti-glucagon antibodies in poly-L-lysine "responder" guinea-pigs, *Nature New Biol.* **230:** 60–61.

CUATRECASAS, P., TELL, G. P. E., SICA, V., PARIKH, I., and CHANG, K.-J., 1974, Noradrenaline binding and the search for catecholamine receptors, *Nature* **247:**92–97.

DEPLAZAS, S. F., and DEROBERTIS, E., 1972, Isolation of a proteolipid from spleen capsule binding (±)-[^{3}H]-norepinephrine, *Biochim. Biophys. Acta* **266:**246–254.

DESBUQUOIS, B., 1974, *Eur. J. Biochem.* (in press).

DESBUQUOIS, B., and AURBACH, G. D., 1971, Use of polyethylene glycol to separate free and antibody-bound peptide hormones in radioimmunoassays, *J. Clin. Endocrinol.* **33:**732–738.

DESBUQUOIS, B., and CUATRECASAS, P., 1972, Independence of glucagon receptors and glucagon inactivation in liver cell membranes, *Nature New Biol.* **236:**202–204.

DESBUQUOIS, B., LAUDET, M. H., and LAUDET, P., 1973, Vasoactive intestinal polypeptide and glucagon stimulation of adenylate cyclase activity via distinct receptors in liver and fat cell membranes, *Biochem. Biophys. Res. Commun.* **53:**1187–1194.

DESBUQUOIS, B., KRUG, F., and CUATRECASAS, P., 1974, Inhibitors of glucagon inactivation: Effect on glucagon–receptor interactions and glucagon-stimulated adenylate cyclase activity in liver cell membranes, *Biochim. Biophys. Acta,* **343:**101–120.

DULAK, N. C., and TEMIN, H. M., 1973a, A partially purified polypeptide fraction from rat liver cell conditioned medium with multiplication stimulating activity for embryo fibroblasts, *J. Cell. Physiol.* **81:**153–160.

DULAK, N. C., and TEMIN, H. M., 1973*b*, Multiplication stimulating activity for chicken embryo fibroblasts from rat liver cell conditioned medium: A family of small polypeptides, *J. Cell. Physiol.* **81**:161–170.

DUNNICK, J. K., and MARINETTI, G. V., 1971, Hormone action at the membrane level. III. Epinephrine interaction with rat liver plasma membrane, *Biochim. Biophys. Acta* **249**:122–134.

EDELMAN, G. M., 1973, personal communication.

EL-ALLAWY, R. M. M., and GLIEMANN, J., 1972, Trypsin treatment of adipocytes: Effect on sensitivity to insulin, *Biochim. Biophys. Acta* **273**:97–109.

ELDEFRAWI, M. E., and O'BRIEN, R. D., 1971, Autoinhibition of acetylcholine binding to *Torpedo* electroplax; A possible molecular mechanism for desensitization, *Proc. Natl. Acad. Sci.* **68**:2006–2007.

FRATI, L., DANIELE, S., DELOGU, A., and COVELLI, I., 1972, Selective binding of the epidermal growth factor and its specific effects on the epithelial cells of the cornea, *Exp. Eye Res.* **14**:135–141.

FREYCHET, P., ROTH, J., and NEVILLE, D. M., Jr., 1971*a*, Insulin receptors in the liver: Specific binding of ^{125}I-insulin to the plasma membrane and its relation to insulin bioactivity, *Proc. Natl. Acad. Sci.* **68**:1833–1837.

FREYCHET, P., ROTH, J., and NEVILLE, D. M., Jr., 1971*b*, Monoiodoinsulin: Demonstration of its biological activity and binding to fat cells and liver membranes, *Biochem. Biophys. Res. Commun.* **43**:400–408.

FREYCHET, P., KAHN, R., ROTH, J., and NEVILLE, D. M., Jr., 1972, Insulin interactions with liver plasma membranes: Independence of binding of the hormone and its degradation, *J. Biol. Chem.* **247**:3953–3961.

GARDNER, J. D., KLAVEMAN, H. L., BILEZIKIAN, J. P., and AURBACH, G. D., 1973, Effect of β-adrenergic catecholamines on sodium transport in turkey erythrocytes, *J. Biol. Chem.* **248**:5590–5597.

GARRAT, C. J., 1964, Effect of iodination on the biological activity of insulin, *Nature* **201**:1324–1325.

GAVIN, J. R., III, ROTH, J., JEN, P., and FREYCHET, P., 1972, Insulin receptors in human circulating cells and fibroblasts, *Proc. Natl. Acad. Sci.* **69**:747–751.

GAVIN, J. R., III, GORDEN, P., ROTH, J., ARCHER, J. A., and BLUELL, D. N., 1973, Characteristics of the human lymphocyte insulin receptor, *J. Biol. Chem.* **248**:2202–2207.

GEY, G. O., and THALHIMER, W., 1924, Observations on the effect of insulin introduced into the medium of tissue culture, *J. Am. Med. Soc.* **82**:1609.

GIACOBINI, G., FILOGARNO, G., WEBER, M., BOQUET, P., and CHANGEUX, J.-P., 1973, Effects of a snake α-neurotoxin on the development of innervated skeletal muscles in chick embryo, *Proc. Natl. Acad. Sci.* **70**:1708–1712.

GIORGIO, N. A., JOHNSON, C. B., and BLECHER, M., 1974, Hormone receptors. III. Properties of glucagon-binding proteins isolated from liver plasma membranes, *J. Biol. Chem.* **249**:428–437.

GLIEMANN, J., OSTERLIND, K., VINTEN, J., and GAMMELTOFT, S., 1972, A procedure for measurement of distribution spaces in isolated fat cells, *Biochim. Biophys. Acta* **286**:1–9.

GOLDFINE, I. D., GARDNER, J. D., and NEVILLE, D. M., Jr., 1972, Insulin action in isolated rat thymocytes. I. Binding of ^{125}I-insulin and stimulation of α-amino isobutyric acid transport, *J. Biol. Chem.* **247**:6919–6926.

GOLDSTEIN, A., LOWNEY, L. I., and PAL, B. K., 1971, Stereospecific and nonspecific interactions of the morphine congener levorphanol in subcellular fractions of mouse brain, *Proc. Natl. Acad. Sci.* **68**:1742–1747.

GREAVES, M. F., and BAUMINGER, S., 1972, Activation of T and B lymphocytes by insoluble phytomitogens, *Nature New Biol.* **235**:67–70.

GREENWOOD, F. C., and HUNTER, W. M., 1963, The preparation of ^{131}I-labelled human growth hormone of high specific activity, *Biochem. J.* **89**:114–123.

HALL, W. Z., 1972, Release of neurotransmitters and their interaction with receptors, *Ann. Rev. Biochem.* **41**:925–952.

HEMBREE, W. C., EHRENKAUFER, R. E., LIEBERMAN, S., and WOLF, A. P., 1973, A general method of tritium labeling utilizing microwave discharge activation of tritium gas methodology and application to biological compounds, *J. Biol. Chem.* **248**:5532–5540.

HENDERSON, P. J. F., 1973, Steady-state enzyme kinetics with high-affinity substrates or inhibitors. *Biochem. J.* **135**:101–107.

HINTZ, R. L., CLEMMONS, D. R., UNDERWOOD, L. E., and VAN WYK, J. J., 1972, Competitive binding of somatomedin to the insulin receptors of adipocytes, chondrocytes and liver membranes, *Proc. Natl. Acad. Sci.* **69**:2351–2355.

HOLLENBERG, M. D., and CUATRECASAS, P., 1973a, Epidermal growth factor: Receptors in human fibroblasts and modulation of action by cholera toxin, *Proc. Natl. Acad. Sci.* **70**:2964–2968.

HOLLENBERG, M. D., and CUATRECASAS, P., 1974a, Hormone receptors and membrane glycoproteins during *in vitro* transformation of lymphocytes, in: *Control of Proliferation in Animal Cells* (B. Clarkson and R. Baserga, eds.), p. 423–434, Cold Spring Harbor, N.Y.

HOLLENBERG, M. D., and CUATRECASAS, P., 1975a, Studies on the interaction of hormones with plasma membrane receptors, in: *Biochemical Actions of Hormones*, Vol. 3 (G. Litwack, ed.), Academic Press, New York, in press.

HOLLENBERG, M. D., and CUATRECASAS, P., 1975b, Insulin and EGF: Human fibroblast receptors related to DNA synthesis and amino acid transport, in preparation *J. Biol. Chem.* (in press).

HOLLENBERG, M. D., O'KEEFE, E. J., and CUATRECASAS, P., 1973, unpublished observations.

HUMMEL, J. P., and DREYER, W. J., 1962, Measurement of protein-binding phenomena by gel filtration, *Biochim. Biophys. Acta* **63**:530–532.

IVERSEN, L. L., 1967, *The Uptake and Storage of Noradrenalin in Sympathetic Nerves*, Cambridge University Press, London.

IZZO, J. L., RONCONE, A., IZZO, M. J., and BALE, W. F., 1964, Relationship between degree of iodination of insulin and its biological, electrophoretic and immunochemical properties, *J. Biol. Chem.* **239**:3749–3784.

KIRSHNER, N., 1962, Uptake of catecholamines by a particulate fraction of the adrenal medulla, *J. Biol. Chem.* **237**:2311–2317.

KRUG, U., and CUATRECASAS, P., 1973, unpublished observations.

KRUG, U., KRUG, F., and CUATRECASAS, P., 1972, Emergence of insulin receptors on human lymphocytes during *in vitro* transformation, *Proc. Natl. Acad. Sci.* **69**:2604–2608.

KRUG, U., HOLLENBERG, M. D., and CUATRECASAS, P., 1973, Changes in the binding of concanavalin A and wheat germ agglutinin to human lymphocytes during *in vitro* transformation, *Biochem. Biophys. Res. Commun.* **52**:305–312.

KUHAR, M. J., PERT, C. B., and SNYDER, S. H., 1973, Regional distribution of opiate receptor binding in monkey and human brain, *Nature* **245**:447–450.

LEFKOWITZ, R. J., and HABER, E., 1971, A fraction of the ventricular myocardium that thas the specificity of the cardiac β-adrenergic receptor, *Proc. Natl. Acad. Sci.* **68**:1773–1777.

LEFKOWITZ, R. J., and LEVEY, G. S., 1972, Norepinephrine—Dissociation and β-receptor binding from adenylate cyclase activation in solubilized myocardium, *Life Sci.* **11**:821–828 (Part 2).

LEFKOWITZ, R. J., HABER, E., and O'HARA, D., 1972, Identification of the cardiac beta-adrenergic receptor protein: Solubilization and purification by affinity chromatography, *Proc. Natl. Acad. Sci.* **69**:2828–2832.

LEFKOWITZ, R. J., O'HARA, D. S., and WARSHAW, J., 1973a, Binding of catecholamines to receptors in cultured myocardial cells, *Nature New Biol.* **244**:79–80.

LEFKOWITZ, R. J., SHARP, G. W. G., and HABER, E., 1973b, Specific binding of β-adrenergic catecholamines to a subcellular fraction from cardiac muscle, *J. Biol. Chem.* **248**:342–349.

LEVINE, S., PICTET, R., and RUTTER, W. J., 1973, Control of cell proliferation and cytodifferentiation by a factor reacting with the cell surface, *Nature New Biol.* **246**:49–51.

LIS, H., and SHARON, N., 1973, The biochemistry of plant lectins, *Ann. Rev. Biochem.* **42**:541–574.

LIVINGSTON, J. N., CUATRECASAS, P., and LOCKWOOD, D. H., 1974, Studies of glucagon resistance in large rat adipocytes: ^{125}I-labeled glucagon-binding and lipolytic capacity, *J. Lipid Res.* **15**:26–32.

MAGUIRE, M. E., GOLMANN, P. H., and GILMAN, A. G., 1974, The reaction of [^{3}H]norepinephrine with particulate fractions of cells responsive to catecholamines, *Molec. Pharmacol.* **10**:563–581.

MARINETTI, G. V., RAY, T. K., and TOMASI, V., 1969, Glucagon and epinephrine stimulation of adenyl cyclase activity in isolated rat liver plasma membranes, *Biochem. Biophys. Res. Commun.* **36**:185–193.

MASSAGLIA, A., ROSA, U., RIALDI, G., and ROSSI, C. A., 1969, Iodination of insulin in aqueous and organic solvents, *Biochem. J.* **115**:11–18.

MELMON, K. L., BOURNE, H. R., WEINSTEIN, J., and SELA, M., 1972, Receptors for histamine can be detected on the surface of selected leukocytes, *Science* **177**:707–709.

MEUNIER, J.-C., OLSEN, R. W., MENEZ, A., FROMAGEOT, P., BOQUET, P., and CHANGEUX, J.-P., 1972, Some physical properties of the cholinergic receptor protein from *Electrophorus electricus* revealed by a tritiated α-toxin from *Naja nigricollis* venom, *Biochemistry* **11**:1200–1210.

MILEDI, R., MOLINOFF, P., and POTTER, L. T., 1971, Isolation of the cholinergic receptor protein of *Torpedo* electric tissue, *Nature* **229**:554–557.

MOLINOFF, P. B., and AXELROD, J., 1971, Biochemistry of catecholamines, *Ann. Rev. Biochem.* **40**:465–500.

OKA, T., and TOPPER, Y. J., 1971, Insulin sepharose and the dynamics of insulin action, *Proc. Natl. Acad. Sci.* **68**:2066–2068.

O'KEEFE, E., HOLLENBERG, M. D., and CUATRECASAS, P., 1974, Epidermal growth factor: characteristics of specific binding in membranes from liver, placenta and other target tissues, *Arch. Biochem. Biophys.* **164**:518–526.

PATON, W. D. M., and RANG, H. P., 1965, The uptake of atropine and related drugs by intestinal smooth muscle of the guinea pig in relation to acetylcholine receptors, *Proc. Roy. Soc. Lond. Ser. B* **163**:1–44.

PERT, C. B., and SNYDER, S. H., 1973a, Opiate receptor: Demonstration in nervous tissue, *Science* **179**:1011–1014.

PERT, C. B., and SNYDER, S. H., 1973b, Properties of opiate–receptor binding in rat brain, *Proc. Natl. Acad. Sci.* **70**:2243–2247.

PIERSON, R. W., Jr., and TEMIN, H. M., 1972, The partial purification from calf serum of a fraction with multiplication-stimulating activity for chicken fibroblasts in cell culture and with nonsuppressible insulin-like activity, *J. Cell. Physiol.* **79**:319–330.

POHL, S. L., KRANS, H. M. J., KOZYREFF, V., BIRNBAUMER, L., and RODBELL, M., 1971, The glucagon-sensitive adenyl cyclase system in plasma membranes of rat liver. VI. Evidence for a role of membrane lipids, *J. Biol. Chem.* **246**:4447–4454.

POHL, S. L., KRANS, H. M. J., BIRNBAUMER, L., and RODBELL, M., 1972, Inactivation of glucagon by plasma membranes of rat liver, *J. Biol. Chem.* **247**:2295–2301.

PORTER, C. W., CHIU, T. H., WIECKOWSKI, J., and BARNARD, E. A., 1973, Types and locations of cholinergic receptor-like molecules in muscle fibres, *Nature New Biol.* **241**:3–7.

RAFTERY, M. A., SCHMIDT, J., CLARK, D. G., and WOLCOTT, R. G., 1971, Demonstration of a specific α-bungarotoxin binding component in *Electrophorus electricus* electroplax membranes, *Biochem. Biophys. Res. Commun.* **45**:1622–1629.

RAFTERY, M. A., SCHMIDT, J., and CLARK, D. G., 1972, Specificity of α-bungarotoxin binding to *Torpedo californica* electroplax, *Arch. Biochem. Biophys.* **152**:882–886.

RODBELL, M., KRANS, H. M. J., POHL, S. L., and BIRNBAUMER, L., 1971a, The glucagon-sensitive adenyl cyclase system in plasma membranes of rat liver. III. Binding of glucagon: method of assay and specificity, *J. Biol. Chem.* **246**:1861–1871.

RODBELL, M., KRANS, H. M. J., POHL, S. L., and BIRNBAUMER, L., 1971b, The glucagon-sensitive adenyl cyclase system in plasma membranes of rat liver. IV. Effects of guanyl nucleotides on binding of ^{125}I-glucagon, *J. Biol. Chem.* **246**:1872–1876.

RODBELL, M., BIRNBAUMER, L., POHL, S. L., and SUNDBY, F., 1971c, The reaction of glucagon with its receptor: Evidence for discrete regions of activity and binding in the glucagon molecule, *Proc. Natl. Acad. Sci.* **68**:909–913.

RONZIO, R. A., and RUTTER, W. J., 1973, Effects of a partially purified factor from chick embryos on macromolecular synthesis of embryonic pancreatic epithelia, *Develop. Biol.* **30**:307–320.

RUBALCAVA, B., and RODBELL, M., 1973, The role of acidic phospholipids in glucagon action on rat liver adenylate cyclase, *J. Biol. Chem.* **248**:3831–3837.

SCATCHARD, G., 1949, The attractions of proteins for small molecules and ions, *Ann. N.Y. Acad. Sci.* **51**:660–672.

SCHRAMM, M., FEINSTEIN, H., NAIM, E., LONG, M., and LASSER, M., 1972, Epinephrine binding to the catecholamine receptor and activation of the adenylate cyclase in erythrocyte membranes, *Proc. Natl. Acad. Sci.* **69**:523–527.

SHIU, R. P. C., KELLY, P. A., and FRIESEN, N. G., 1973, Radioreceptor assay for prolactin and other lactogenic hormones, *Science* **180**:968–971.

SHORE, P. A., 1972, Transport and storage of biogenic amines, *Ann. Rev. Pharmacol.* **12**:209–226.

SIMON, E. J., HILLER, J. M., and EDELMAN, I., 1973, Stereospecific binding of the potent narcotic analgesic [^{3}H]etorphine to rat brain homogenate, *Proc. Natl. Acad. Sci.* **70**:1947–1949.

SNYDER, S. H., 1973, personal communication.

SODERMAN, D. D., GERMERSHAUSEN, J., and KATZEN, M., 1973, Affinity binding of intact fat cells and their ghosts to immobilized insulin, *Proc. Natl. Acad. Sci.* **70**:792–796.

SONENBERG, M., 1971, Interaction of human growth hormone and human erythrocyte membranes studied by intrinsic fluorescence, *Proc. Natl. Acad. Sci.* **68**:1051–1055.

STADIE, W. C., HAUGAARD, N., and VAUGHAN, M., 1952, Studies of insulin binding with isotopically labelled insulin, *J. Biol. Chem.* **199**:729–739.

STADIE, W. C., HAUGAARD, N., and VAUGHAN, M., 1953, The quantitative relation between insulin and its biological activity, *J. Biol. Chem.* **220**:745–751.

STJARNE, L., 1964, Studies of catecholamine uptake storage and release mechanisms, *Acta Physiol. Scand* **62**:1–97 (Suppl. 228).

SUZUKI, F., DAKUHARA, Y., ONO, M., and TAKEDA, Y., 1972, Studies on the mode of action of insulin: Properties and biological activity of an insulin–dextran complex, *Endocrinology* **90**:1220–1230.

SYTKOWSKI, A. J., VOGEL, Z., and NIRENBERG, M. W., 1973, Development of acetylcholine receptor clusters on cultured muscle cells, *Proc. Natl. Acad. Sci.* **70**:270–274.

TELL, G. P. E., and CUATRECASAS, P., 1974, β-Adrenergic receptors: Stereo-specificity and lack of affinity for catechols, *Biochem. Biophys. Res. Commun.*, **57**:793–800.

TEMIN, H. M., PIERSON, R. W., Jr., and DULAK, N. C., 1972, The role of serum in the control of multiplication of avian and mammalian cells in culture, in: *Growth, Nutrition and Metabolism of Cells in Culture*, Vol. I, (V. I. Cristofalo and G. Rothblat, eds.), pp. 50–81, Academic Press, New York.

THORELL, J. I., and JOHANSSON, B. G., 1971, Enzymatic iodination of polypeptides with ^{125}I to high specific activity, *Biochim. Biophys. Acta* **251**:363–369.

TOMASI, V., KORETZ, S., RAY, T. K., DUNNICK, J., and MARINETTI, G. V., 1970, Hormone action at the membrane level. II. The binding of epinephrine and glucagon to the rat liver plasma membranes, *Biochim. Biophys. Acta* **211**:31–42.

TSUSHIMA, T., and FRIESEN, H. G., 1973, Radioreceptor assay for growth hormone, *J. Clin. Endocrinol. Metab.* **37**:334–337.

ULOTH, R. H., KIRK, J. R., GOULD, W. A., and LARSEN, A. A., 1966, Sulfonanilides. I. Monoalkyl-and arylsulfonamidophenethanolamines, *J. Med. Chem.* **9:**88–97.

VENTER, J. C., DIXON, J. E., MAROKO, P. R., and KAPLAN, N. O., 1972, Biologically active catecholamines covalently bound to glass beads, *Proc. Natl. Acad. Sci.* **69:**1141–1145.

VENTER, J. C., ROSS, J., Jr., DIXON, J., MAYER, S. E., and KAPLAN, N. D., 1973, Immobilized catecholamine and cocaine effects on contractibility of cardiac muscle, *Proc. Natl. Acad. Sci.* **70:**1214–1217.

WEINSTEIN, Y., MELMON, K. L., BOURNE, H. R., and SELA, M., 1973, Specific leukocyte receptors for small endogenous hormones: Detection by cell binding to insolubilized hormone derivatives, *J. Clin. Invest.* **52:**1349–1361.

WOLFE, B. B., ZIRROLLI, J. A., and MOLINOFF, P. B., Binding of [^{3}H]epinephrine to proteins of rat ventricular muscle: Nonidentity with beta adrenergic receptors, *Molec. Pharmacol.* **10:**582–596.

YALOW, R. S., and BERSON, S. A., 1966, Purification of ^{131}I parathyroid hormone with microfine granules of precipitated silica, *Nature* **212:**357–358.

YOUNG, A. B., and SNYDER, S. H., 1973, Strychnine binding associated with glycine receptors of the central nervous system, *Proc. Natl. Acad. Sci.* **70:**2832–2836.

ZULL, J. E., and REPKE, D. W., 1972, Studies with tritiated polypeptide hormones. The preparation and properties of an active, highly tritiated derivative of parathyroid hormone: Acetamidino-parathyroid hormone, *J. Biol. Chem.* **247:**2183–2188.

6

STRUCTURE–ACTIVITY RELATIONS FOR NEUROTRANSMITTER RECEPTOR AGONISTS AND ANTAGONISTS

A. S. Horn

1. INTRODUCTION

Until fairly recently, the only way of discovering anything about the nature of postsynaptic receptors for neurotransmitters was the time-honored method of studying the structure–activity relationships of agonists and antagonists. This information was usually incidental to the main practical preoccupation of finding compounds that were pharmacologically more active and specific. The nature of the information obtainable about receptors by this method is, of course, limited. One may show, for example, that in a particular drug certain chemical groups are essential for activity. Depending on the nature of these groups, it is possible to hypothesize binding via ionic or hydrogen bonds and van der Waals or hydrophobic interactions. However, the nature of the receptor components through which these interactions occur is in most cases totally unknown. There is also the problem that unless one works with conformationally rigid moelcules the actual shape of the drug on interaction with the receptor is uncertain. In recent years, more direct attempts have been made to learn something of the chemical

A. S. Horn ● MRC Neurochemical Pharmacology Unit, Department of Pharmacology, University of Cambridge, Cambridge, England

nature of various receptors by actual isolation of the macromolecules thought to comprise the receptor material. An extensive review of earlier work in this area using a variety of reversible and irreversible agonists and antagonists has been published (Ehrenpreis *et al.*, 1969). More recent studies are dealt with elsewhere in this series (Hollenberg and Cuatrecasas, Chap. 5, this volume; Changeux, Chap. 7, Vol. 6; Snyder, Chap. 6, Vol. 5).

Ariens (1971) has suggested that in the production of an effect by a drug on a specific receptor two essential parameters are distinguishable: the *affinity* and the *intrinsic activity* of the drug for the receptor. The affinity of the molecule is the initial tendency of the drug and receptor to interact, whereas the intrinsic activity is the ability of the bound drug to induce in the receptor the conformational changes required for production of a stimulus and hence an effect. Thus agonists possess both affinity and intrinsic activity, while antagonists have affinity but lack intrinsic activity, i.e., do not have the ability to bring about the conformational changes required to produce a stimulus. This dual concept is sometimes useful in the analysis of structure–activity relationships. In some instances, it is possible to show that certain moieties in the compound are of significance for the affinity of the drug while others are crucial for its intrinsic activity. The interaction between drug and receptor is thus seen as a mutual molding process similar to the "induced fit" concept for enzymes proposed by Koshland (1958).

The compounds whose structure–activity relationships at their respective receptor sites that are to be discussed are the biogenic amines

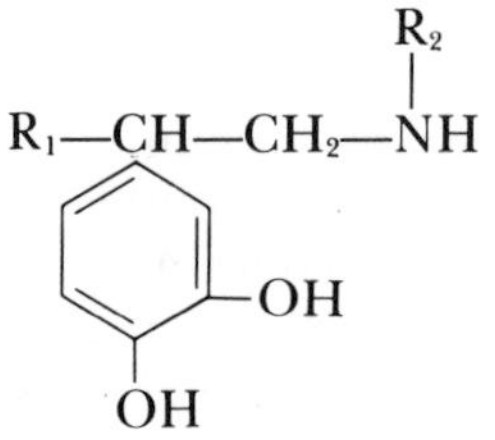

$$R_1—CH—CH_2—NH—R_2$$

Dopamine $R_1 = R_2 = H$
Norepinephrine $R_1 = OH$ $R_2 = H$
Epinephrine $R_1 = OH$ $R_2 = CH_3$

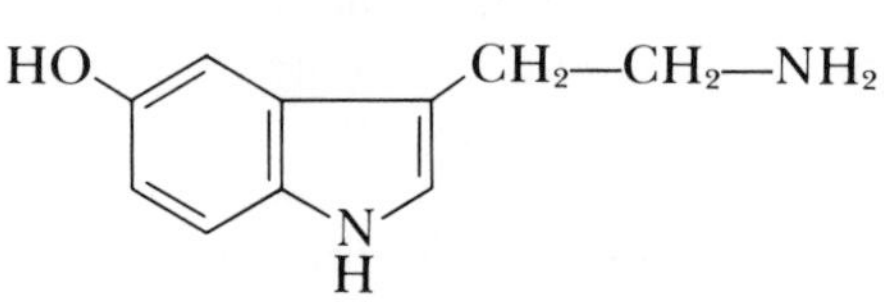

5-Hydroxytryptamine

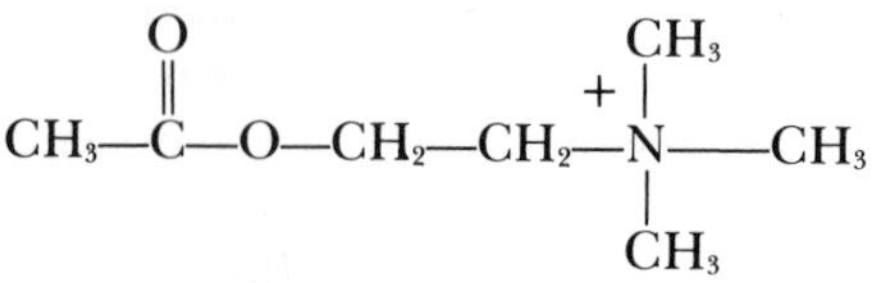

Acetylcholine

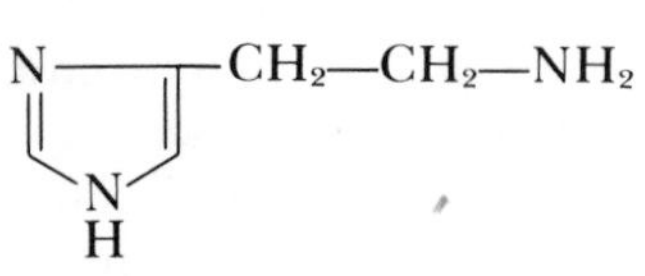

Histamine

FIG. 1. The biogenic amines.

norepinephrine . (NE), dopamine (DA), 5-hydroxytryptamine (5-HT), acetylcholine (ACh), and histamine (Fig. 1). Studies from both the peripheral and the central nervous systems will be included. The receptors for the amino acids, peptides, and opiates are dealt with elsewhere (Ryall, Chap. 3, Vol. 4; Kelly, Chap. 4, Vol. 4; McLennan, Chap. 5, Vol. 4; Nicoll, Chap. 6, Vol. 4; Snyder, Chap. 6, Vol. 5).

2. NOREPINEPHRINE

2.1. Peripheral Nervous System

In the peripheral sympathetic nervous system, there are two types of receptors with which norepinephrine and related substances can react. These were classified by Ahlquist (1948) as α- and β-receptors on the basis of their responses to various sympathomimetic amines. The effect on α-receptors is generally excitatory (vasoconstriction, myometrial contraction, contraction of dilator muscle of the pupil and splenic smooth muscle) and that on β-receptors is inhibitory (vasodilation, relaxation of the smooth muscle of bronchi, intestine, and uterus). There are, however, some exceptions to this general rule. The receptor site is merely responsible for the combination of the drug and not for the subsequent tissue response. Binding of a sympathomimetic agonist with similar types of receptors in different tissues can lead to diametrically opposite effects depending on the event sequence that the initial combination has set in motion. More recent work has shown that there may be subdivisions of these two main classes in some tissues (Furchgott, 1972).

2.1.1. α- and β-Agonists

The α- and β-agonists to be considered are all derivatives of the basic phenethylamine structure (Fig. 2). As both receptor types often occur in the same tissue, in order to obtain meaningful structure–activity relationships it is necessary to employ selective adrenergic blocking agents. A further complication is the fact that certain phenethylamines may bring about a sympathomimetic effect by an indirect action due to the release of norepinephrine, but this can be circumvented by the use of reserpine. The various possible sites of loss of a sympathomimetic amine in a test system,

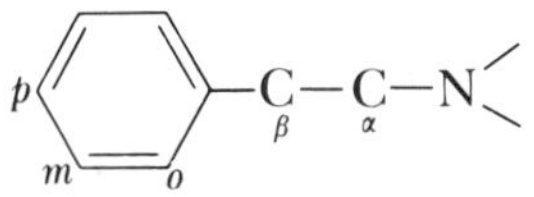

FIG. 2. Basic phenethylamine structure.

such as by uptake and enzymic inactivation, that may also affect agonist responses are described in a review by Furchgott (1972). Results from isolated muscles, perfused organs, and complete organ systems have resulted in the following generalizations (Ariens, 1967; Lands and Brown, 1967; Goodman and Gilman, 1970; Triggle, 1971).

a. *Length of the Side Chain.* Compounds with the highest α- and β-agonist activity have two carbon side chains separating the aromatic ring from the amino group.

b. *Amino Group Substitution (Tables 1 and 2).* Substitution of N-alkyl groups of increasing size produces a fall in the α-adrenergic activity and a rise in the β-adrenergic activity. However, N-methylation of a primary amine such as NE to produce epinephrine increases α-activity but further N-alkylation decreases it. Compounds with bulky substituents on the amino function such as aralkyl groups act as α-adrenergic blocking agents. This implies that they have an affinity for the α-receptors but lack intrinsic activity. In the case of β-adrenergic activity, amino group substitution leads to an increase in affinity while intrinsic activity is maintained. As it is known that at the β-carbon atom the stereochemical demands of the β-receptor are higher than those of the α-receptor, it has been suggested (Triggle, 1970)

TABLE 1

Effects of Various Sympathomimetic Amines on the Blood Pressure and Heart Rate in Reserpinized Cats

$$\text{CH—CH—NH}$$
$$\quad R_1 \quad R_2 \quad R_3$$

Compound	R_1	R_2	R_3	m	p	Relative effectiveness Blood pressure	Heart rate
Norepinephrine	OH	H	H	OH	OH	1000.0	1000.0
Epinephrine	OH	H	CH_3	OH	OH	144.0	1700.0
Phenylephrine	OH	H	CH_3	OH	H	49.0	8.6
Synephrine	OH	H	CH_3	H	OH	3.0	2.8
Metaraminol	OH	CH_3	H	OH	H	10	2.4
Phenylpropanolamine	OH	CH_3	H	H	H	1.8	0.8
Ephedrine	OH	CH_3	CH_3	H	H	0.6	5.0
m-Tyramine	H	H	H	OH	H	1.0	2.5
Tyramine	H	H	H	H	OH	inactive	

Data from Lands and Brown (1967) and Trendelenburg *et al.* (1962).

TABLE 2

Effect of N-Substituents in Norepinephrine Analogues on β-Mimetic Activity

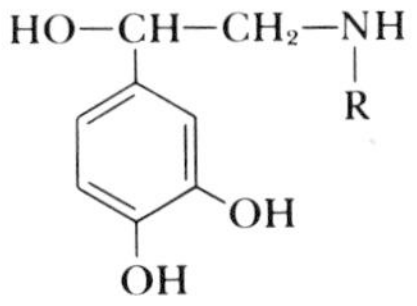

HO—CH—CH$_2$—NH
|
R

OH

OH

R	Relative vasodepressor activity
CH(CH$_3$)$_2$	100
CH(CH$_3$)C$_2$H$_5$	50
C$_2$H$_5$	50
Cyclopentyl	25
(CH$_2$)$_2$CH$_3$	20
CH$_2$CH(CH$_3$)$_2$	8
(CH$_2$)$_3$CH$_3$	6
n-C$_5$H$_{11}$	6
CH(C$_2$H$_5$)$_2$	4
CH(CH$_3$)CH(CH$_3$)$_2$	4
Cyclohexyl	3

Data from Lands and Tainter (1953).

that the increased bulk of the *N*-substituent may cause progressively greater structural changes in the receptor macromolecules, hence increasing stereoselectivity. At physiological pH, these *N*-alkyl homologues will all exist predominantly as the protonated species and it is unlikely that the small variations in pK are responsible for the large variations in activity (Triggle, 1971). It appears likely that the charged amine function interacts with its binding site through a cationic–anionic interaction and/or hydrogen bonding.

c. Substitution on the Aromatic Nucleus (Table 1). The presence of hydroxyl groups in the *m*- and *p*-positions produces the maximum α- and β-activity. Progressive elimination of the phenolic hydroxyl groups of catecholamines demonstrates that the *m*-hydroxyl group is more important than the *p*-hydroxyl for activity on both receptor types. Teleologically, this seems reasonable as it is the *m*-hydroxyl group that is methylated by COMT to produce metabolites that are weaker agonists, especially on β-receptors (Langer and Rubio, 1973). Removal of both hydroxyl groups produces a strong decrease in affinity for the α-receptor and a decrease in the intrinsic activity on the β-receptor. Phenylethanolamines, in fact, act as weak β-blocking agents. One of the phenolic hydroxyls of the catechol grouping can be replaced by an alkyl- or arylsulfonamide function which possess an acidic proton with a pK$_a$ similar to that of phenols and has a relatively similar steric disposition. For agonist activity, it is necessary for the sulfonamide group to be in the *m*-position (Larsen *et al.*, 1967). The methoxylated derivative, methoxamine (2,5-dimethoxyphenylpropanolamine), is a selective α-agonist which in large doses blocks β-receptors. 6-Methylepinephrine is less active on the blood pressure of the spinal cat than the parent compound (Singh Grewal, 1952). Lands (1952*a,b*) has studied the effects of a number of *m*-amino and *m*-fluoro analogues of epinephrine on the blood pressure of anesthetized dogs and has shown that they are weaker than the *m*-hydroxyl compound.

 d. Substitution on the α-Carbon Atom (Table 1). The compounds with substitutions on the α-carbon atom that have been studied were usually racemic mixtures. Substitution of α-alkyl groups in epinephrine and NE leads to a decrease in α-adrenergic agonist activity similar to that observed in the case of *N*-alkyl substitution (Lands and Tainter, 1953). α-Ethylnorepinephrine, however, is a potent agonist for both α- and β-receptors (Ahlquist, 1968). α-Methyl group substitution also seems to reduce β-adrenergic activity.

 e. Substitution on the β-Carbon Atom (Table 1). The naturally occurring epinephrine and NE have hydroxyl groups at the β-carbon atom and occur as the levorotatory isomers having the D or R configuration (Pratesi *et al.*, 1958, 1959). Utilizing the separate stereoisomers and racemates of epinephrine, NE, and isoproterenol, Ariens (1963) has shown that the stereoselectivity is much higher at the β- than at the α-receptor. NE and epinephrine exhibited D:L ratios of 4 and 8, respectively, at the α-receptor (rat vas deferens), while at the β-receptor (guinea pig atrium) the ratios were increased to 20 and 50, respectively. The D:L ratio for isoproterenol at the β-receptor was estimated to be greater than 500. Removal of the β-hydroxyl group leads to a decrease in activity on both receptor types (Barger and Dale, 1910; Cameron and Tainter, 1936; Lands *et al.*, 1947*a*, 1948). Removal of the β-hydroxyl group from isoproterenol leads to a compound that does not increase bronchodilation. β-Keto and β-amino compounds that have been studied appear to have activity similar to that of the catecholamines (Barger and Dale, 1910; Lands *et al.*, 1948; Lehmann and Randall, 1948).

 f. Absence of the Benzene Ring. Studies of the effects of replacement of the benzene ring by the nonaromatic, nonplanar cyclohexane ring on the blood pressure in anesthetized dogs have shown that the cyclohexane analogues are consistently less active than the aromatic compounds (Gunn and Gurd, 1940; Lands and Grant, 1972). Long-chain aliphatic amines have been found to possess only weak pressor activity (Barger and Dale, 1910; Swanson and Chen, 1946; Marsh *et al.*, 1951). In both the cyclohexyl and long-chain aliphatic series of amines, there is only a small degree of stereoselectivity (Lands *et al.*, 1947*b*; Swanson *et al.*, 1945).

 The structures of several agonists that are relatively selective for either α- or β-adrenergic receptors are shown in Fig. 3.

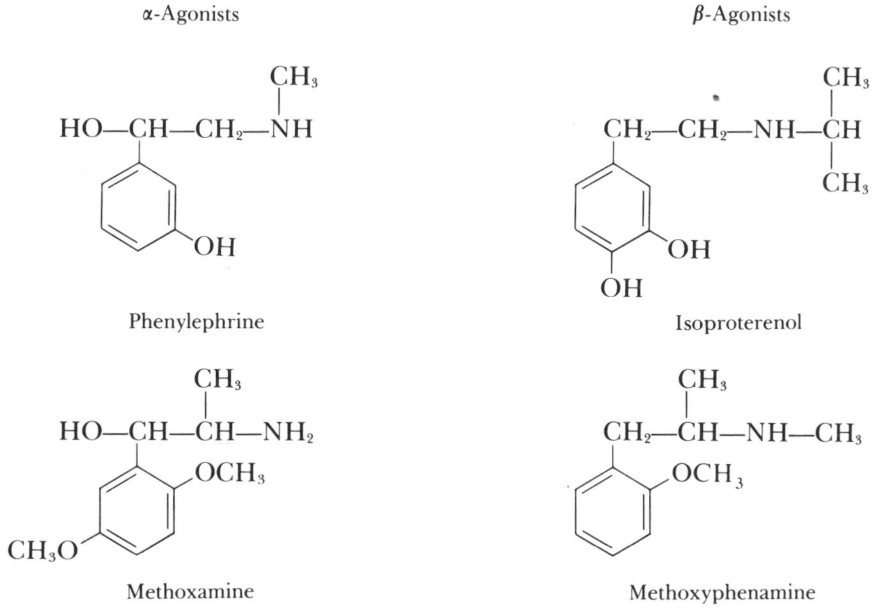

α-Agonists   β-Agonists

$$CH_3$$
$$HO—CH—CH_2—NH$$

$$OH$$

Phenylephrine

$$CH_3$$
$$CH_2—CH_2—NH—CH$$
$$CH_3$$

$$OH$$
$$OH$$

Isoproterenol

$$CH_3$$
$$HO—CH—CH—NH_2$$
$$OCH_3$$
$$CH_3O$$

Methoxamine

$$CH_3$$
$$CH_2—CH—NH—CH_3$$
$$OCH_3$$

Methoxyphenamine

FIG. 3. Selective α- and β-adrenergic agonists.

2.1.2. α- and β-Antagonists

Unlike the agonists that have just been dealt with, structure–activity analyses for the α- and β-antagonists are more difficult, as in many cases only a small number of compounds have been studied and their sites and mechanisms of action remain to be elucidated. These antagonists, or "adrenolytics" as they are sometimes called, were developed in the hope that they might be useful as antihypertensive agents. In some instances, compounds of clinical value have been discovered.

a. α-Antagonists. As can be seen from Fig. 4, the α-antagonists are comprised of a rather diverse group of molecular structures which often bear little structural resemblance to the catecholamines. It is possible that information gained from structure–activity studies is not related to the α-adrenoceptor site but to some other site of interaction in the sequence of events initiated by normal agonist–receptor combination.

In 1906, Dale showed that ergot alkaloids antagonize the pressor effects of epinephrine and sympathetic nerve stimulation. These alkaloids are peptide derivatives of lysergic acid. Reduction of the 9,10-double bond yields compounds such as dihydroergocornine, which is a more potent α-antagonist than the unsaturated compound. Derivatives of 2-(2-methoxyphenoxy)ethylamine where R is allyloxypropanol, p-methoxyphenylbutyl, or 2,5-dimethoxyphenoxypropyl have undergone

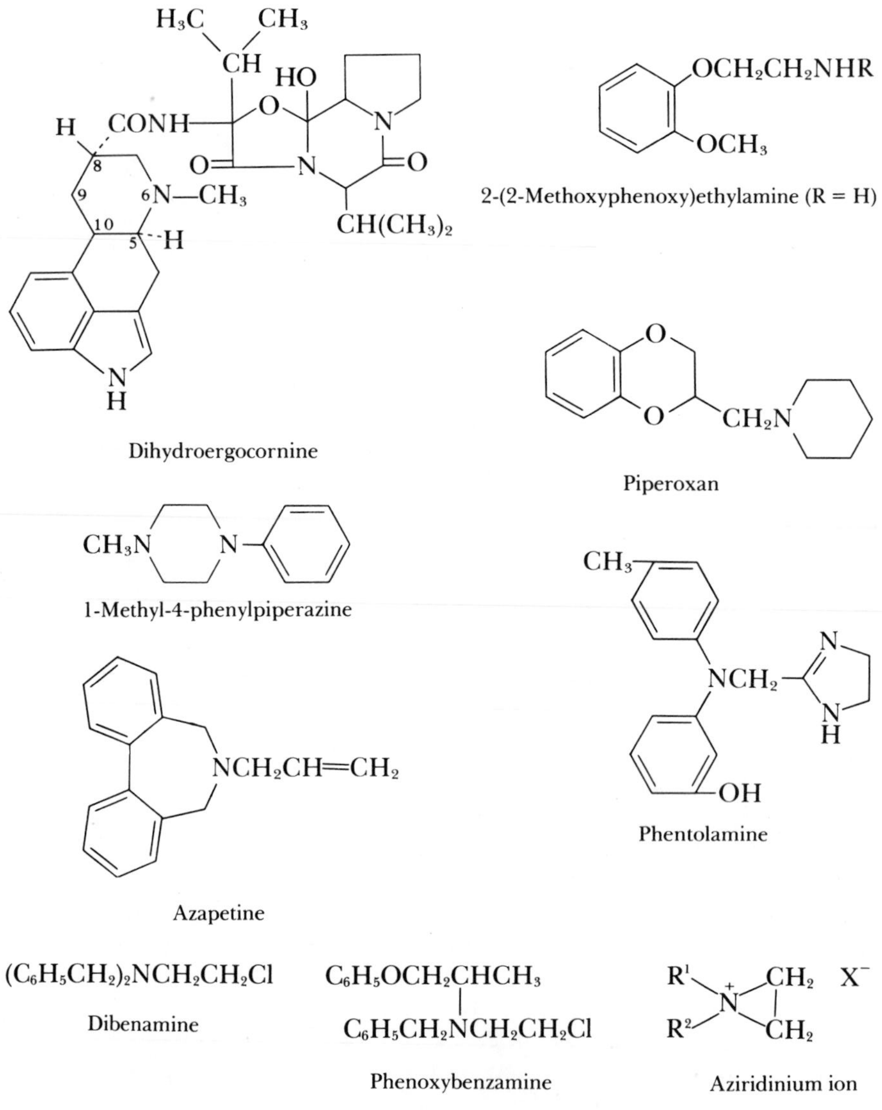

FIG. 4. Structures of various α-adrenergic antagonists.

clinical trial and were shown to produce short-lived reductions in blood pressure. Benzodioxanes such as piperoxan have been studied quite extensively (Werner and Barrett, 1967). In general, aromatic substituents decrease activity and secondary amines are as effective as the tertiary compounds. 1-Methyl-4-phenylpiperazine was shown by Bovet and Bovet-Nitti (1948) to possess weak adrenolytic properties. The phenyl group is essential for activity, but more potent compounds have resulted from varying the substituent on the other nitrogen atom (Werner and Barrett, 1967). The imidazoline derivative phentolamine is a potent α-adrenolytic (Urech *et al.*, 1950) and is used for peripheral vascular disease. Azapetine is also a potent α-adrenergic blocker that has clinical value. Dibenamine and phenoxybenzamine are well-known examples of the class of potent irreversible α-blockers. These compounds form aziridinium ions (Fig. 4) under physiological conditions. This three-membered ring is highly reactive and can be opened by suitable nucleophilic groups, leading to covalent attachment. Structure–activity relationships in this area have been reviewed (Triggle, 1971).

   b. β-Receptor Antagonists. The structural similarity between β-receptor agonists and antagonists is much closer than was evident for agents acting at α-receptors (Fig. 5). For example, removal of the catechol grouping in isoproterenol or its replacement by chorine atoms leads to compounds that are β-adrenergic blocking agents (Powell and Slater, 1958). Various aspects of β-receptor antagonists have been dealt with in reviews (Ariens, 1967;

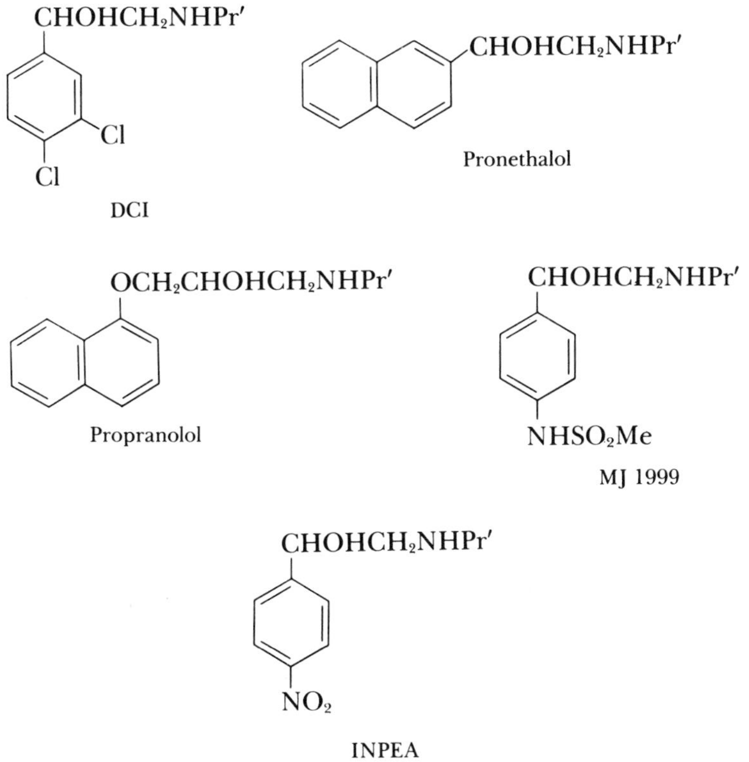

CHOHCH$_2$NHPr′

Cl
Cl

DCI

CHOHCH$_2$NHPr′

Pronethalol

OCH$_2$CHOHCH$_2$NHPr′

Propranolol

CHOHCH$_2$NHPr′

NHSO$_2$Me

MJ 1999

CHOHCH$_2$NHPr′

NO$_2$

INPEA

FIG. 5. Structures of various β-adrenergic antagonists.

Ahlquist, 1968; Dollery *et al.*, 1969; Harrison, 1971). The action of dichloroisoproterenol (DCI), the first drug shown to produce a specific blockade of β-adrenergic receptors, was complicated by the fact that it is also a partial agonist. This fact led to the development of pronethalol and then propranolol, which is largely without intrinsic activity (Black *et al.*, 1965; Blinks, 1967). The analysis below will deal mainly with variations in the dichloroisoproterenol molecule (Ariens, 1967; Corrodi *et al.*, 1863).

Amino group substitution: As in the case of the β-agonists, there is an increase in affinity for the β-receptor in a series of antagonists based on the dichloroisoproterenol and pronethalol molecules with increasing N-alkyl substitution. Branched alkyl groups such as isopropyl and tertiary butyl are more effective than unbranched groups (Ariens, 1967).

Substitution on the aromatic nucleus: It was mentioned previously that removal of both phenolic hydroxyl groups from catecholamines results in phenylethanolamines that act as weak β-adrenergic blocking agents. Introduction of a chlorine atom or a methyl group in the *m-* or *p*-position in compounds having an N-isopropyl group results in an increase in the affinity for β-receptors by these antagonists. Introduction of ethyl and larger alkyl groups produces less active compounds (Corrodi *et al.*, 1963).

Substitution on the α-carbon atom: Substitution in the side chain of α-methyl groups results in a decrease in β-blocking activity (Corrodi *et al.*, 1963).

Substitution on the β-carbon atom: The presence of a hydroxyl group in the β-position is important for antagonist activity. Where the separate stereoisomers have been studied, large ratios for the separate activities have been found (Burns *et al.*, 1964; Howe, 1963; Kvam *et al.*, 1965). Certain of the most active isomers have been shown to have the R configuration (Howe, 1963). It is of interest that although these antagonists do have local anesthetic action there are no essential differences between the stereoisomers in this respect. Desoxy analogues of propranolol possess only weak blocking activity.

Barrett (1972) has reviewed the design of β-adrenergic receptor blocking agents.

2.2. Adrenergic Receptors in the CNS

Microiontophoretic studies of adrenergic receptor types in the central nervous system using a variety of antagonists in areas such as the spinal cord (Biscoe *et al.*, 1966) and thalamus (Phillis and Tebecis, 1967) and agonists and antagonists in the brain stem (Boakes *et al.*, 1971) of the cat have led to the conclusion that in these areas the central adrenergic receptors differ in their drug sensitivity from those in the peripheral nervous system and are not readily defined as α and β types. In the olfactory bulb, however, the

NE-induced slowing of the firing rate of cells was antagonized by the α-adrenergic blocking agents dibenamine and phentolamine while β-antagonists were ineffective (Bloom *et al.*, 1964). On neurons of the lateral vestibular nucleus of Deiters, NE produced excitation that was antagonized by the β-adrenolytic DCI but not by the α-adrenolytics dibenamine and phentolamine (Yamamoto, 1967). Recent extensive studies of an adrenergic receptor on the Purkinje cells of the rat cerebellum are dealt with elsewhere (Bloom, Chap. 1, Vol. 6).

2.3. Possible Modes of Action

2.3.1. The β-Adrenoceptor

The catecholamines are known to exert a regulatory action on the turnover and cellular levels of cyclic AMP by alterations in the catalytic activity of adenylate cyclase (Robison *et al.*, 1967). To date, the best-characterized β-receptor-mediated response via stimulation of adenylate cyclase is the acceleration of glycogenolysis in skeletal muscle (Mayer and Stull, 1971). Bloom and Goldman (1966) and Belleau (1967) have suggested that the β-receptor could be part of the active center of the adenylate cyclase system. The former authors consider the receptor to be composed of "adenylate cyclase–ATP," the enzyme–substrate complex. The binding of the agonist at the active center of the complex is thought to result in the hydrolysis of the terminal phosphate group by the mechanism shown in Fig. 6. Robison *et al.* (1967) have suggested that the adenylate cyclase consists of two types of subunits; a regulatory unit directed toward the exterior of the cell and a catalytic unit whose active site is directed to the cell interior. It is

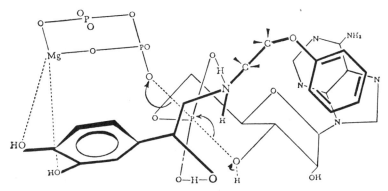

Fɪɢ. 6. A possible mechanism for the intramolecular hydrolysis by β-adrenergic agonists of ATP bound to adenylate cyclase. From Bloom and Goldman (1966); reproduced with permission.

possible that either of these subunits could possess different hormonal specificities in different tissues. One of the difficulties in testing these proposals is that of solubilizing and purifying the membrane-bound adenylate cyclase.

2.3.2. The α-Adrenergic Receptor

It has been suggested that α-adrenoceptor effects could result from a fall in the level of cyclic AMP (Robison *et al.*, 1971), and there is some evidence for this proposal (Turtle and Kipnis, 1967; Burns *et al.*, 1971). In blood platelets, however, there is little evidence to link α-receptor activation with changes in cyclic AMP (Born, 1971; Cole *et al.*, 1971).

Bloom and Goldman (1966) and Belleau (1967) have suggested that the α-adrenergic receptor consists of an enzyme–substrate complex of ATPase and ATP. Thus excitatory α-adrenergic responses, such as smooth muscle contraction, involve the catecholamine-mediated enzymatic hydrolysis of ATP to ADP via a specific magnesium-activated ATPase. It has been shown that α-adrenergic activation results in a change in the ionic permeability of

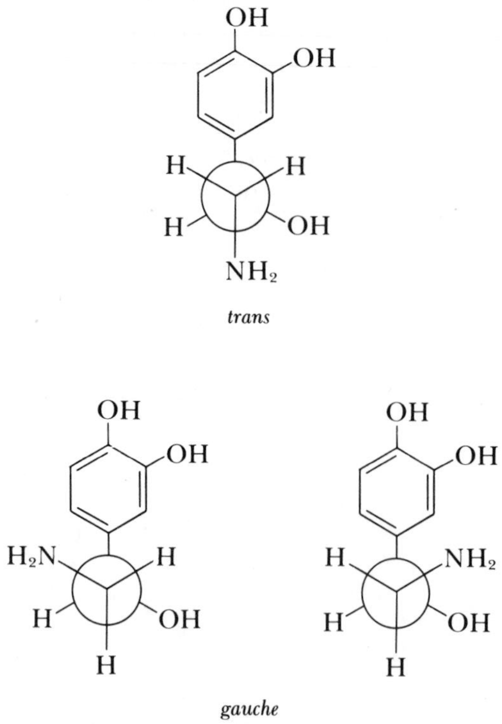

FIG. 7. Newman projections of the staggered conformers of norepinephrine.

the cell membrane of several tissues, such as intestinal smooth muscle and guinea pig liver (Haylett and Jenkinson, 1972). It is also possible that α-receptors may initiate contraction in smooth muscle by releasing intracellular calcium (Triggle, 1972). Further aspects of the action of catecholamines on cyclic AMP in the CNS are dealt with elsewhere (Daly, Chap. 2, Vol. 5).

2.4. Crystallographic, NMR, and Theoretical Studies of the Conformation of NE

The X-ray structure of norepinephrine HCl has been determined (Carlstrom and Bergin, 1967). The preferred conformation in the solid state is *trans* (Fig. 7). The crystal structures of various sympathomimetic amines have been reviewed by Carlstrom *et al.* (1973). Nuclear magnetic resonance (NMR) analysis of NE has also shown that the *trans* conformer is the preferred form in solution (Ison *et al.*, 1973). Theoretical calculations have led to similar results (Kier, 1968a; Pederson *et al.*, 1971; Pullman *et al.*, 1972). Some workers, however, have suggested that the *gauche* form is the preferred conformation (Katz *et al.*, 1973).

3. DOPAMINE

3.1. Dopamine Receptors in the Mammalian Peripheral and Central Nervous Systems

To date, no neurons containing solely DA have been reported in the periphery of higher animals. In the renal artery of the dog, however, low doses of DA cause an increase in renal blood flow (McNay *et al.*, 1965), and more recent work has supported the possible existence of DA receptors in the renal vasculature (Goldberg *et al.*, 1968; Bell and Lang, 1973).

In the mammalian CNS, histochemical fluorescence (Fuxe, 1965; Ungerstedt, 1971) and pharmacological studies (for review, see Hornykiewicz, 1966) have provided evidence for DA being located in specific neuronal tracts, the most prominent being that between the substantia nigra and the caudate nucleus. The two other prominent dopaminergic systems are the mesolimbic and tuberoinfundibular pathways. Biochemical quantitation of the amounts of DA in certain nuclei in these two pathways has been reported (Cuello *et al.*, 1973; Horn *et al.*, 1974). Electrophysiological studies have provided evidence that DA is probably an inhibitory transmitter in the nigrostriatal system (see York, Chap. 2, Vol. 6).

3.2. Dopamine Receptors in Invertebrates

The stretch receptor of the crayfish *Pacifastacus leniusculus* is strongly inhibited by DA, which is about 10 times more active than epinephrine or NE in this system (McGeer *et al.*, 1961). In the brain of the snail *Helix aspersa*, DA has been shown to inhibit the spontaneous firing of certain neurons and there is increasing evidence that it is an inhibitory transmitter in this invertebrate (Kerkut and Walker, 1961; Kerkut, 1973; Woodruff, 1971). In *Aplysia*, DA receptors occur on the axons of certain neurons and DA elicits both excitation and inhibition in this system (see Ascher and Kehoe, Chap. 7, Vol. 4).

3.3. Structure-Activity Relationships of DA Receptor Agonists and Antagonists in the Mammalian Peripheral Nervous System

Goldberg *et al.* (1968) investigated the structural requirements for DA-like activity in the renal artery of the dog (Table 3). Of the 45 compounds examined, only *N*-methyldopamine (epinine) had definite dopaminergic activity. Although apomorphine also produced renal vasodilation, it was not certain that the two compounds had the same mechanism of action. *N*-Ethyldopamine and *N*-isopropyldopamine were classified as mainly β-adrenergic. The stereoisomers of α-methyldopamine were inactive. It was concluded that the structural requirements for DA-like activity in this preparation are more specific than are those for activity at α- and β-adrenergic receptors. The effect of DA on the renal artery can be blocked by haloperidol (Yeh *et al.*, 1969) and chlorpromazine (Brotzu, 1970), which supports the concept of a DA receptor being involved in this effect.

3.4. Structure-Activity Relationships of DA Receptor Agonists and Antagonists in Invertebrates

Woodruff and Walker (1969) have conducted a structure–activity study of DA agonists and antagonists of neurons of *Helix aspersa*. It was found, as in the renal artery of the dog, that only epinine had a potency comparable to that of DA. Epinephrine, NE, 5-HT, and α-methyldopamine were 10–100 times less potent. Even in doses of up to 1000 times that of DA, other analogues were without dopaminergic activity (Table 4). Hydroxyl groups in the *m*- and *p*-positions of the benzene ring were required for activity; a single *p*-hydroxyl group was not sufficient. Methylation of the *m*-hydroxyl group resulted in an inactive compound. A β-hydroxyl group in the side chain reduced DA-like activity. It was concluded that the action of DA on these neurons is mediated by a specific DA receptor rather than by either an α- or a β-adrenergic receptor. The structural requirements for activity were found

TABLE 3

Relationship Between Chemical Structure and Actions of Phenethylamines on the Renal Vascular Bed

Compound	Predominant type of activity
Dopamine	Dopamine-like
Epinine	β-Adrenergic
Isoproterenol	β-Adrenergic
l-Epinephrine	β-Adrenergic
l-Norepinephrine	β-Adrenergic
Kephrine	β-Adrenergic
Isopropyldopamine	β-Adrenergic
Ethyldopamine	β-Adrenergic
d-Norepinephrine	β-Adrenergic
d-Amphetamine	Nonselective
Ephedrine	Nonselective
Pseudoephedrine	Nonselective
Mephentermine	Nonselective
Dimethyldopamine	Inactive
N-Acetyldopamine	Inactive
l-α-Methyldopamine	Inactive
d-α-Methyldopamine	Inactive
Cobefrin	Inactive
Tyramine	Inactive
Sympatol	Inactive
Paredrine	Inactive
Metatyramine	Inactive
Phenylephrine	Inactive
Metaraminol	Inactive
Phenylethylamine	Inactive
Fenfluramine	Inactive

Data from Goldberg *et al.* (1968).

to be a catechol grouping in the *m*- and *p*-positions and the presence of a terminal amino group either unsubstituted or having one methyl group.

Derivatives of lysergic acid such as LSD and ergometrine are potent antagonists of DA's action on this receptor, while chlorpromazine and haloperidol are inactive.

3.5. DA Receptor Agonists and Antagonists in the Mammalian CNS

3.5.1. Introduction

In the rat, amphetamine increases spontaneous locomotor activity and induces stereotyped motor responses such as compulsive gnawing and sniffing. That amphetamine's action is indirect is shown by the fact that these

TABLE 4

Effect of Various Phenethylamine Analogues on Dopaminergic Neurons
of Helix aspersa

Compound	Ratio agonist/dopamine[a]
Dopamine	1
N-Methyldopamine	0.5–2.2
5-Methoxydopamine	16.5
(−)-Noradrenaline	17.3
(+)-α-Methyldopamine	30.7
(−)-Adrenaline	91.8
Isoprenaline	
Orciprenaline	
(±)-Octopamine	
Tyramine	
(−)-Metaraminol	
(±)-Oxedrine	>1000
Hydroxyamphetamine	
3-Methoxydopamine	
Methoxytyramine	
3,4-Dimethoxydopamine	
Methoxamine	
Apomorphine	

Data from Woodruff and Walker (1969).
[a]Equipotent molar doses (for dopamine: approximately 0.005 μmol). Experiments
were performed on the parietal ganglion of the isolated brain of *Helix aspersa*.

effects are blocked by the catecholamine synthesis inhibitor α-methyl-*p*-
tyrosine (Randrup and Munkvad, 1970; Weisman *et al.*, 1966). It is thought
that amphetamine induces these effects by releasing and/or inhibiting the
uptake of NE and DA (Carlsson *et al.*, 1966; Scheel-Kruger, 1972; Carr and
Moore, 1970; Glowinski, 1970; Horn *et al.*, 1974). By using relatively specific
inhibitors of dopamine β-hydroxylase such as diethyldithiocarbamate
(DDC), it has been possible to show that the stereotyped behavior is probably
due to activity in a dopaminergic system (Randrup and Scheel-Kruger,
1966). Apomorphine also produces stereotypy in rats, but unlike amphetamine its mode of action is most probably by direct receptor stimulation
(Anden *et al.*, 1967; Ernst, 1967). The clinically efficacious neuroleptics such
as chlorpromazine and haloperidol are able to specifically block these
stereotyped effects (Randrup *et al.*, 1963; Janssen *et al.*, 1967). *In vivo* studies
have further shown that the neuroleptic drugs accelerate the synthesis and
turnover of DA formed from [14C]tyrosine in the brains of rats and mice
(Nyback and Sedvall, 1968; Nyback, 1971). It is thought that this accelerated
turnover is probably due to a dopaminergic receptor blockade which results
in a compensatory feedback mechanism of a biochemical or neuronal nature

activating the presynaptic neurons (Carlsson and Lindqvist, 1963; Anden *et al.*, 1964; Laverty and Sharman, 1965; Da Prada and Pletscher, 1966; see also Sedvall, Chap. 5, Vol. 6). Studies using metabolites of chlorpromazine have shown that desmethyl-, didesmethyl-, and 7-hydroxychlorpromazine as well as chlorpromazine N-oxide all accelerate accumulation and disappearance of [^{14}C]DA to about the same extent as chlorpromazine, while chlorpromazine sulfoxide is inactive (Nyback and Sedvall, 1972). Studies on the antagonism of amphetamine-induced stereotyped behavior in rats by chlorpromazine metabolites have shown that at 50 mg/kg chlorpromazine blocks this effect while chlorpromazine N-oxide and desmethyl-, and 7-hydroxychlorpromazine are all less potent. Chlorpromazine sulfoxide, 6-hydroxy-, 8-hydroxy-, and didesmethylchlorpromazine were all inactive (Lal and Sourkes, 1972). Using a variety of test procedures based on functional, biochemical, and histochemical techniques, Anden *et al.* (1970) have examined the specificity of various neuroleptics as blockers of either neostriatal DA or spinal NE receptors. It was shown that pimozide and fluspirilene blocked only DA receptors. Spiroperidol, perphenazine, fluphenazine, clopenthixol, flupenthixol, haloperidol, and methylperidol were predominantly DA receptor blockers and had only a small effect on NE receptors. However, chlorpromazine, thioridazine, and chlorprothixene blocked both DA and NE receptors. Phenoxybenzamine was shown to block only NE receptors. A common complication in the clinical use of the neuroleptics is the production of extrapyramidal motor disorders (Klein and Davis, 1969). It is thought that this may be due in some cases to a

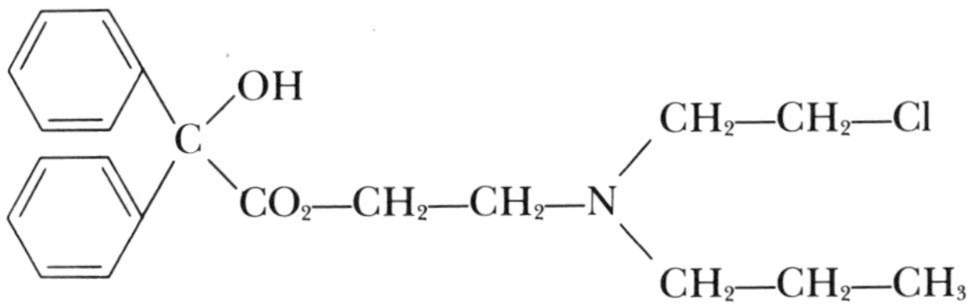

N-Propylbenzilylcholine mustard

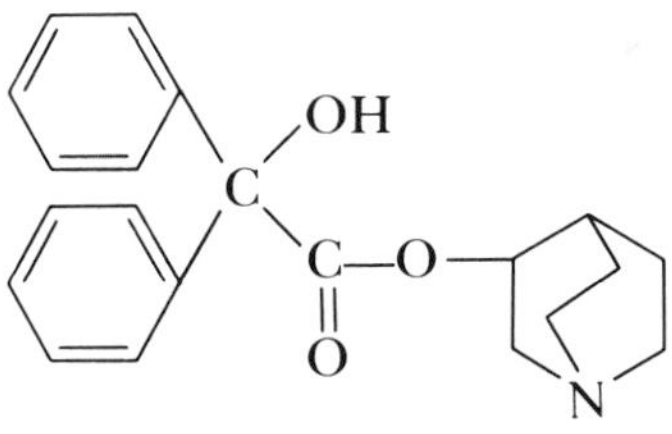

3-Quinuclidinyl benzilate

FIG. 8. Muscarinic antagonists.

TABLE 5

Dissociation Equilibrium Constants of Various Drugs for Cortical Muscarinic Receptors

Drug	Dissociation equilibrium constant[a] (M)	IC$_{50}$ for striatal dopamine-sensitive adenylate cyclase[b] (M)
Atropine	$5.2 \pm 0.3 \times 10^{-10}$	—
Benztropine	$1.3 \pm 0.1 \times 10^{-8}$	$>10^{-4}$
Ethopropazine	$1.0 \pm 0.1 \times 10^{-8}$	—
Thioridazine	$2.5 \pm 0.1 \times 10^{-8}$	3.0×10^{-6}
Clozapine	$5.5 \pm 1.0 \times 10^{-8}$	4.5×10^{-6}
Chlorpromazine	$3.5 \pm 0.2 \times 10^{-7}$	1.0×10^{-6}
Pimozide	$1.6 \pm 0.1 \times 10^{-6}$	4.5×10^{-6}
Trifluoperazine	$4.0 \pm 0.4 \times 10^{-6}$	4.0×10^{-7}
Flupenthixol	$2.2 \pm 0.8 \times 10^{-6}$	7.0×10^{-8}
Spiroperidol	$1.2 \pm 0.1 \times 10^{-5}$	2.0×10^{-6}

[a]Data from Miller and Hiley (1974).
[b]Data from Miller and Iversen (1974).

blockade of dopamine receptors leading to a predominance of cholinergic activity in the basal ganglia. Certain of these side effects are usually alleviated by the use of centrally acting anticholinergic drugs (Freyhan, 1961). The neuroleptics differ quite considerably, however, in the degree to which they produce extrapyramidal disorders; for example, clozapine and thioridazine produce fewer side effects than trifluoperazine and haloperidol (Klein and Davis, 1969; Shader and DiMascio, 1970). Several workers have suggested that those neuroleptics that produce fewer extrapyramidal effects owe this to their anticholinergic activity (Miller and Hiley, 1974; Snyder *et al.*, 1974). By use of the irreversible muscarinic antagonist N-propylbenzilylcholine mustard (Miller and Hiley, 1974) (Fig. 8) and the reversible antagonist quinuclidinyl benzilate (Snyder *et al.*, 1974) (Fig. 8), it has been shown that the tendency to produce extrapyramidal side effects is inversely proportional to the neuroleptic's affinity for the muscarinic receptor (Table 5).

3.5.2. The Neuroleptics

The four main classes of neuroleptics now in clinical use are the phenothiazines (chlorpromazine), the thioxanthenes (flupenthixol), the butyrophenones (haloperidol), and the diphenylbutyl piperidines (pimozide) (Fig. 9). Although they exhibit a range of pharmacological activity, there is increasing evidence, as previously discussed, that their ability to block dopamine receptors in the CNS may be related to their antipsychotic effects (Anden *et al.*, 1970; Matthysse, 1973; Snyder, 1972; Horn and Snyder, 1971). The structure–activity relationships that will be

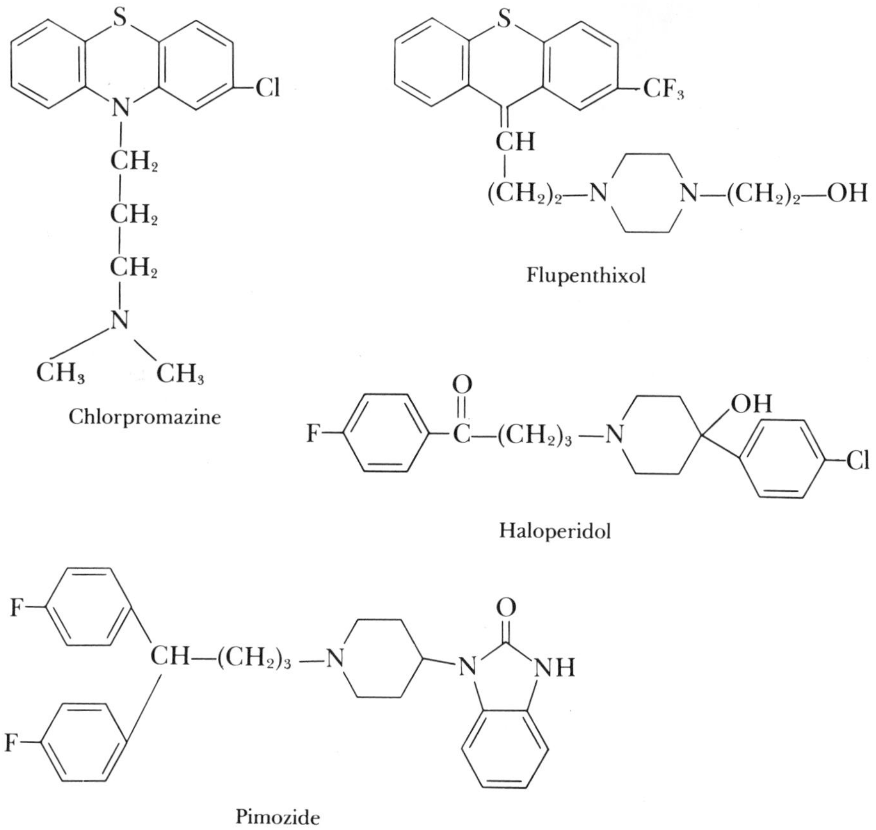

Chlorpromazine

Flupenthixol

Haloperidol

Pimozide

FIG. 9. The neuroleptics.

discussed below have been obtained from a variety of screening procedures (Janssen, 1965, 1973; Janssen *et al.*, 1967; Gordon, 1967; Zirkle and Kaiser, 1970; Petersen and Møller-Nielsen, 1964).

a. Phenothiazines. The side Chain (Table 6A): In general, a basic amino group separated by three carbon atoms from the phenothiazine nucleus is optimal for antipsychotic activity. Shortening or branching of the side chain decreases neuroleptic activity and produces compounds that are predominantly antihistamines.

The basic amino group (Table 6A): A basic tertiary amino group provides maximum potency. The compounds containing secondary and primary amines are generally less potent. Activity is also decreased when the dimethylamino group in chlorpromazine is replaced by pyrrolidino, morpholino, or thiomorpholino groups. Substitution of a 4-methyl-1-piperazino

TABLE 6A

Effect of Various Side Chains and 2-Substituents in Phenothiazines on the Antiapomorphine Test

Compound	X	R	Antiapomorphine test (chlorpromazine index[a])
Promazine	H	b	0.03
Methopromazine	OCH$_3$	b	0.25
Acepromazine	COCH$_3$	b	1.0
Chlorpromazine	Cl	b	1.0
Propionylpromazine	COC$_2$H$_5$	b	1.0
Triflupromazine	CF$_3$	b	4.0
Perazine	H	c	0.3
Prochlorperazine	Cl	c	2.2
Thiethylperazine	SC$_2$H$_5$	c	4.0
Trifluoperazine	CF$_3$	c	25
Butyrylperazine	CO-n-C$_3$H$_7$	c	40
Thioperazine	SO$_2$N(CH$_3$)$_2$	c	250
Perphenazine	Cl	d	50
Acetophenazine	COCH$_3$	d	100
Carphenazine	COC$_2$H$_5$	d	125

[a]The potency of various phenothiazines relative to chlorpromazine, which is assigned a value of 1, in antagonizing the emesis produced by apomorphine in dogs. Data from Zirkle and Kaiser (1970).
[b]R = (CH$_2$)$_3$N(CH$_3$)$_2$.

[c]R = (CH$_2$)$_3$N⟨⟩NCH$_3$.

[d]R = (CH$_2$)$_3$N⟨⟩N(CH$_2$)$_2$OH.

group (*cf.* trifluoperazine) in the side chain leads to a significant enhancement in activity. Potency is further increased by introduction of a 2-hydroxyethyl group on the 4-position of the piperazino ring (*cf.* fluphenazine).

Aromatic ring substituents (Table 6B): For maximum neuroleptic potency, a substituent in the 2-position is necessary. Some of the 2-substituents in the more potent neuroleptics are —CF$_3$, —SO$_2$CF$_3$, —SCF$_3$, —Cl, and —Br. Substitution in the 3-position also increases the activity of the compound in comparison to that of the parent molecule, but this effect is less significant

TABLE 6B

Effect of Aryl Substituents in Promazine on Neuroleptic Potency

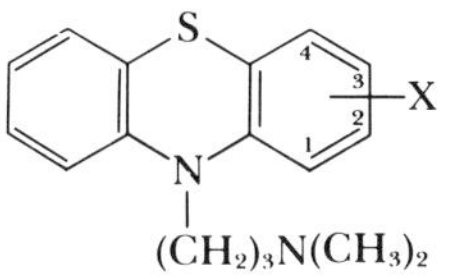

$(CH_2)_3N(CH_3)_2$

X	Relative potency in blocking conditioned response in rats[a]
H	0.07
2-Cl	1
3-Cl	0.18
2-OCH$_3$	0.07
2-CO$_2$CH$_3$	0.49
2-CONHNH$_2$	0.07
2-CF$_3$	1.7
3-CF$_3$	0.43
4-CF$_3$	0.06
2-CH$_3$	0.28
2-CH(CH$_3$)$_2$	0.32
2-C(CH$_3$)$_3$	0.18

[a]Intraperitoneal dose (mg/kg) blocking conditioned reflex in 50% of rats compared with a similar dose of chlorpromazine. Data from Zirkle and Kaiser (1970).

than for the 2-position. Introduction of substituents in the 1- or 4-position of an unsubstituted phenothiazine or in the 7- or 8-position of chlorpromazine produces a fall in activity. The decrease in potency when the substituent on position 2 is moved to other positions is apparently not due to an alteration in such physical properties as membrane activity, ionization constants, lipid solubility, or the ability to penetrate the blood–brain barrier (Green, 1967).

Other aromatic ring systems: Replacement of one benzene ring by a pyridine system has an adverse effect on neuroleptic activity. Substitution of the sulfur atom in phenothiazines by an oxygen atom produces the phenoxazines, which are less potent neuroleptics. Introduction of selenium instead of sulfur yields the phenoselenazines, which are intermediate in potency between the phenothiazines and the phenoxazines. Replacement of the sulfur bridge by a saturated carbon atom yields the acridans, which have a neuroleptic potency similar to that of the phenoselenazines. The need for an "angled" tricyclic ring system is shown by the fact that phenothiazine analogues having flat, fully aromatic ring systems such as the acridines and anthracenes are generally very weak or inactive as neuroleptics.

b. *Thioxanthenes (Table 7).* The thioxanthenes may be regarded as analogues of the phenothiazines in which the nitrogen atom of the phenothiazine nucleus has been replaced by an unsaturated carbon atom. As a result of the unsaturated side chain, if there is a 2-substituent on the aromatic nucleus there is the possibility of *cis–trans* geometrical isomerism (Petersen and Møller-Nielsen, 1964). If the 2-substituent and the side chain are on the same side of the double bond, this isomer is designated as the *cis* form. Where the isomers have been separated, one form has been found to be much more active than the other (Møller-Nielsen *et al.*, 1962, 1973). In the case of chlorprothixene and thiothixene, X-ray crystallographic analysis has shown that the active compound has the *cis* configuration (Dunitz *et al.*, 1964; Schaefer, 1967; Post *et al.*, 1974). Far fewer thioxanthenes than phenothiazines have been synthesized. In general, however, the structural requirements for activity are as follows:

1. The presence of a double bond at carbon 9. Reduction of this bond leads to a decrease in activity.
2. A substituent at the 2-position. This can take the form of a halogen, $-OCH_3$, $-CF_3$, etc.
3. The 2-substituent and the side chain in a *cis* configuration to each other. It is only for chlorprothixene and thiothixene, however, that the configuration is known with certainty. The original claim for the active isomer having the *trans* configuration was based on less accurate physical measurements.

TABLE 7

Comparison of Various Thioxanthenes Against Other Neuroleptics

	Test			
	Apomorphine stereotypy, rat	Apomorphine stereotypy, dog	Apomorphine vomiting, dog	Amphetamine stereotypy, rat
	ED_{50} mg/kg i.p.	ED_{50} mg/kg s.c.	ED_{50} mg/kg s.c.	ED_{50} mg/kg s.c.
α,β-Flupenthixol	0.5	0.08	0.02	0.2
α-Flupenthixol	0.3	0.06	0.01	0.07
β-Flupenthixol	>80	—	3.5	>160
Clopenthixol	30	3.2	0.04	0.2
Chlorprothixene	45	6.0	0.9	0.5
Fluphenazine	0.2	0.02	0.01	0.08
Perphenazine	0.5	0.6	0.06	0.09
Chlorpromazine	59	>20	0.6	0.6
Haloperidol	2.6	0.2	0.01	0.02

Data from Møller-Nielsen *et al.* (1973).

TABLE 8

Effect of Various Side Chains in Butyrophenones on the Antiapomorphine and Antiamphetamine Tests

$$F\text{—}\underset{}{\bigcirc}\text{—}CO(CH_2)_3NR$$

Compound	NR	Potency[a]	
		Antiapomorphine test, dog[b]	Antiamphetamine test, rat[c]
Haloperidol		47	35
Spiroperidol		2800	33
Benperidol		1400	33
Droperidol		700	33
Trifluperidol		140	33

Data from Zirkle and Kaiser (1970).

[a] Relative potency compared (ED_{50} mg/kg) with that of chlorpromazine, which is arbitrarily assigned a value of 1.

[b] Dogs given subcutaneous doses of experimental compounds are challenged with an emetic dose of apomorphine at various time intervals thereafter.

[c] Ability of subcutaneously administered compounds to inhibit compulsory gnawing and chewing responses to an intravenous dose of 10 mg/kg of amphetamine is determined.

TABLE 8 (continued)

Compound	NR	Potency[a]	
		Antiapomorphine test, dog[b]	Antiamphetamine test, rat[c]
Methylperidol	(structure) OH, CH_3	47	33
Paraperidide	(structure) $CON(CH_3)_2$, Cl	70	10
Haloperidide	(structure) CON, Cl	350	10
Methylperidide	(structure) CON, CH_3	350	10
Butropipazone	(structure) NC_6H_5	$\frac{1}{2}$	1
Fluanisone	(structure) CH_3O	5	3
Floropipamide	(structure) $CONH_2$	$\frac{1}{2}$	$\frac{1}{5}$
Anisoperidone[d]	(structure) C_6H_5	$\frac{1}{2}$	1
Aceperone	(structure) $CH_2NHCOCH_3$, C_6H_5	1	$< \frac{1}{160}$
Chlorpromazine		1	1

[d]The 4′-F-substituent of the butyrophenone is replaced by CH_3.

c. Butyrophenones (Table 8). The butyrophenones, which are structurally dissimilar to the two previous groups, were developed from studies originally aimed at increasing the morphine-like potency of a series of 4-phenylpiperidines related to meperidine (Janssen, 1965, 1967). Clinically they are more potent on a milligram basis than the phenothiazines. The structure–activity relationships are as follows:

The benzene ring: In all cases, the highest neuroleptic potency is associated with a fluorine substituent in the *p*-position of the benzene ring.

The carbonyl group: Potency is generally lost by replacement of the carbonyl group. In some cases, however, a hydroxyl or cyano group can replace it with no loss in potency.

The propylene side chain: Shortening, lengthening, or branching of the propylene side chain markedly decreases the potency.

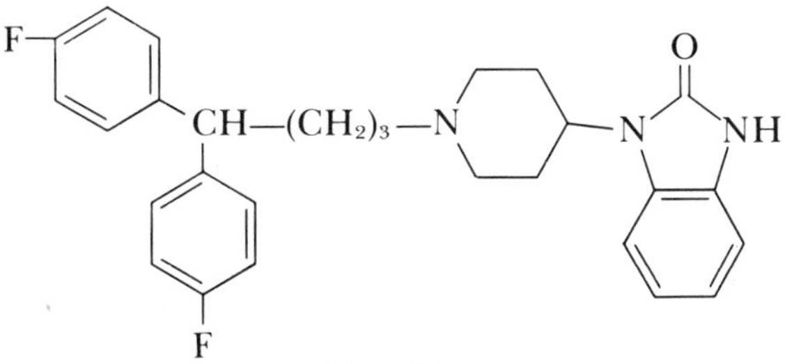

Pimozide

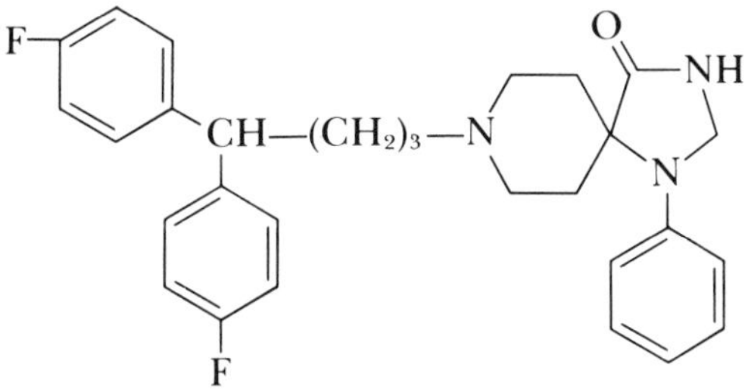

Fluspirilene

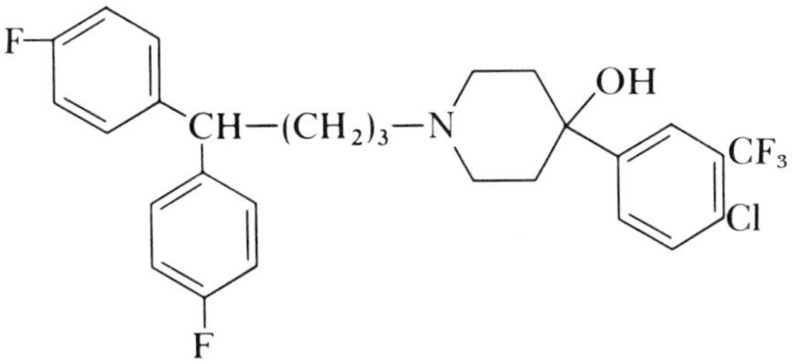

Penfluridol

FIG. 10. The diphenylbutyl piperidines.

The basic amino group: Considerable variation in the basic amino group is possible without loss of activity. Generally, maximum potency is obtained with 4-substituted piperidines, 1,2,3,6-tetrahydropyridino, or piperazino derivatives, i.e., where the nitrogen atom is part of a six-membered ring. Replacement by larger or smaller rings or uncyclized amines results in a decrease in potency. When the amino group is a piperidine ring, 2- or 3-substitution markedly decreases activity from the maximum associated with 4-substitution. Decreasing the basicity of the nitrogen atom by amide formation leads to a fall in activity. Some of the most potent compounds have a disubstitution pattern at the 4-position, e.g., phenyl and hydroxyl, cyclized ureas, or amides. For maximum activity, piperazine derivatives require an aromatic group at the 4-position. The crystal and molecular structures of several butyrophenones have been determined (Koch and Germain, 1972; Reed and Schaefer, 1973).

d. *The Piperidines Diphenylbutyl (Fig. 10).* The diphenylbutyl piperidines are the newest class of neuroleptic drugs, and only a few compounds such as pimozide, fluspirilene, and penfluridol have been studied in detail (Janssen *et al.*, 1968, 1970). Structurally this class has similarities to both the phenothiazines and the butyrophenones. Clinically they have a more prolonged mode of action. Certain structure–activity relationships for this group of compounds have been reported (Janssen, 1973)and they include requirements for:

1. *p*-Fluorine substituents on both phenyl rings.
2. An unbranched propyl chain between the basic nitrogen and the benzhydryl moiety.
3. A substituted piperidine ring.

The conformation of penfluridol in the solid state has been determined (Koch, 1973).

3.5.3. Adenylate Cyclase and the Dopamine Receptor

An adenylate cyclase that can be stimulated by low concentrations of DA has been demonstrated in homogenates of the rat caudate nucleus (Kebabian *et al.*, 1972), olfactory tubercle, and nucleus accumbens (Horn *et al.*, 1974) as well as in homogenates of bovine retina (Brown and Makman, 1972). In all these preparations, low concentrations of apomorphine also stimulate the activity of the enzyme. These results suggest that the DA-sensitive adenylate cyclase in brain homogenates may represent a model for biochemical studies of DA receptors in the brain. In a structure–activity study (Sheppard *et al.*, 1973), it was shown that mono- or dimethylation of DA's amino group led to a small reduction in the ED_{50}, whereas N-isopropyl or N-propyl derivatives were inactive. The ED_{50} was reduced more than thirtyfold by *dl*-α-methyl and 5- or 6-methyl substitutions. Substitution of a methyl group in the *o*-position of the ring had no effect. The authors suggested that the conformation of DA required for stimulation of the adenylate cyclase is similar to that of the DA skeleton in apomorphine. It is known that the stimulation of the enzyme by DA in DA-rich rat brain areas and bovine retina can be antagonized by the neuroleptics (Kebabian *et al.*, 1972; Horn *et al.*, 1974; Brown and Makman, 1973). Miller and Iversen (1974) have reported on more extensive studies of the effects of various neuroleptics and other psychotropic drugs on the DA-sensitive adenylate cyclase in rat corpus striatum (Table 9). The two most active compounds, flupenthixol and fluphenazine, have the same 2-substituent (—CF$_3$) and the same basic side chain (2-hydroxyethyl-piperazinyl). Substitution of a methyl group for the 2-hydroxyethyl group yields trifluoperazine, which is less active. Changing the 2-substituent and the amine side chain to produce chlorpromazine reduces activity still further. It is of interest that the clinically less efficacious neuroleptic promazine, which lacks a 2-substituent, only weakly antagonizes this DA-stimulated response. Chlorimipramine, a tricyclic antidepressant which has a 2-substituent but has a dimethylene bridge between the two aromatic rings rather than a sulfur atom, is also weakly active. Benztropine, which is known to act presynaptically as a potent inhibitor of DA uptake in the corpus striatum (Coyle and Snyder, 1969), is a very weak antagonist. Spiroperidol and pimozide, which are among the most potent neuroleptics in clinical use, were found to be weaker antagonists then chlorpromazine in this assay system. It is possible that the *in vivo* potency of

TABLE 9

Inhibition of Dopamine-Sensitive Adenylate Cyclase Activity in Rat Corpus Striatum by Drugs

Drug	Class	IC$_{50}$[a] (M)
Flupenthixol ($\alpha + \beta$)	Thioxanthene neuroleptic	7.0×10^{-8}
Fluphenazine	Phenothiazine neuroleptic	9.5×10^{-8}
Trifluoperazine	Phenothiazine neuroleptic	4.0×10^{-7}
Chlorpromazine	Phenothiazine neuroleptic	1.0×10^{-6}
Spiroperidol	Butyrophenone neuroleptic	2.0×10^{-6}
Prochlorperazine	Phenothiazine neuroleptic	2.5×10^{-6}
Thioridazine	Phenothiazine neuroleptic	3.0×10^{-6}
Clozapine	Dibenzodiazepine neuroleptic	4.5×10^{-6}
Pimozide	Diphenylbutylamine neuroleptic	4.5×10^{-6}
Chlorimipramine	Tricyclic antidepressant	9.0×10^{-6}
Promazine	Phenothiazine (weak neuroleptic)	4.5×10^{-5}
Morphine	Opiate analgesic	1.0×10^{-4}
Benztropine	Anticholinergic	$>1 \times 10^{-4}$
Promethazine	Phenothiazine, antihistamine	$>1 \times 10^{-4}$

Data from Miller and Iversen (1974).
[a]Drug concentration required to produce 50% inhibition of adenylate cyclase activity evoked by 100 μM dopamine.

spiroperidol and pimozide may be due to a more specific localization of these compounds in the CNS. In support of this, when chlorpromazine is injected it is found to be evenly distributed in rat brain whereas pimozide shows a selective accumulation in the caudate nucleus (Soudijn and Van Wijngaarden, 1972).

3.5.4. Conformational Studies on DA and Chlorpromazine

Based on the X-ray crystallographic results for the conformation of chlorpromazine (McDowell, 1969) and DA (Bergin and Carlstrom, 1968), a possible molecular mechanism for the blockade of the DA receptor by chlorpromazine has been suggested (Horn and Snyder, 1971) (Fig. 11). It can be seen that DA can be readily superimposed on a portion of the chlorpromazine molecule. The aromatic ring of DA lies over ring *a* of chlorpromazine such that the *m*-hydroxyl group overlies the sulfur atom of chlorpromazine. The primary amine function of the extended side chain of DA would then be superimposed on the tertiary amine group of chlorpromazine. Thus chlorpromazine could bind in this fashion and inhibit the attachment of DA to its receptor site. The question arises as to the significance of a solid-state conformation to the actual conformation at the receptor site. The situation is complicated by the fact that the conformation of the free base of chlorpromazine (McDowell, 1969) differs from that of the more recently determined hydrochloride (Dorignac-Calas and Marsau, 1972). At physiological pH, the chlorpromazine side chain amino group will carry a positive charge. Nevertheless, it is felt that the particular conformation of chlorpromazine described by McDowell may be relevant to the conformation at the receptor site because it is similar in overall conformation to the molecular structures reported for the active geometrical isomers of the two conformationally more rigid thioxanthenes, chlorprothixene (Dunitz *et al.*, 1964) and thiothixene (Schaefer, 1967); i.e., the 2-substituent and the side chain are on the same side of the molecule. The importance of a 2-substituent in clinically efficacious phenothiazines has already been mentioned. This substituent may be playing any of a number of roles. It is known, for example, that several tricyclic ring systems are not rigidly held in an "angled" conformation but have a certain amount of conformational freedom (Aroney *et al.*, 1968; Nogradi *et al.*, 1970; Aizenshtat *et al.*, 1972). In certain cases, it has been suggested that polar substituents can influence the conformation of the parent ring system (Aizenshtat *et al.*, 1972). This flexibility of the ring system will, of course, affect, the conformation of the attached side chain; thus it is possible that the 2-substituent could affect the conformation of the side chain by influencing the conformation of the ring system. It is unlikely that the 2-substituent could actually interact significantly with the amino group through space as the distances are rather large. A further possibility is that the 2-substituent may provide additional binding

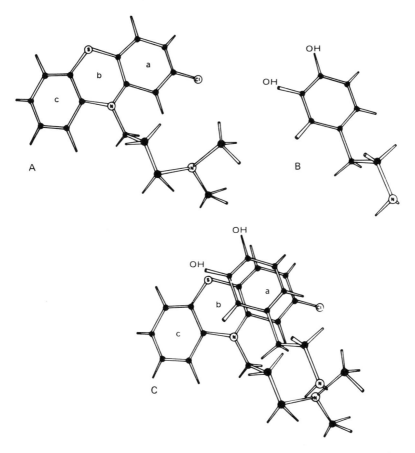

FIG. 11. Drawings of Dreiding models of the molecular structures of chlorpromazine (A) and dopamine (B) based on X-ray crystallographic analysis. (C) How dopamine may be superimposed on a portion of the chlorpromazine molecule. From Horn and Snyder (1971); reproduced with permission.

force or facilitate a favorable conformational change in the receptor that increases binding.

In the case of DA, X-ray crystallographic and quantum mechanical calculations indicate that the preferred conformation of DA is with the ethylamine side chain extended and perpendicular to the ring system, i.e., the *trans* conformation (Bergin and Carlstrom, 1968; Carlstrom *et al.*, 1973; Pullman *et al.*, 1972) (Fig. 12). The idea that this conformation may be related to the one occurring at the receptor is supported by the fact that apomorphine, which is a rigid molecule whose conformation has been determined by X-ray analysis (Giesecke, 1973), is readily seen to have a portion of the extended DA molecule in its structure (Fig. 12).

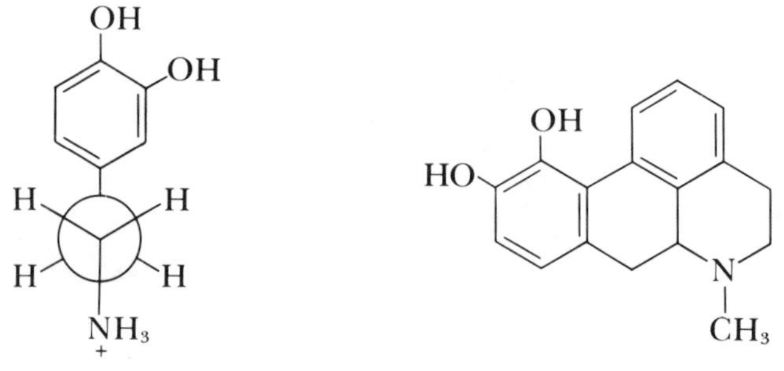

trans conformation of Dopamine   Apomorphine

FIG. 12. Fully extended *trans* conformation of dopamine and structure of apomorphine.

4. 5-HYDROXYTRYPTAMINE

Serotonin (5-HT) occurs widely in nature in nervous and nonnervous tissue as well as in fruits and vegetables (Erspamer, 1966). In mammals, the highest concentration occurs in the pineal gland, and there are also large amounts in the raphe nucleus, the hypothalamus, and the enterochromaffin cells of the intestinal tract (Erspamer, 1966; Saavedra *et al.*, 1974). In man, only about 1–2% of the total 5-HT occurs in the CNS. There is between 8 and 10% in the blood platelets, and the rest occurs in the gastrointestinal tract. In rats and mice, 5-HT also occurs in mast cells. The biochemical and neurophysiological effects of 5-HT in the CNS are dealt with elsewhere (Green and Grahame-Smith, Chap. 4, Vol. 3; Aghajanian, Chap. 3, Vol. 6).

4.1. 5-HT Receptors in the Mammalian Peripheral Nervous System and Other Preparations

5-HT produces contractions of mammalian smooth muscle, and this fact has been used in the past to quantify this amine (Erspamer, 1966; Garattini and Valzelli, 1965). The preparations that have been most commonly used are the rat uterus (Erspamer, 1940), colon (Dalgliesh *et al.*, 1953), and fundus of the stomach (Vane, 1957) as well as the guinea pig ileum (Gaddum and Hameed, 1954). The fundal strip of the rat stomach is one of the most sensitive bioassays for 5-HT, being sensitive to concentrations as low as 50 pg. Other preparations sensitive to 5-HT include the mollusc heart (Gaddum and Paasonen, 1955) and the isolated rabbit ear (Gaddum and Hameed, 1954). Certain cells in the salivary gland of the blowfly are stimulated to secrete fluid by low concentrations of 5-HT (Berridge and Patel, 1968). Gaddum and Picarelli (1957) showed, on the basis of differing pharmacological behavior in the isolated guinea pig ileum, that there were two classes of 5-HT receptors. Certain receptors were postulated to be nervous (M) receptors sensitive to such blocking agents as morphine, cocaine, and atropine, while a second class was defined as muscular (D) receptors sensitive to blockade by LSD, phenoxybenzamine, and benzyloxygramine. Receptors having similar properties to those of the M class have also been reported in the cat superior cervical ganglion (Trendelenburg, 1956, 1957) and in the cat inferior mesenteric ganglion (Gyermek and Bindler, 1962).

4.2. Structure–Activity Relationships of 5-HT Agonists

Large numbers of 5-HT analogues have been prepared and tested in a variety of serotonin-sensitive assay systems, and some of these results are shown in Table 10. The following discussion will deal mainly with results from the rat uterus and stomach preparations, as they behave in a fairly similar manner (Erspamer, 1966).

1. Substitution of the phenolic hydroxyl group in positions other than 5 produces a fall in activity. This is most marked for substitution in position 6 or 7, while 4-hydroxyl substitution produces only a moderate decrease in activity.
2. Methylation of the 5-hydroxyl group or replacement by other substituents reduces activity. The fall in activity is moderate in the case of an amino group but quite large for halogen atoms or benzyloxy groups.
3. Conjugation of the 5-hydroxyl group with sulfuric or glucuronic acid yields compounds that are practically inactive.
4. Removal of the phenolic hydroxyl group, as in tryptamine, produces a sharp fall in activity. It is of interest, however, that this effect is less than that due to a shift of the 5-hydroxyl group to position 6 or 7.
5. Shortening or lengthening of the side chain by one carbon atom results in a fall in biological activity. The one-carbon side chain compounds are weaker than the three-carbon analogues.
6. Substitution of the side chain in position 2 rather than 3 produces compounds lacking activity.
7. Introduction of an α-methyl group into the side chain leads to either an increase or a moderate decrease in activity depending on the other substituents in the molecule. Substitution of two methyl groups or an ethyl group produces a larger fall in activity.
8. Substitution of a β-hydroxyl group into the side chain results in a practically inactive compound when tested on the rat uterus preparation.

TABLE 10
Equipotent Molar Ratios of Indolealkylamines Estimated on Five Isolated Smooth Muscle Preparations[a]

Ring substituent	Side chain	Stimulant action				
		Rat uterus[b,c]	Rat stomach[b,d]	Molluscan heart[c,e]	Rabbit ear[c]	Guinea pig ileum[c]
5—OH	3—CH_2—CH_2—NH_2 (5-Hydroxytryptamine)	1	1	1	1	1
5—OH	3—CH_2—CH_2—$NHCH_3$	1	6.3	=	1.4	7
5—OH	3—CH_2—CH_2—$N(CH_3)_2$ (Bufotenine)	4	10	0.3 (0.028)	11	4
5—OH	3—CH_2—CH_2—$N(C_2H_5)_2$	9	18:20	=	=	=
5—OH	3—CH_2—CH_2—$N(C_3H_7$ iso$)_2$	16	4.5	=	=	=
5—OH	3—CH_2—CH_2—$N(C_3H_7)_2$	39	16:4	=	=	=
5—OH	3—CH_2—CH_2—$N(C_4H_9)_2$	540;1100	151	0	0	450
5—OH	3—CH_2—CH_2—$N(CH_3)_3$ (Bufotenidine)	>1000[f]	=	=	=	=
5—OH	3—CH_2—$CH(CH_3)$—NH_2	1.3;2	1.4;1.7	8.2 (6)	3.3	8
5—OH	3—CH_2—$C(CH_3)_2$—NH_2	310	=	170	0	24
5—OH	3—CH_2—$CH(C_2H_5)$—NH_2	50	7	50	40	44
5—OH	3—CH_2—CH_2—$NHCOCH_3$	+−[g]	=	=	=	=
5—OH	3—$CHOH$—CH_2—$N(CH_3)_2$	0	=	0	0	0
5—OH	3—CH_2—$C(N)$—NH_2	0	=	=	108	=
5—OH, 2,3-dihydro	3—CH_2—CH_2—NH_2	10[h]	=	=	=	=
5—OH	2—CH_2—CH_2—NH_2	0	=	0	0	190
5—OCH_3	3—CH_2—CH_2—NH_2 (5-Methoxytryptamine)	9.6;8	20;39	0.5	5.4	9
5—OCH_3	3—CH_2—CH_2—$NHCH_3$	150	=	=	=	=
5—OCH_3	3—CH_2—CH_2—$N(CH_3)_2$	150	=	=	=	=
5—OCH_3	3—CH_2—CH_2—$N(C_4H_9)_2$	0	=	540	0	0
5—OCH_3	3—CH_2—$CH(CH_3)$—NH_2	1.5;4.3	2.9;1.4	4.6	1.5	43
5—OCH_3	3—CH_2—CH_2—$NHCOCH_3$ (Melatonin)	0	=	=	345	0
5—$OCOCH_3$	3—CH_2—CH_2—NH_2	=	=	(+)[i]	=	=
5—CH_3	3—CH_2—CH_2—NH_2	173	184;620	=	=	=
5—CH_3	3—CH_2—$CH(CH_3)$—NH_2	1300;240	14;22	190	340	0
5—Cl	3—CH_2—CH_2—NH_2	=	100	=	=	=
5—NH_2	3—CH_2—CH_2—NH_2	11	=	1.3	23	22
5—OC_7H_7	3—CH_2—CH_2—$N(CH_3)_2$	20,000	625	=	=	=
5—OC_7H_7	3—CH_2—CH_2—$N(C_2H_5)_2$	10,000	470	=	=	=
5—OC_7H_7	3—CH_2—CH_2—$N(C_3H_7)_2$	20,000	614	=	=	=
5—OC_7H_7	3—CH_2—CH_2—$N(C_4H_9)_2$	20,000	20,000	=	=	=
5—OC_7H_7	3—CH_2—$CH(CH_3)$—NH_2	20,000	63	=	=	=
5—O-sulfate	3—CH_2—CH_2—$N(CH_3)_2$ (Bufoviridine)	500	=	=	0	1000
5—O-glucuronide	3—CH_2—CH_2—NH_2	0	=	0	=	0
5—O-glucuronide	3—CH_2—CH_2—$N(CH_3)_2$	0	=	0	=	0
5—OH, 2—CH_3	3—CH_2—CH_2—NH_2	=	=	(31.4)	=	=
5—OCH_3, 2—CH_3	3—CH_2—CH_2—NH_2	=	=	(43.8)	=	=
5—OCH_3, 2—CH_3, 1—C_7H_7 (BAS)	3—CH_2—CH_2—NH_2	=	=	(30)[j]	=	=
5—OH, 2—CH_3, 1—C_7H_7 (BAS-phenol)	3—CH_2—CH_2—NH_2	=	=	(300)[j]	=	=

TABLE 10 (continued)

Ring substituent	Side chain	Stimulant action				
		Rat uterus[b,c]	Rat stomach[b,d]	Molluscan heart[c,e]	Rabbit ear[c]	Guinea pig ileum[c]
5,6—(OH)$_2$	3—CH$_2$—CH$_2$—NH$_2$	=	$\simeq 1^k$	=	=	=
5,6—(OCH$_3$)$_2$	3—CH$_2$—CH$_2$—NH$_2$	58	300	4	140	300
5,6,7—(OCH$_3$)$_3$	3—CH$_2$—CH$_2$—NH$_2$	110	=	130	560	145
6—OH	3—CH$_2$—CH$_2$—NH$_2$	0	460	47	155	0
6—OCH$_3$	3—CH$_2$—CH$_2$—NH$_2$	0	1520	174	480	400
4—OH	3—CH$_2$—CH$_2$—NH$_2$	11	1.8	15	22	26
4—OH	3—CH$_2$—CH$_2$—N(CH$_3$)$_2$ (Psilocin)	10–20^l	0^l	=	=	=
4—O-phosphate	3—CH$_2$—CH$_2$—N(CH$_3$)$_2$ (Psilocybin)	330; 50–100^l	3–1000^l	18	0	760
7—OH	3—CH$_2$—CH$_2$—NH$_2$	0	=	0	1300	0
2—CH$_3$	3—CH$_2$—CH$_2$—N(CH$_3$)$_2$	20,000	1200;6600	=	=	=
2—CH$_3$	3—CH$_2$—CH$_2$—N(C$_2$H$_5$)$_2$	1000	280	=	=	=
2—CH$_3$	3—CH$_2$—CH$_2$—N(C$_3$H$_7$)$_2$	630	70	=	=	=
1—CH$_3$	3—CH$_2$—CH$_2$—NH$_2$	142	=	0	330	520
1—CH$_3$	3—CH$_2$—CH(CH$_3$)—NH$_2$	1350	69	=	=	=
	3—CH$_2$—CH$_2$—NH$_2$ (Tryptamine)	176;210	408;933	22 (9.9)	20	280
	3—CH$_2$—CH$_2$—NHCH$_3$	128;2000	1120;2400	(3.7)	17	48
	3—CH$_2$—CH$_2$—NHC$_2$H$_5$	2000	250;350	(9.1)	=	=
	3—CH$_2$—CH$_2$—NHC$_3$H$_7$	0;2000	330;490	0	0	0
	3—CH$_2$—CH$_2$—N(CH$_3$)$_2$	200;1000	196;350	107 (10.7)	35	58
	3—CH$_2$—CH$_2$—N(C$_2$H$_5$)$_2$	160;500	83;112	650 (7.9)	0	0
	3—CH$_2$—CH$_2$—N(C$_3$H$_7$)$_2$	95;200	34;40	59	0	0
	3—CH$_2$—CH$_2$—N(C$_3$H$_7$ iso)$_2$	520	53	=	=	=
	3—CH$_2$—CH$_2$—N(C$_4$H$_9$)$_2$	720;500	244	810	0	870
	3—CH$_2$—CH(CH$_3$)—NH$_2$	0;800	31;60	0 (8.6)	0	0
	3—CH$_2$—CH(C$_2$H$_5$)—NH$_2$	20,000	4600	=	=	=
	3—CH$_2$—C(CH$_3$)$_2$—NH$_2$	=	1400	=	=	=
	3—CH$_2$—CH$_2$—NHCOCH$_3$	0	=	=	=	=
	3—CHOH—CH$_2$—NHCH$_3$	0	=	23	370	0
	3—CH$_2$—C(N)—NH$_2$	0	=	=	120	=
	3—CH$_2$—CH$_2$—CH$_2$—NH$_2$	=	1920	=	=	=
	3—CH$_2$—CH$_2$—CH$_2$—N(CH$_3$)$_2$	=	=	(2000)	=	=
	3—CH$_2$—NH$_2$	=	29,000	=	=	=
	3—CH$_2$—N(CH$_3$)$_2$ (Gramine)	0	=	0 (0)	0	400

[a]5-HT taken as unity. Values in parentheses have been obtained on the heart of *Venus mercenaria* (Greenberg, 1960), the others on the heart of *Helix luconum* (Bertaccini and Zamboni, 1961). Data from Erspamer (1966).
References: [b]Barlow and Kahn (1959a,b). [c]Bertaccini and Zamboni (1961). [d]Vane (1959). [e]Greenberg (1960). [f]Erspamer (1954), [g]McIsaac and Page (1958). [h]Fellman *et al.* (1962). [i]Osborne *et al.* (1962). [j]Woolley (1959). [k]Colhoun (1963). [l]Woolley and Campbell (1962).

9. Alkylation of the side chain amino group produces variable results; generally an increase in both the size and number of the alkyl group leads to a fall in activity.

Changes within the indole nucleus have also been examined for their effects on activity. The nuclei that have been examined are shown in Fig. 13. Indazolealkylamines display serotonin-like activity, particularly the 5-HT analogue, which has about one-fifth the activity of the natural agonist in both the rat uterus and guinea pig ileum preparations (Table 11). Studies in the

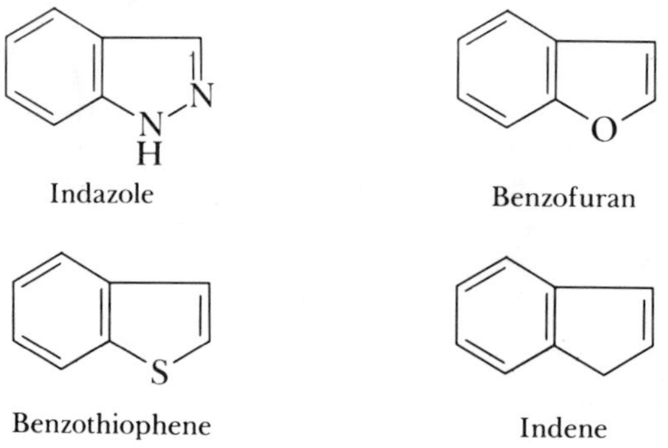

Indazole

Benzofuran

Benzothiophene

Indene

FIG. 13. Nuclei of indole analogues.

benzofuran series have shown that on the rat uterus the 5-HT and tryptamine analogues were 10 and 10,000 times less active, while on the rat fundus strip they were 100 and 1000 times weaker. Comparisons of substituted tryptamines and indenes on the rat fundus strip preparations indicate that activity is greatest in the primary amines and tends to decline in the order $N(i\text{-}Pr)_2 > NH\text{-}n\text{-}Pr > N(Et)_2 < N(Me)_2$. There is a close similarity in activity for the indole and indene series when unsubstituted in the

TABLE 11

Equipotent Molar Ratios of Indazolealkylamines Estimated on Four Isolated Smooth Muscle Preparations (Bertaccini and Zamboni, 1961)[a]

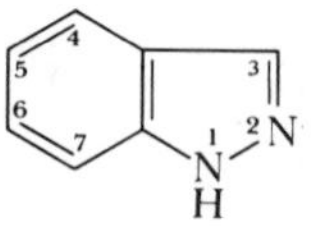

Ring substituent	Side chain	Stimulant action			
		Rat uterus	*Helix* heart	Rabbit ear	Guinea pig ileum
5—OH	3—CH$_2$—CH$_2$—NH$_2$	4.3–5[b]	3.9	27	5.3
5—OH	3—CH$_2$—CH$_2$—NHCH(CH$_3$)$_2$	227	172	0	0
5—OC$_7$H$_7$	3—CH$_2$—CH$_2$—NH$_2$	0	0	0	0
5—OC$_7$H$_7$	3—CH$_2$—CH$_2$—N(CH$_3$)$_2$	0	0	0	0
5—OC$_7$H$_7$	3—CH$_2$—CH$_2$—NHCH(CH$_3$)$_2$	0	0	0	0
	3—CH$_2$—CH$_2$—NH$_2$	360	335	134	0
	3—CH$_2$—CH$_2$—N(CH$_3$)$_2$	39	7.2	85	20
	3—CH$_2$—CH$_2$—NHCH(CH$_3$)$_2$	0	0	0	0
	2—CH$_2$—CH$_2$—NH$_2$	0	0	700	570
	1—CH$_2$—CH$_2$—NH$_2$	870	0	66	185

[a] 5-HT taken as unity. Data from Erspamer (1966).
[b] Ainsworth (1958).

benzene ring. The chemistry and pharmacology of the benzothiophene analogues of serotonin have been reviewed by Campaigne *et al.* (1970). Recently a structure–activity study has been carried out for 5-HT analogues on the salivary gland of the blowfly (Berridge, 1972).

Information about the molecular structures of various indolealkylamines is contained in a review by Carlstrom *et al.* (1973). The preferred conformation of serotonin and a postulate on the nature of important interatomic distances at its receptor site have been presented by Kier (1968a) based on molecular orbital calculations.

4.3. 5-HT Antagonists

A wide variety of drugs are known to antagonize the action of 5-HT on smooth muscle and nerve elements (Gyermek, 1961, 1966). These include various indole compounds such as derivatives of gramine, tryptamine, harmine, quaternary ammonium salts of N,N-dialkyltryptamines, and indoleacetamidines. Some of the ergot alkaloids were among the early 5-HT antagonists discovered. Certain lysergic acid derivatives such as LSD, 2-bromo-LSD, and methysergide are potent antagonists. Various other groups of drugs such as the phenothiazines (chlorpromazine), antihistamines (cyproheptadine), and β-haloalkylamines (phenoxybenzamine) also act as serotonin antagonists. The two antagonists most commonly used clinically in this capacity are methysergide and cyproheptadine (Fig. 14).

5. ACETYLCHOLINE

Acetylcholine has the distinction of being the first specific chemical substance that was demonstrated to be released in response to stimulation of a

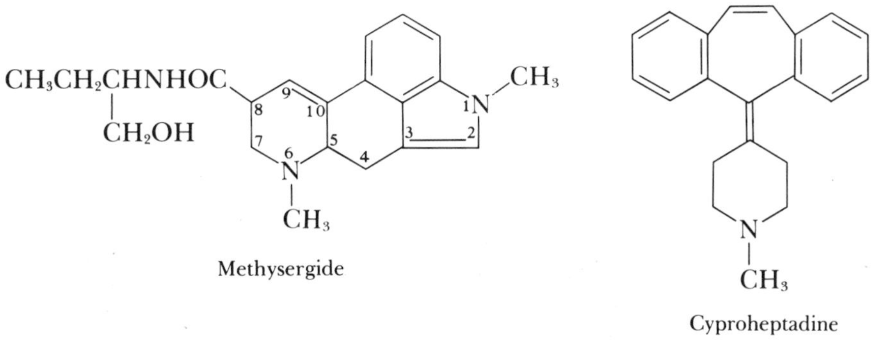

Methysergide

Cyproheptadine

FIG. 14. 5-HT antagonists.

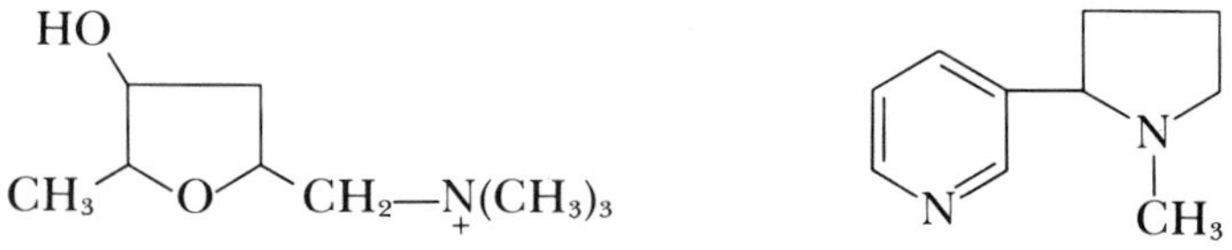

Muscarine   Nicotine

FIG. 15. The alkaloids muscarine and nicotine.

nerve. This was shown by Loewi in 1921. The history of the discovery and significance of ACh in cholinergic nerves has been reviewed (Dale, 1953; Hebb and Krnjević, 1962). In other volumes of this series, the topics of the biochemistry of cholinergic nerves (Marchbanks, Chap. 5, Vol. 3), cholinergic receptors in the CNS (Krnjević, Chap. 4, Vol. 6), and attempts to isolate and purify the cholinergic receptor (Changeux, Chap. 7, Vol. 6) are reviewed.

Cholinergic receptors in the peripheral nervous system are divided, on the basis of their pharmacological responses, into muscarinic and nicotinic receptors.

5.1. Muscarinic Actions of ACh

The "muscarinic" actions of ACh were named after the alkaloid muscarine (Fig. 15), which was shown to possess pharmacological properties similar to the responses obtained by stimulation of the parasympathetic nervous system. Thus they include stimulation of such smooth muscle–containing organs as the gastrointestinal tract, bronchi, and gallbladder. Exocrine glands such as the sweat, salivary, mucous, and tear glands are also stimulated. Conversely, the heart is slowed and the sphincters in the gastrointestinal, biliary, and urinary tracts are relaxed, as is the musculature of the blood vessels.

5.2. Nicotinic Actions of ACh

The "nicotinic" actions of ACh are so called because they are similar to the pharmacological actions of the alkaloid nicotine (Fig. 15). These effects occur in the autonomic ganglion cell and at the motor end plate of striated muscle. Thus nicotinic activity results in the contraction of skeletal muscle and the stimulation of sympathetic and parasympathetic ganglia. The nicotinic receptors of skeletal muscle and of autonomic ganglia are not identical, however, as they respond differently to certain agonists and antagonists. Thus dimethylphenylpiperazinium and phenyltrimethylammonium (Fig. 16) are highly selective stimulants of autonomic ganglion cells

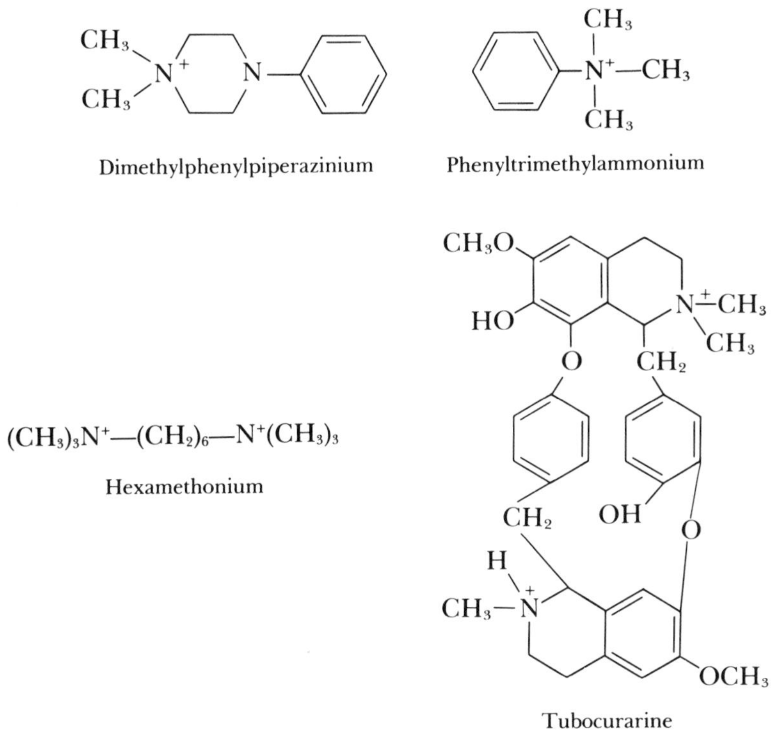

Dimethylphenylpiperazinium   Phenyltrimethylammonium

$(CH_3)_3N^+—(CH_2)_6—N^+(CH_3)_3$

Hexamethonium

Tubocurarine

FIG. 16. Compounds which act at nicotinic receptors.

and of skeletal muscle end plates, respectively. Hexamethonium (Fig. 16) is a selective ganglionic blocking agent, whereas *d*-tubocurarine (Fig. 16) blocks transmission at both motor end plates and autonomic ganglia.

5.3. Cholinergic Agonists

The possible structural changes of ACh that have been examined are variations in the nature of the quaternary ammonium group, the ester and acyl groups, and the alkyl chain connecting the ester and quaternary ammonium groups.

5.3.1. The Quaternary Ammonium Group (Tables 12 and 13)

The carbon isostere of ACh, 3,3-dimethylbutyl acetate, has 1/3000 the activity of ACh (Burgen, 1965). Replacement of the nitrogen atom by arsenic, phosphorus, or sulfur atoms leads to compounds that are also

TABLE 12

Effect of Variations in the Onium Atom[a]

$$Me_nXCH_2CH_2OAC$$

Me$_n$X	Potency	Test preparation	Reference
Me$_3$P$^+$	8.3	Rabbit ileum	b
Me$_3$As$^+$	1.1	Rabbit ileum	b
Me$_2$S$^+$	3.3	Guinea pig ileum	c
Me$_3$C	negligible	Guinea pig ileum	d
	0.03	Guinea pig ileum	e

[a]Acetylcholine has a relative potency of 100. Data from Friedman (1967).
References: [b]Ing (1949). [c]Ing *et al.* (1952). [d]Banister and Whittaker (1951). [e]Burgen (1965).

TABLE 13

Effect of Variations in the Onium Group[a]

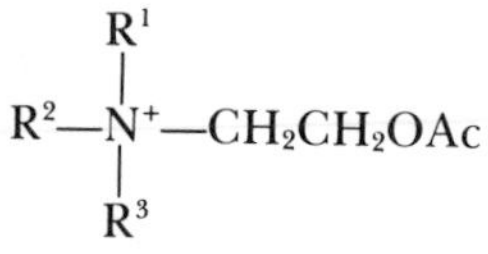

$$R^2\!-\!\overset{\displaystyle R^1}{\underset{\displaystyle R^3}{N^+}}\!-\!CH_2CH_2OAc$$

R^1	R^2	R^3	Potency	Test preparation	Reference
H	H	H	0.005	Rabbit ileum	b
H	H	Me	0.1	Rabbit ileum	b
H	Me	Me	2.5	Rabbit ileum	b
H	Me	Me	0.33	Rabbit ileum	c
H	Et	Et	1.7	Rabbit ileum	d
Me	Me	Et	25.0	rat jejunum	e
Me	Me	Et	33.0	Guinea pig ileum	f
Me	Et	Et	0.33	Rat jejunum	e
Me	Et	Et	0.25	Guinea pig ileum	f
Me	Et	Et	0.14	Guinea pig ileum	b
Me	Et	Et	6.3	Rabbit ileum	g
Me	Me	NH$_2$	12.5	Guinea pig ileum	h
Me	Me	n-Pr	0.33	Rabbit ileum	i
Me	Me	n-Bu	weak	Guinea pig ileum	j
Me	Me	CH$_2$CH$_2$COOMe	1.0	Guinea pig ileum	k
Et	Et	Et	0.25	Rat jejunum	e
Et	Et	Et	0.33	Guinea pig ileum	f
Et	Et	Et	0.06	Guinea pig ileum	b
Et	Et	Et	inactive	Dog blood pressure lowering	l
Me	Me	OCH$_3$	50.0	Guinea pig ileum	m
CD$_3$	CD$_3$	CD$_3$	100.0	Dog blood pressure lowering	n

[a]Acetylcholine has a relative potency of 100. Data from Friedman (1967).
References: [b]Ing (1949). [c]Van Rossum (1962). [d]Nachod and Lands (1953). [e]Ariens and Simonis (1964). [f]Barlow *et al.* (1963). [g]Lands (1951). [h]Schueler and Hanna (1951). [i]Schueler (1953). [j]Ing *et al.* (1952). [k]Schueler and Keasling (1951). [l]Renshaw and Hunt (1929). [m]Burks *et al.* (1965). [n]Belleau (1965).

considerably weaker (Welch and Roepke, 1935; Ing *et al.*, 1952). A comparison of the acetate esters of ethanolamine, *N*-methylethanolamine, and *N,N*-dimethylethanolamine with ACh showed that these analogues lack nicotinic activity and retain only a small muscarinic effect (Stehle *et al.*, 1936). Replacement of the quaternary methyl groups by ethyl groups also results in a loss of activity (Holton and Ing, 1949).

5.3.2. The Acyl and Ester Groups (Table 14)

Changes within the acyl methyl group usually result in less potent compounds. Polar groups such as —OH or —NH$_2$ markedly reduce potency. Effective replacements for the acyl methyl group are —NH$_2$ (carbachol), CH$_2$=CH—, and CH$_3$—C=O. Choline possesses some nicotinic and muscarinic activity, but it is much weaker than ACh. Esterification of choline by a variety of organic and inorganic acids has been examined. Propionylcholine is less active than ACh, although resembling it in action (Hunt and Taveau, 1906; Chang and Gaddum, 1933). Isobutyrylcholine resembles ACh in being a vasodepressant, while the *n*-butyryl analogue is a vasostimulant (Hunt and Taveau, 1906). Higher homologues in the fatty acid series yield less potent compounds or ones possessing a different range of activity. None of the above changes has yielded clinically useful compounds. Carbachol, the carbamate ester of choline, has stronger nicotinic effects than ACh and is resistant to enzymatic hydrolysis. The dimethylphosphate ester of choline has powerful nictotinic but little muscarinic activity (Renshaw and Hopkins, 1929). The nitrate ester of choline is also active (Hunt and Renshaw, 1925). Replacement of the oxygen atom of choline by sulfur decreases the nicotinic effect, leaves the muscarinic effect largely unchanged, but increases the curare-like action (Renshaw *et al.*, 1938; Hunt and Renshaw, 1932). Acetylation of thiocholine produces a compound that is 300 times less active as a muscarinic agent (Scott and Mautner, 1967). Replacement of the ester group by ketone, ether, or hydroxyl groups does not abolish activity (Simonart, 1932; Welsh and Taub, 1951). Generally, the ethers are less active than the reference compounds. Substitution by nitro, nitrile, or carboxamido groups produces active compounds; however, the nicotinic and muscarinic activities are markedly reduced (Hunt and Renshaw, 1933).

5.3.3. The Dimethylene Bridge (Table 15)

The distance between the quaternary ammonium and ester groups appears to be critical. Acetyl-β-methylcholine is 20 times more potent in its muscarinic action than ACh but has weaker nicotinic activity (Simonart, 1932; Wurzel, 1959). However, the α-methyl analogue has stronger nicotinic

TABLE 14

Effect of Variations in the Ester Group[a]

$$\overset{\displaystyle O}{\underset{\displaystyle \parallel}{}}$$

$$RCOCH_2CH_2N^+Me_3$$

R	Potency	Test preparation	Reference
H	0.4	Rat jejunum	b
H	10.0	Rabbit ileum	c
H_2N	33.3	Rat jejunum	d
FCH_2	6.6	Guinea pig ileum	e
$HOCH_2$	0.25	Guinea pig ileum	f
H_2NCH_2	0.22	Rabbit ileum	c
$EtOCH_2$	inactive	Rabbit ileum	c
D_3C	76.9	Cat blood pressure lowering	g
CH_3CH_2	3.0	Rabbit ileum	f
CH_3CH_2	6.6	Guinea pig ileum	h
CH_3CH_2	0.25	Rat jejunum	b
$CH_2{=}CH{-}$	20.0	Guinea pig ileum	h
CH_3CHOH	($\pm$) 0.71	Guinea pig ileum	i
CH_3CHOH	($-$) 0.11	Guinea pig ileum	i
CH_3CHOH	($+$) 0.02	Guinea pig ileum	i
$CH_2OHCHOH$	($\pm$) 0.04	Guinea pig ileum	i
CH_3CO	14.28	Rabbit ileum	f
$CH_3CH_2CH_2$	0.25	Rabbit ileum	f
$CH_3\underset{\displaystyle \mid}{\overset{}{C}}H$ $\quad CH_3$	0.03	Rat jejunum	b
$H_2NCH_2CH_2CH_2$	0.05	Guinea pig ileum	h
$CH_3CHOHCH_2$	($\pm$) 0.06	Guinea pig ileum	i
$CH_3CH_2CH_2CH_2$	0.01	Rat jejunum	b
$CH_3CH_2CH_2CH_2$	0.20	Rabbit ileum	f
$H_3C{\diagdown}{\atop}C{=}CH{\diagup}H_3C$	0.10	Guinea pig ileum	h

[a] Acetylcholine has a relative potency of 100. Data from Friedman (1967).
References: [b] Ariens and Simonis (1964). [c] Bovet and Bovet-Nitti (1948). [d] Van Rossum and Ariens (1959). [e] Salle (1952). [f] Chang and Gaddum (1933). [g] Erlenmeyer and Lobeck (1937). [h] Whittaker (1963). [i] Sastry et al. (1960).

than muscarinic activity. Acetate esters of β-propyl- and β-butylcholine possess weak muscarinic activity (Hunt and Taveau, 1909; Simonart, 1934). Acetyl-β-methylcholine is more resistant to enzymatic hydrolysis than the parent compound. It is of interest that the introduction of a double or triple bond into the weakly active butane analogue enhances activity. The *trans* isomer of the butane compound is 16 times more potent than the *cis* isomer.

TABLE 15

Effect of Variations in the Alkylene Chain[a]

R_3N^+-alkylene-OAc

N^+R_3	Alkylene group	Potency	Test preparation	Reference
N^+Me_3	absent	2.0	Guinea pig ileum	b
N^+Me_3	CH_2	0.02	Guinea pig ileum	b
		0.08	Cat blood pressure lowering	c
N^+Me_3	$CHCH_2$ $\mid$ CH_3	(±)5.0	Cat blood pressure lowering	d
		(±)2.0	Guinea pig ileum	e
		(−)0.4	Guinea pig ileum	e
		(+)3.3	Guinea pig ileum	e
N^+Me_3	CH_2CH $\mid$ CH_3	(±)100	Cat blood pressure lowering	d
		(±)66.7	Rat jejunum	f
		(±)62.5	Guinea pig ileum	e
		(−)0.4	Guinea pig ileum	e
		(−)0.2	Rat jejunum	g
		(+)100	Guinea pig ileum	e
		(+)76.9	Rat jejunum	g
N^+Me_2H	CH_2CH $\mid$ CH_3	(±)0.07	Rat jejunum	f
N^+Me_2Et	CH_2CH $\mid$ CH_3	(±)16.7	Rabbit ileum	h
N^+Me_3	CH_2CH $\mid$ Et	0.5	Cat blood pressure lowering	i
N^+Me_3	CH_2CH $\mid$ Et	5.0	Rabbit ileum	h
N^+Me_3	$(CH_2)_3$	0.11	Rabbit ileum	j
N^+Me_3	$(CH_2)_4$	0.13	Rabbit ileum	j
		1.00	Rabbit ileum	k
N^+Me_3	$CH_2CH{=}CHCH_2$			
	cis	2.0	Dog heart inhibition	l
	trans	33.3	Dog heart inhibition	l
N^+Me_3	$CH_2C{\equiv}CCH_2$	50.0	Rabbit ileum	k
N^+Me_3	$CH_2C{\equiv}CCH_2CH_2$	10.0	Rabbit ileum	k
N^+Me_3	$CH_2C{\equiv}CCH$ $\mid$ CH_3	25.0	Rabbit ileum	k

[a]Acetylcholine has a relative potency of 100. Data from Friedman (1967).
References: [b]Geiger and Alpers (1964). [c]Hunt and Renshaw (1925). [d]Simonart (1932). [e]Beckett *et al.* (1961). [f]Van Rossum (1962). [g]Ellenbroek and Van Rossum (1960). [h]Schueler (1953). [i]Simonart (1934). [j]Lands and Cavallito (1954). [k]Jacob *et al.* (1952). [l]Marszak *et al.* (1954).

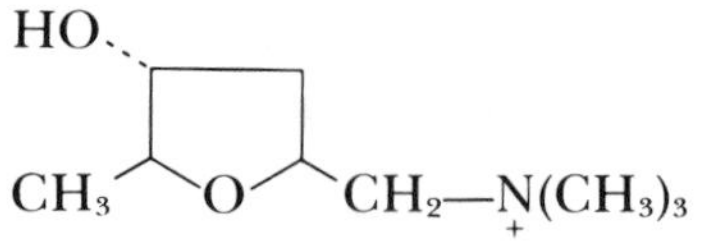

L(+)-Muscarine

FIG. 17. The active stereoisomer of muscarine.

5.3.4. Cyclic Analogues

There are several compounds with cholinergic activity that may be regarded as cyclic analogues of ACh. One of the most well known is muscarine, whose parasympathomimetic effects were first described in 1869 by Schmiedeberg and Koppe but whose structure was not settled until 1957 (Wilkinson, 1961). This compound is of particular interest because the muscarinic activity is stereospecific, nearly all the activity being confined to the L(+) stereoisomer (Fig. 17). It is also essentially devoid of nicotinic activity. The ring methyl group is essential for high activity, as its removal or the substitution of a larger group results in a significant decrease in activity (Waser, 1961; Eugster, 1959). The activity is also lowered by substitution of a thiophene ring for a furan system (Gyermek and Unna, 1958). Various other cyclic ethers with cholinergic activity have been prepared, and their value in studying the structural and conformational requirements of the cholinergic receptor will be discussed later.

5.4. Antagonists at the Nicotinic Receptor

Nicotinic receptor antagonists are divided into those acting at neuromuscular junctions and those acting at autonomic ganglia.

5.4.1. Neuromuscular Blocking Agents

Neuromuscular blocking agents are further divided, depending on their mode of action, into competitive (stabilizing) agents, of which d-tubocurarine (Fig. 16) is the best-known example, or depolarizing agents, such as decamethonium (Fig. 18). It should be noted in passing that the previously accepted structure for (+)-tubocurarine has been shown to be incorrect (Everett et al., 1970); the correct structure is shown in Fig. 16.

$$(CH_3)_3N^+ \text{—} (CH_2)_{10} \text{—} N^+(CH_3)_3$$

FIG. 18. The depolarizing agent decamethonium.

Although there have been several review articles on this class of drugs (Bovet *et al.*, 1959; Lewis and Muir, 1967; Stenlake, 1963; Hunt and Kuffler, 1950; Taylor and Nederguard, 1965), it is difficult to propose meaningful structure–activity generalizations. More recently, however, Pauling and Petcher (1973) have examined several compounds in this class whose conformations have been derived either from X-ray diffraction analysis or from atomic model building. It was suggested that for a compound to display potent curariform activity it should possess

1. Two quaternary nitrogen atoms separated by 1080 ± 30 pm.
2. Rigidity of molecular conformation.
3. A sufficient degree of lipophilicity on the concave side to promote subsidiary hydrophobic interaction with the receptor in the area between the cationic centers.
4. Oxygen atoms suitably disposed about the molecule to aid orientation.

It was also pointed out that the main structural feature of depolarizing agents such as decamethonium and succinylcholine is their flexibility. This is in contrast to the rigidity of the curariform drugs. Hydrophilic groups appear to be important in curariform agents, while they do not seem to be essential in depolarizing blocking agents.

5.4.2. Ganglionic Blocking Agents

The drugs that block transmission in autonomic ganglia exhibit a wide diversity of chemical structure. One of the best-known examples is hexamethonium (Fig. 16). The structure–activity relationships of this class of compounds have been reviewed (Ing, 1936; Moe and Freyburger, 1950; Paton and Zaimis, 1952; Ing, 1956) and will not be discussed here.

5.4.3. Antagonists at the Muscarinic Receptor

Atropine (Fig. 19), which is a belladonna alkaloid, is the classical example of a muscarinic receptor antagonist. The antimuscarinic properties of atropine are due to its being an ester of tropic acid and to the presence of a tertiary amino alcohol; the tropine base itself is relatively inactive. Substitution of other aromatic acids for tropic acid modifies but does not always

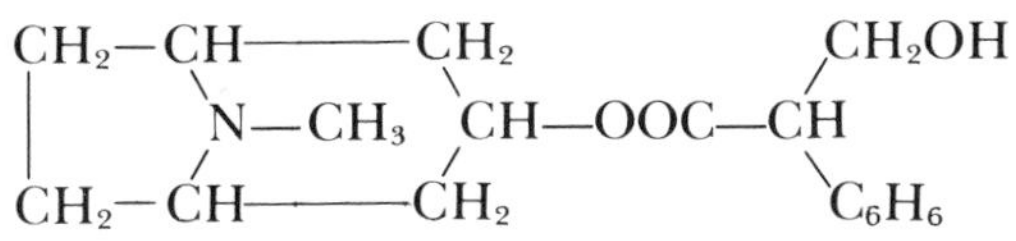

$$
\begin{array}{l}
\mathrm{CH_2-CH\!-\!\!-\!\!-\!\!-CH_2} \qquad\quad \mathrm{CH_2OH} \\
\quad\quad \mathrm{N-CH_3 \ \ CH-OOC-CH} \\
\mathrm{CH_2-CH\!-\!\!-\!\!-\!CH_2} \qquad\quad\quad \mathrm{C_6H_6}
\end{array}
$$

FIG. 19. The belladonna alkaloid atropine.

abolish activity. Atropine is a mixture of d- and l-hyoscyamine. The l-isomer is twice as potent as the racemic mixture in its antimuscarinic activity. It has been suggested (Cannon and Long, 1967) that the molecular skeleton shown in Fig. 20 defines the structural features that are common to many series of antimuscarinic compounds. In general, R_1 is a planar unsaturated ring such as phenyl, furanyl, or thienyl, and R_2 is usually alkyl, aryl, or hydrogen. Substitution with groups larger than a phenyl ring (e.g., p-bromophenyl) usually results in a sharp drop in activity. The R_3 group is one capable of hydrogen bonding (e.g., hydroxyl, amide). The nitrogen atom is positively charged due either to its quaternary alkyl substitution or to its being a protonated tertiary amine. For a quaternary ammonium group, optimal activity usually occurs with groups larger than methyl; however, substitution with groups larger than isopropyl results in a fall in activity. Introduction of heterocyclic rings also yields compounds with high activity. The carbon-to-nitrogen portion of the compound may have an ester linkage. In a number of series, however, this function is absent, clearly indicating that it is not essential for activity. Other examples of structure–activity correlations for this group of drugs are available (Gyermek and Nador, 1957; Bachrach, 1958; Ing, 1946; Stoll, 1948; Lands, 1951; Lands and Luduena, 1956).

Various muscarinic antagonists with high degrees of specificity and affinity have been used to characterize the muscarinic receptor in the peripheral and central nervous systems. These include the irreversible antagonists benzilylcholine mustard (Gill and Rang, 1966; Fewtrell and Rang, 1973) and its N-propyl analogue (Hiley et al., 1972; Cuthbert and Young, 1973; Hiley and Burgen, 1974; Burgen et al., 1974a,b) and the reversible antagonist quinuclidinyl benzilate (Yamamura and Snyder, 1974) (Fig. 8). It was shown that the area with the highest binding capacity in the rat brain is the corpus striatum (Yamamura and Snyder, 1974), while in the dog it was localized to the caudate nucleus (Hiley and Burgen, 1974). These studies have also demonstrated that the binding of these labeled antagonists is inhibited by atropine and other muscarinic antagonists and agonists

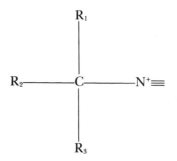

FIG. 20. Molecular skeleton of antimuscarinic compounds.

TABLE 16

Relative Potencies of Drugs in Reducing [³H]QNB Binding to Rat Brain Homogenates[a]

Drug	ED_{50}[b] (M)
Quinuclidinyl benzilate (QNB)	7×10^{-10}
Scopolamine	8×10^{-10}
Isopropamide	1×10^{-9}
Atropine	2×10^{-9}
Oxotremorine	1×10^{-6}
Pilocarpine	7×10^{-6}
d-Chlorpheniramine	1×10^{-5}
d-Brompheniramine	1×10^{-5}
l-Brompheniramine	1×10^{-5}
Arecoline	1×10^{-5}
Acetylcholine	2×10^{-5}
Carbamylcholine	3×10^{-5}
Acetyl-β-methylcholine	7×10^{-5}

[a]No effect at 1×10^{-5} M: Aspartic acid, γ-aminobutyric acid, glutamic acid, proline, naloxone, methylphenidate, glycine, pempidine, levorphanol, dextrorphan, purified corticotoxin and neurotoxin from the cobra (*Naja naja*), hexamethonium, d-tubocurarine, mecamylamine, Δ^9-tetrahydrocannabinol, neostigmine, and physostigmine. Data from Yamaura and Snyder (1974).

[b]Concentration of drug which displaced specific [³H]QNB binding by 50%.

(Table 16) but that nicotinic and noncholinergic drugs have little affinity for these binding sites (Hiley *et al.*, 1972; Burgen *et al.*, 1974a,b; Yamamura and Snyder, 1974).

5.5. Possible Modes of Action

As ACh has been the most extensively studied neurotransmitter, it is to be expected that more theories attempting to explain its mode of action at the receptor site have been advanced than for any other biogenic amine. The interested reader is referred to various reviews dealing with these early theories (Ehrenpreis *et al.*, 1969; Korolkovas, 1970; Gearien, 1970; Triggle, 1971). Because ACh is a flexible molecule, information about its possible conformations at various receptor sites can be obtained only by a combined application of nuclear magnetic resonance spectroscopy (NMR), theoretical calculations, and X-ray analysis of less flexible, though active, analogues.

5.6. NMR Studies

A NMR study of ACh in D_2O has shown that a *gauche* orientation (Fig. 21) is the preferred conformation in solution (Culvenor and Ham, 1966).

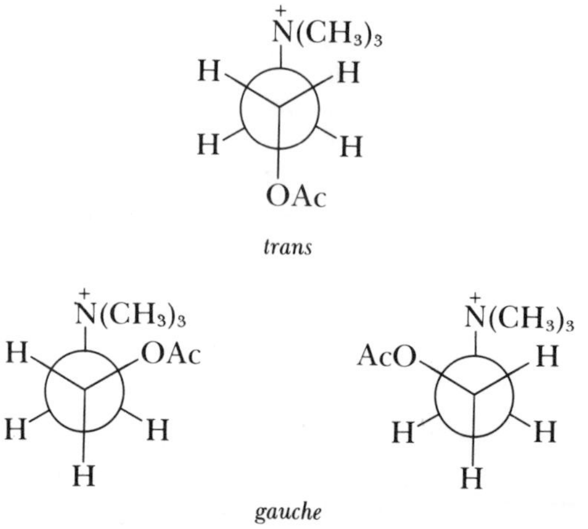

$$\overset{+}{N}(CH_3)_3$$

H⤳⤳H

H⤳⤳H

OAc

trans

$$\overset{+}{N}(CH_3)_3$$

H⤳OAc

H⤳H

H

$$\overset{+}{N}(CH_3)_3$$

AcO⤳H

H⤳H

H

gauche

FIG. 21. Conformers of acetylcholine.

However, similar studies on the analogues acetylthiocholine and acetylselenocholine showed that the *trans* conformation was the preferred form (Cushley and Mautner, 1970). Nicotine has also been the subject of NMR (Simpson *et al.*, 1967) and circular dichroism studies (Testa and Jenner, 1973).

5.7. Theoretical Studies

In a molecular orbital study on ACh, muscarine, and muscarone, Kier (1967) has shown that the minimum-energy conformations for all three compounds are essentially *gauche*. In the case of muscarine, this result was supported by other workers (Liquori *et al.*, 1968a). However, other studies on ACh have shown the presence of four conformations, two *gauche* and two *trans*, having energies separated by less than 1 kCal/mol. (Liquori *et al.*, 1968b). More recent studies using theoretical modifications of the above methods have examined ACh and its analogues and have stressed various other aspects of conformation and electronic structure (Pullman *et al.*, 1971; Beveridge and Radna, 1971).

5.8. X-Ray Crystallographic Studies

A possible way to circumvent the difficulties of working with a flexible agonist such as ACh is to examine the molecular structures of potent rigid and semirigid muscarinic and nicotinic agents. This approach has been used extensively by Chothia, Pauling, and coworkers (Canepa *et al.*, 1966; Chothia

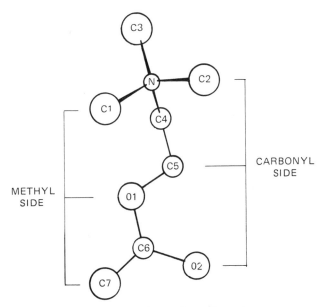

FIG. 22. Acetylcholine in the conformation relevant to muscarinic and nicotinic nerve receptors. From Chothia (1970a);
reproduced with permission.

and Pauling, 1968, 1970; Chothia, 1970a; Baker et al., 1971). Chothia has
proposed, on the basis of the crystal structures of cyclic muscarinic and
nicotinic agonists, that the conformation of ACh relevant to both types of
receptors is similar to that shown in Fig. 22. It is suggested that the "methyl
side" of ACh activates muscarinic receptors and that blockage of this side
removes muscarinic activity. It was concluded that the carbonyl side of ACh
interacts with nicotinic receptors and that blockage of this function occurs in
muscarinic agonists, hence explaining their lack of nicotinic activity. This
explanation of muscarinic activity has been questioned by workers who have
examined other ACh analogues (Shefter and Triggle, 1970). The original
claim has also been defended (Chothia, 1970b). By conformational analysis
of several rigid and semirigid ACh agonists and antagonists of known and
unknown crystal structure, Beers and Reich (1970) have proposed different
requirements for nicotinic and muscarinic activity. In the case of nicotinic
agents, specific binding is suggested to be mediated by (1) a coulombic
interaction involving the alkyl ammonium moiety and (2) a hydrogen bond
formed approximately 5.9 Å from the center of the positive charge. For
muscarinic agents, the binding is hypothesized to be mediated by (1) a
quaternary ammonium group or its equivalent and (2) an unshared pair of
electrons that can take part in H-bond formation approximately 4.4 Å from
the positive charge center. Some support for these proposals has come from
the theoretical studies of Pullman et al. (1971).

6. HISTAMINE

Compared to the putative transmitters that have already been discussed, less is known about the role of histamine in the brain. This was due in the past to the lack of a sensitive and specific assay. However, this shortcoming has been overcome and the topic is discussed by Taylor (Chap. 6, Vol. 3). The structure–activity studies reported here will therefore be from the peripheral nervous system.

6.1. Physiological Effects

There are important species differences in the response to injected histamine. Man and the guinea pig are very sensitive, whereas the rat is relatively resistant. There are also some differences in the response to histamine of similar organs in different species. A fall in blood pressure, followed by a rise, is produced by intravenous histamine. The former effect is due to dilation of the arterioles, the latter to a release of catecholamines from the adrenal medulla. Histamine produces a contraction in many smooth muscles. The guinea pig ileum is very sensitive to this amine and has been used in its quantification. Bronchiolar musculature is also sensitive to histamine, particularly in guinea pigs. Histamine acts directly to produce hydrochloric acid secretion in the stomach. The salivary and various other exocrine glands are stimulated by this amine.

6.2. Histamine Receptors

Black *et al.* (1972) have provided evidence for at least two subtypes of histamine receptors. It was shown that 4-methylhistamine, relative to histamine, had more activity as an agonist on rat gastric acid secretion and contraction of rat uterus and guinea pig atrium than on the H_1-receptor preparations of guinea pig ileum and rat stomach strip. However, the analogue 2-methylhistamine had more activity on H_1-receptors. It was

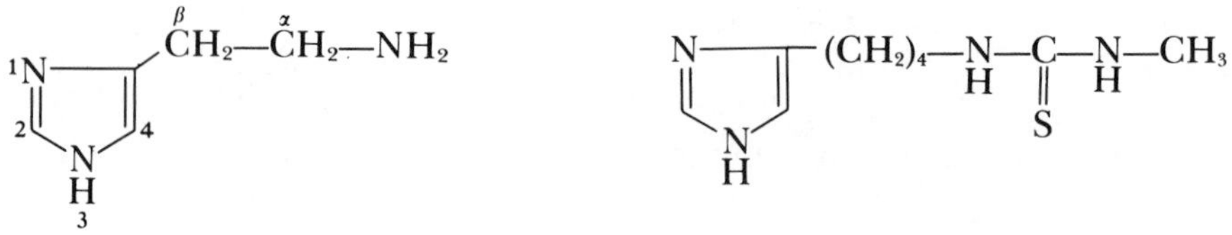

Histamine   Burimamide

FIG. 23. Histamine and its antagonist burimamide.

further shown that burimamide N-methyl-N'-[4-(4(5)-imidazolyl)-butyl]thiourea (Fig. 23), was a specific competitive antagonist of histamine on the rat uterus and guinea pig atrium and on gastric acid production in rats. These workers have therefore proposed that the receptors for these effects of histamine should be classed as H_2-receptors.

6.3. Structure–Activity Relationships

Histamine is 4-(2-aminoethyl)imidazole (Fig. 23). Jones (1966) has extensively reviewed the activity of more than 200 compounds on histamine receptors on the guinea pig ileum and their effects on blood pressure and gastric acid secretion. The results for the guinea pig ileum will be discussed first.

The side chain: Lengthening the side chain by one or two carbon atoms eliminates activity. Shortening the side chain by one carbon atom also reduces potency. Substitution of alkyl groups in the side chain lowers but does not eliminate activity.

Substitution on the amino group: Replacement of one or both of the hydrogens of the amino group with small alkyl substituents produces compounds that are less active. As the size of the group(s) increases, a compound's activity as an agonist decreases.

Position of attachment of the side chain to the imidazole nucleus: When the side chain is moved to position 1 or 2, activity is completely lost.

Methyl substituents on the nucleus: Substitution of methyl groups in the 1, 2, or 5 position of the imidazole ring yields less active analogues.

Replacement of the imidazole nucleus: Certain other heterocyclic ring systems such as pyrazole, triazole, pyridine, and thiazole (Fig. 24) may be substituted for the imidazole nucleus to produce analogues possessing histamine-like activity on the guinea pig ileum. Unlike the imidazole ring,

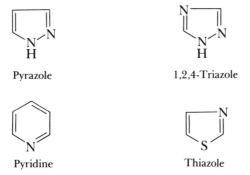

Pyrazole   1,2,4-Triazole

Pyridine   Thiazole

FIG. 24. Heterocyclic ring systems that have been incorporated into histamine analogues.

the pyrazole nucleus may have an aminoethyl side chain substituted at position 1, 3, or 4 without loss of histamine-like activity.

6.4. Structure–Activity Relationships for Histamine-like Activity on Gastric Acid Secretion and Inhibition of the Rat Uterus

The aminoethyl side chain is necessary for histamine-like activity on gastric acid secretion and inhibition of the rat uterus. Changes in the side chain produce similar results on activity to those found for the guinea pig ileum. There is a marked fall in activity on modification of the imidazole ring. The relationship of the side chain and the basic atom in the ring appears to be less critical in these preparations as 2- and 4-(2-aminoethyl)pyridines are approximately equiactive whereas the 2-isomer is a hundredfold more potent than the 4-isomer on guinea pig ileum (Ash and Schild, 1966).

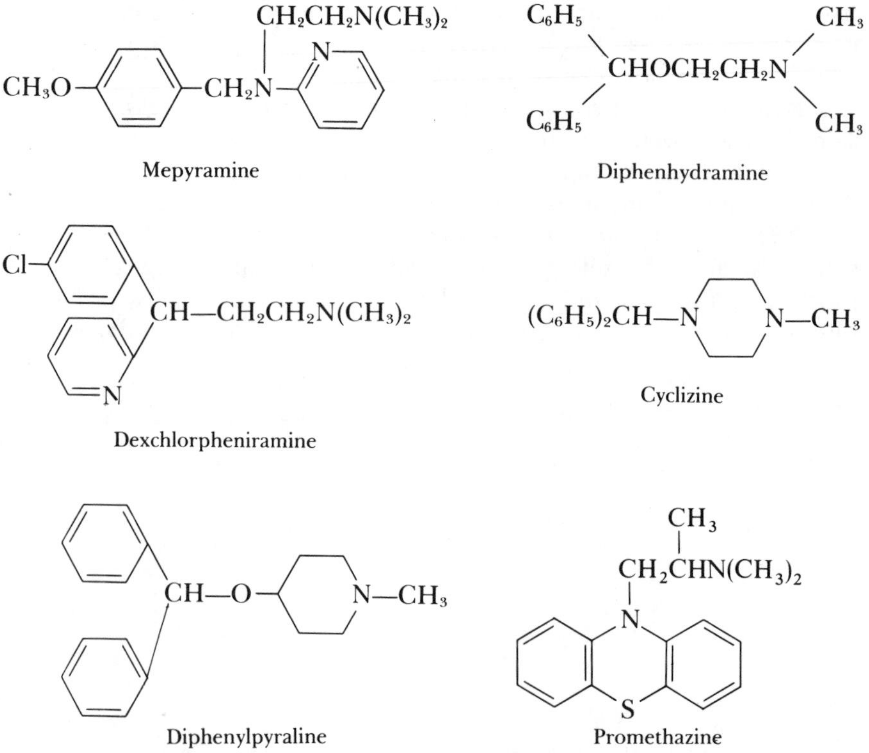

Mepyramine

Diphenhydramine

Dexchlorpheniramine

Cyclizine

Diphenylpyraline

Promethazine

FIG. 25. Structures of various antihistamines.

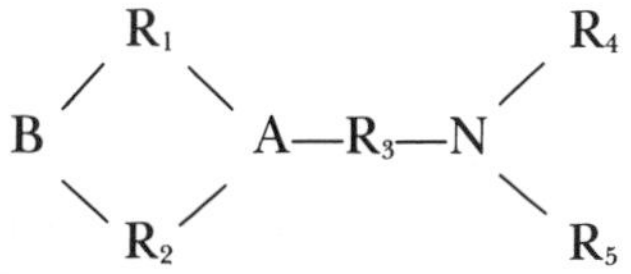

$$B \diagup\diagdown \begin{matrix} R_1 \\ \\ R_2 \end{matrix} \diagdown\diagup A—R_3—N \begin{matrix} \diagup R_4 \\ \\ \diagdown R_5 \end{matrix}$$

FIG. 26. General structure of antihistamine compounds having greatest activity.

6.5. Structure–Activity Relationships of Antihistamines

The structure–activity relationships of the antihistamines have been reviewed by several authors (Loew, 1947; Huttrer, 1947; Bovet, 1950; Idson, 1950; Melville, 1973; Leonard and Huttrer, 1950; Barlow, 1964). Compounds possessing antihistamine activity belong to many chemical classes, but for convenience they may be divided into drugs containing the following moieties (Fig. 25): ethylenediamines, —N—C—C—N— (mepyramine); aminoethyl ethers, O—C—C—N— (diphenhydramine); propylamines, —C—C—C—N— (dexchlorpheniramine); piperazines (cyclizine); piperidines (diphenylpyraline); and phenothiazines (promethazine). In general, maximum activity is found in compounds having the general structure shown in Fig. 26. R_1 and R_2 are aromatic or heterocyclic rings, one of which can be separated from A by a methylene group (A can be CO, N, or C); R_3 is usually a dimethylene chain or a two-carbon fragment of a nitrogen-containing heterocyclic ring. It is only in the case of tricyclic compounds, such as the piperidylalkyl phenothiazines, that a three-carbon chain at R_3 produces antihistamine activity greater than that occurring in the two-carbon analogue. The two aromatic rings R_1 and R_2 are sometimes bridged by a carbon or heteroatom (B) at the *ortho* position. The groups R_4 and R_5 can be small planar cyclic systems or methyl groups. Maximum activity is observed if both rings are not coplanar. From an analysis of several groups of antihistamines, it is concluded that the most significant intramolecular distance is that between the center of the aromatic rings and the terminal nitrogen atom. The most potent antagonists appear to have an intramolecular distance of 5–6 Å between these two moieties. In the antihistamines having an asymmetrical center or a suitably substituted double bond, it has been possible to show that stereoselective activity occurs (Jarrousse and Regnier, 1951; Adamson *et al.*, 1951; Harms and Nauta, 1960). It is of interest that although the antihistamines can antagonize to various degrees most of the effects of histamine on the different organs and systems of the body, they are mostly without effect on histamine-induced gastric secretion. An exception to this is the previously mentioned compound burimamide (Black *et al.*, 1972).

6.6. Possible Mechanisms of Action

It has been suggested (Rocha e Silva, 1960) that histamine binds to its receptor by the imino group of the imidazole ring and the free amino group of the side chain. It was further hypothesized that the imino group forms a transitory bond with a polarized carbonyl group of a peptide link in the receptor while the amino group forms a hydrogen bond with a protein residue of histidine or arginine. Bloom and Goldman (1966) proposed that the histamine–receptor interaction involves a phosphoryl group transfer process. Nauta *et al.* (1968) have put forward a detailed model of the histamine receptor. It is postulated to consist of a polypeptide chain in the form of a α-helix. The binding of receptor and antihistamine drug is claimed to occur at three points:

1. A phenyl group of a phenylalanylhistidyl residue of the α-helix interacts with an aromatic ring of the drug.
2. An imidazole ring of the same residue attaches to the amino group of the drug.
3. A hydroxyl group of the neighboring serine of the receptor forms a hydrogen bond with the ether oxygen of the drug.

Barlow (1964) has suggested how certain antihistamines might bind to their receptors via a combination of Van der Waals, electrostatic, and ionic binding. Hückel molecular orbital calculations (Kier, 1968*b*) have shown that there are two conformations of histamine of nearly equal energy. In one conformation, the ring nitrogen atom adjacent to the side chain and the terminal amino group nitrogen atom are 4.55 Å apart. This is similar to the internitrogen distance in the antihistamine triprolidine. Kier therefore proposed that this conformation of the molecule is specific for H_1-receptors. The other low-energy conformation of histamine has an internitrogen distance of 3.60 Å. A more extensive theoretical study of histamine and its analogues by Periti (1970) has supported and extended the initial work of Kier. NMR studies have also supported Kier's suggestions, as it was found that there are approximately equal proportions of the *trans* and *gauche* rotamers (Casy *et al.*, 1970). In the solid state, however, X-ray analysis has shown that histamine acid phosphate exists in the *trans* conformation. It is of interest that a semirigid analogue of the *trans* form of histamine, 2-(4-imidazolyl)cyclopropylamine, was only weakly active in producing gastric acid secretion *in vivo* (Burger *et al.*, 1970). Various aspects of the crystal and molecular structure of histamine and histidine are dealt with by Carlstrom *et al.* (1973). The crystal and molecular structure of burimamide has recently been reported (Kamenar *et al.*, 1973).

7. REFERENCES

ADAMSON, D. W., BARRETT, P. A., BILLINGHURST, J. W., GREEN, A. F., and JONES, T. S. G., 1951, Geometrical isomers in a series of antihistamines, *Nature* **168**:204–205.

AHLQUIST, R. P., 1948, A study of adrenotropic receptors, *Am. J. Physiol.* **153**:586–600.

AHLQUIST, R. P., 1968, Agents which block adrenergic β-receptors, in: *Annual Review of Pharamacology*, Vol 8 (H. W. Elliott, ed.), pp. 259–272, Annual Reviews, Inc., Palo Alto, Calif.

AINSWORTH, C., 1958, Substituted β-aminoethylindazoles, *J. Am. Chem. Soc.* **80**:965–967.

AIZENSHTAT, Z., KLEIN, E., WEILER-FEILCHENFELD, H., and BERGMANN, E. D., 1972, Conformational studies on xanthene, thioxanthene and acridan, *Israel J. Chem.* **10**:753–763.

ANDEN, N. E., ROOS, B. E., and WERDINIUS, B., 1964, Effects of chlorpromazine, haloperidol and reserpine on the levels of phenolic acids in rabbit corpus striatum, *Life Sci.* **3**:149–158.

ANDEN, N. E., RUBENSON, A., FUXE, K., and HOKFELT, T., 1967, Evidence for dopamine receptor stimulation by apomorphine, *J. Pharm. Pharmacol.* **19**:627–629.

ANDEN, N. E., BUTCHER, S. G., CORRODI, H., FUXE, K., and UNGERSTEDT, U., 1970, Receptor activity and turnover of dopamine and noradrenaline after neuroleptics, *Eur. J. Pharmacol.* **11**:303–314.

ARIENS, E. J., 1963, in: *First International Pharmacological Meeting Stockholm 1961*, Vol. 7, p. 247, Macmillan, New York.

ARIENS, E. J., 1967, The structure–activity relationships of β-adrenergic drugs and β-adrenergic blocking drugs, *Ann. N.Y. Acad. Sci.* **139**:606–631.

ARIENS, E. J., 1971, A general introduction to the field of drug design, in: *Drug Design*, Vol. 1 (E. J. Ariens, ed.), pp. 1–270, Academic Press, New York.

ARIENS, E. J., and SIMONIS, A. M., 1964, A molecular basis for drug action, *J. Pharm. Pharmacol.* **16**:137–157.

ARONEY, M. J., HOSKINS, G. M., and LEFEVRE, R. J. W., 1968, Molecular polarisability: The conformations as solutes of phenothiazine and of N-methyl and N-phenylphenothiazine, *J. Chem. Soc. (B)* **1968**:1206–1208.

ASH, A. S. F., and SCHILD, H. O., 1966, Receptors mediating some actions of histamine, *Brit. J. Pharmacol.* **27**:427–439.

BACHRACH, W. H., 1958, Anticholinergic drugs: Survey of the literature and some experimental observations, *Am. J. Digest. Dis.* **3**:743–799.

BAKER, R. W., CHOTHIA, C. H., PAULING, P., and PETCHER, T. J., 1971, Structure and activity of muscarinic stimulants, *Nature* **230**:439–445.

BANISTER, J., and WHITTAKER, V. P., 1951, Pharmacological activity of the carbon analogue of acetylcholine, *Nature* **167**:605–606.

BARGER, G., and DALE, H. H., 1910, Chemical structure and sympathomimetic action of amines, *J. Physiol.* **41**:19–59.

BARLOW, R. B., 1964, *Introduction to Chemical Pharamacology*, 2nd ed., pp. 344–377, Wiley, New York.

BARLOW, R. B., and KAHN, I., 1959a, Actions of some analogues of tryptamine on the isolated rat uterus and on the isolated rat fundus strip preparations, *Brit. J. Pharmacol.* **14**:99–107.

BARLOW, R. B., and KAHN, I., 1959b, Actions of some analogues of 5-hydroxytryptamine on the isolated rat uterus and the rat fundus strip preparations, *Brit. J. Pharmacol.* **14**:265–272.

BARLOW, R. B., SCOTT, K. A., and STEPHENSON, R. P., 1963, An attempt to study the effects of chemical structure on the affinity and efficacy of compounds related to acetylcholine, *Brit. J. Pharmacol.* **21**:509–522.

BARRETT, A. M., 1972, Design of β-blocking drugs, in: *Drug Design*, Vol. III (E. J. Ariens, ed.), pp. 205–228, Academic Press, New York.

BECKETT, A. H., HARPER, N. J., CLITHEROW, J. W., and LESSER, E., 1961, Muscarinic receptors, *Nature* **189**:671–673.

BEERS, W. H., and REICH, E., 1970, Structure and activity of acetylcholine, *Nature* **228**:917–922.

BELL, C., and LANG, W. J., 1973, Neural dopaminergic vasodilator control in the kidney, *Nature* **246**:27–29.

BELLEAU, B., 1965, in: *Isotopes in Pharmacology* (L. Roth, ed.), p. 469, University of Chicago Press, Chicago.

BELLEAU, B., 1967, Stereochemistry of adrenergic receptors: Newer concepts on the molecular mechanism of action of catecholamines and antiadrenergic drugs at the receptor level, *Ann. N.Y. Acad. Sci.* **139**:580–605.

BERGIN, R., and CARLSTROM, D., 1968, The crystal structure of dopamine hydrochloride, *Acta Crystallog.* **B24**:1506–1510.

BERRIDGE, M. J., 1972, The mode of action of 5-hydroxytryptamine, *J. Exp. Biol.* **56**:311–321.

BERRIDGE, M. J., and PATEL, N. E., 1968, Insect salivary glands: Stimulation of fluid secretion by 5-hydroxytryptamine and adenosine 3′,5′-monophosphate, *Science* **162**:462–463.

BERTACCINI, G., and ZAMBONI, P., 1961, The relative potency of 5-hydroxytryptamine-like substances, *Arch. Int. Pharmacodyn.* **133**:138–156.

BEVERIDGE, D. L., and RADNA, R. J., 1971, A quantum theoretical study of the molecular electronic structure of acetylcholine, *J. Am. Chem. Soc.* **93**:3759–3764.

BISCOE, T. J., CURTIS, D. R., and RYALL, R. W., 1966, An investigation of catecholamine receptors of spinal interneurones, *Int. J. Neuropharmacol.* **5**:429–434.

BLACK, J. M., DUNCAN, W. A. M., and SHANKS, R. G., 1965. Comparison of some properties of pronethalol and propranolol, *Brit. J. Pharmacol.* **25**:577–591.

BLACK, J. W., DUNCAN, W. A. M., DURANT, C. J., GANELLIN, C. R., and PARSONS, E. M., 1972, Definition and antagonism of histamine H_2-receptors, *Nature* **236**:385–390.

BLINKS, J. R., 1967, Evaluation of the cardiac effects of several β-adrenergic blocking agents, *Ann. N.Y. Acad. Sci.* **139**:673–685.

BLOOM, B. M., and GOLDMAN, I. M., 1966, The nature of catecholamine–adenine mononucleotide interactions in adrenergic mechanisms, in: *Advances in Drug Research*, Vol. 3 (N. J. Harper and A. B. Simmonds, eds.), pp. 121–169, Academic Press, London.

BLOOM, F. E., COSTA, E., and SALMOIRAGHI, G. C., 1964, Analysis of individual rabbit olfactory bulb neuron responses to the microelectrophoresis of acetylcholine, norepinephrine and serotonin synergists and antagonists, *J. Pharmacol. Exp. Ther.* **146**:16–23.

BOAKES, R. J., BRADLEY, P. B., BROOKES, N., CANDY, J. M., and WOLSTENCROFT, J. H., 1971, Actions of noradrenaline, other sympathomimetic amines and antagonists on neurones in the brain stem of the cat, *Brit. J. Pharmacol.* **41**:462–479.

BORN, G. V. R., 1971, in: *Effects of Drugs on Cellular Control Mechanisms* (B. R. Rabin and R. B. Freedman, eds.), pp. 237–257, Macmillan, London.

BOVET, D., 1950, Introduction to antihistamine agents and antergan derivatives, *Ann. N.Y. Acad. Sci.* **50**:1089–1126.

BOVET, D., and BOVET-NITTI, F., 1948, in: *Medicaments du Systeme Nerveux Vegetatif*, pp. 222–237, Karger, Basel.

BOVET, D., BOVET-NITTI, F., and MARINI-BETTOLO, G. B. (eds.), 1959, *Curare and Curare-like Agents*, Elsevier, Amsterdam.

BROTZU, G. 1970, Inhibition by chlorpromazine of the effects of dopamine on the dog kidney, *J. Pharm. Pharmacol.* **22**:664–667.

BROWN, J. H., and MAKMAN, M. H., 1972, Stimulation by dopamine of adenylate cyclase in retinal homogenates and of adenosine 3′,5′-cyclic monphosphate formation in intact retina, *Proc. Natl. Acad. Sci.* **69**:539–543.

BROWN, J. H., and MAKMAN, M. H., 1973, Influence of neuroleptic drugs and apomorphine on dopamine-sensitive adenylate cyclase of retina, *J. Neurochem.* **21**:477–479.

BURGEN, A. S. V., 1965, The role of ionic interaction at the muscarinic receptor, *Brit. J. Pharmacol.* **25**:4–17.

BURGEN, A. S. V., HILEY, C. R., and YOUNG, J. M., 1974a, The binding of ³H-propylbenzilylcholine mustard by longitudinal muscle strips from guinea-pig small intestine, *Brit. J. Pharmacol.* **50**:145–151.

BURGEN, A. S. V., HILEY, C. R., and YOUNG, J. M., 1974b, The properties of muscarinic receptors in mammalian cerebral cortex, *Brit. J. Pharmacol.*, **51**:279–285.

BURGER, A., BERNABE, M., and COLLINS, P. W., 1970, 2-(4-Imidazolyl)cyclopropylamine, *J. Med. Chem.* **13**:33–35.

BURKS, T. F., LONG, J. P., DARKO, L. L., and CANNON, J. G., 1965, Evaluation of N-methoxy substitution in cholinergic agents, *Fed. Proc.* **24**:611.

BURNS, J. J., COLVILLE, K. I., LINDSAY, L. A., and SALVADOR, R. A., 1964, Blockade of some metabolic effects of catecholamines by N-isopropyl methoxamine (B. W. 61–43), *J. Pharmacol. Exp. Ther.* **144**:163–171.

BURNS, T. W., LANGLEY, P. E., and ROBISON, G. A., 1971, Adrenergic receptors and cyclic AMP: Regulation of human adipose tissue lipolysis, *Ann. N.Y. Acad. Sci.* **185**:115–128.

CAMERON, W. M., and TAINTER, M. L., 1936, Comparative actions of sympathomimetic compounds: Bronchiodilator actions in bronchial spasms induced by histamine, *J. Pharmacol. Exp. Ther.* **57**:152–169.

CAMPAIGNE, E., KNAPP, D. R., NEISS, E. S., and BOSIN, T. R., 1970, Biologically active benzothiophene derivatives, in: *Advances in Drug Research*, Vol. 5 (N. J. Harper and A. B. Simmonds, eds.), pp. 1–54, Academic Press, London.

CANEPA, F. G., PAULING, P. J., and SORUM, H., 1966, Structure of acetylcholine and other substrates of cholinergic systems, *Nature* **210**:907–909.

CANNON, J. G., and LONG, J. P., 1967, Postganglionic parasympathetic depressants, in: *Drugs Affecting the Peripheral Nervous System* (A. Burger, ed.), pp. 133–148, Dekker, New York.

CARLSSON, A., and LINDQVIST, M., 1963, Effect of chlorpromazine or haloperidol on formation of 3-methoxytyramine and normetanephrine in mouse brain, *Acta Pharmacol. Toxicol.* **20**:140–144.

CARLSSON, A., FUXE, K., HAMBERGER, B., and LINDQVIST, M., 1966, Biochemical and histochemical studies of the effects of imipramine-like drugs and (+)-amphetamine on central and peripheral catecholamine neurons, *Acta Physiol. Scand.* **67**:481–497.

CARLSTROM, D., and BERGIN, R., 1967, The crystal structure of noradrenaline hydrochloride, *Acta Crystallog.* **23**:313–319.

CARLSTROM, D., BERGIN, R., and FALKENBERG, G., 1973, Molecular characteristics of biogenic monoamines and their analogs, *Quart. Rev. Biophys.* **6**:257–310.

CARR, L. A., and MOORE, K. E., 1970, Effects of amphetamine on the contents of norepinephrine and its metabolites in the effluent of perfused cerebral ventricles of the cat, *Biochem. Pharmacol.* **19**:2361–2374.

CASY, A. F., ISON, R. R., and HAM, N. S., 1970, The conformation of histamine in solution: 'H Nuclear magnetic resonance study, *Chem. Commun.* **1970**:1343–1344.

CHANG, H. C., and GADDUM, J. H., 1933, Choline esters in tissue extracts, *J. Physiol.* **79**:255–285.

CHOTHIA, C., 1970a, Interaction of acetylcholine with different cholinergic nerve receptors, *Nature* **225**:36–38.

CHOTHIA, C., 1970b, Structure–activity relationships of some muscarinic agonists: A reply to Shefter and Triggle, *Nature* **227**:1355–1356.

CHOTHIA, C., and PAULING, 1968, Conformations of acetylcholine, *Nature* **219**:1156–1157.

CHOTHIA, C., and PAULING, P., 1970, The conformation of cholinergic molecules at nicotinic nerve receptors, *Proc. Natl. Acad. Sci.* **65**:477–482.

COLE, B., ROBISON, G. A., and HARTMANN, R. C., 1971, Studies on the role of cyclic AMP in platelet function, *Ann. N.Y. Acad. Sci.* **185**:477–487.

COLHOUN, E. H., 1963, Synthesis of 5-hydroxytryptamine in the American cockroach, *Experientia* **19**:9–10.

CORRODI, H., PERSSON, H., CARLSSON, A., and ROBERTS, J., 1963, A new series of substances which block the adrenergic β-receptors, *J. Med. Chem.* **6**:751–755.

COYLE, J. T., and SNYDER, S. H., 1969, Antiparkinsonian drugs: Inhibition of dopamine uptake in the corpus striatum as a possible mechanism of action, *Science* **166**:899–901.

CUELLO, A. C., HORN, A. S., MACKAY, A. V. P., and IVERSEN, L. L., 1973, Catecholamines in the median eminence: New evidence for a major noradrenergic input, *Nature* **243**:465–467.

CULVENOR, C. C. J., and HAM, N. S., 1966, The proton magnetic resonance spectrum and conformation of acetylcholine, *Chem. Commun.* **1966**:537–539.

CUSHLEY, R. J., and MAUTNER, H. G., 1970, N.M.R. studies on the conformation of acetylcholine isologues, *Tetrahedron* **26**:2151–2159.

CUTHBERT, A. W., and YOUNG, J. M., 1973, The number of muscarinic receptors in chick amnion muscle, *Brit. J. Pharmacol.* **49**:498–505.

DALE, H. H., 1906, On some physiological actions of ergot, *J. Physiol.* **34**:163–206.

DALE, H. H., 1953, *Adventures in Physiology*, Pergamon Press, London.

DALGLIESH, C. E., TOH, C. C., and WORK, T. S., 1953, Fractionation of the smooth muscle stimulants present in extracts of gastro-intestinal tract: Identification of 5-hydroxytryptamine and its distinction from substance P, *J. Physiol.* **120**:298–310.

DAPRADA, M., and PLETSCHER, A., 1966, Acceleration of cerebral dopamine turnover by chlorpromazine, *Experientia* **22**:465–466.

DOLLERY, C. T., PATERSON, J. W., and CONOLLY, M. E., 1969, Clinical pharmacology of beta receptor blocking drugs, *Clin. Pharmacol. Ther.* **10**:765–799.

DORIGNAC-CALAS, M. R., and MARSAU, P., 1972, Structure cristalline du chlorhydrate de chloro-3 (dimethylamino-3'propyl)-10-phenothiazine, *Comp. Rend. Acad. Sci. Paris* **274**:1806–1809.

DUNITZ, J. D., ESER, H., and STRICKLER, P., 1964, Die Konfiguration des physiologisch Wirksamen 2-Chloro-9-(w-dimethylaminopropyliden)-thioxanthens, *Helv. Chim. Acta* **47**:1897–1902.

EHRENPREIS, S., FLEISCH, J. H., and MITTAG, T. W., 1969, Approaches to the molecular nature of pharmacological receptors, *Pharmacol. Rev.* **21**:131–181.

ELLENBROEK, B. W. J., and VAN ROSSUM, J. N., 1960, Absolute configuration and parasympathomimetic activity—Chemistry and pharmacology of acetyl-β-methyl choline, *Arch. Int. Pharmacodyn.* **125**:216–220.

ERLENMEYER, H., and LOBECK, H., 1937, Darstellung und Eigenschaften des Acetyl-d3-cholin, *Helv. Chim. Acta* **20**:142–150.

ERNST, A. M., 1967, Mode of action of apomorphine and *d*-amphetamine for gnawing compulsion in rats, *Psychopharmacologia* **10**:316–323.

ERSPAMER, V., 1940, Pharmakologische Studien uber Enteramin. I, *Naunyn-Schmiedberg's Arch. Exp. Pathol. Pharmakol.* **196**:343–365.

ERSPAMER, V., 1954, Il sistema cellulare enterocromaffine e l'enteramina (5-idrossitriptamina), *Rend. Sci. Farm.* **1**:1–193.

ERSPAMER, V., 1966, Bioassay of indoleaklyamines, in: *5-Hydroxytryptamine and Related Indolealkylamines* (O. Elchler and A. Farah, eds.), pp. 132–181, Vol. 19 of *Handbook of Experimental Pharmacology*, Springer, Berlin.

EUGSTER, C. H., 1959, Synthese and pharmakologische Eigenschaften des Desmethylmuscarones und der stereoisomeren Desmethylmuscarine Die Basen starken der isomeren Normuscarine, *Helv. Chim. Acta* **42**:1177–1189.

EVERETT, A. J., LAUE, L. A., and WILKINSON, S., 1970, Revision of the structures of (+)-tubocurarine chloride and (+)-chondrocurine, *Chem. Commun.* **1970**:1020–1021.

FELLMAN, J. H., FUJITA, T. S., and BELBER, C. J., 1962, 2,3-Dihydro-5-hydroxytryptamine, *Biochem. Pharmacol.* **11**:557–561.

FEWTRELL, C. M. S., and RANG, H. P., 1973, Labelling cholinergic receptors in smooth muscle, in: *Drug Receptors* (H. P. Rang, ed.), pp. 211–224, Macmillan, London.

FREYHAN, F. A., 1961, in: *Extrapyramidal System and Neuroleptics* (J. M. Bordeleau, ed.), pp. 483–486, Editions Psychiatriques, Montreal.

FRIEDMAN, H. L., 1967, Postganglionic parasympathetic stimulants, in: *Drugs Affecting the Peripheral Nervous System* (A. Burger, ed.), pp. 79–131, Dekker, New York.

FURCHGOTT, R. F., 1972, The classification of adrenoceptors (adrenergic receptors): An evaluation from the standpoint of receptor theory, in: *Catecholamines*, (H. Blaschko and E. Muscholl, eds.), pp. 283–335, Vol. 33 of *Handbook of Experimental Pharmacology*, Springer, Berlin.

FUXE, K., 1965, Evidence for the existence of monoamine neurons in the central nervous system. IV. Distribution of monamine nerve terminals in the central nervous system, *Acta Physiol. Scand.* **64:**37–85 (Suppl. 247).

GADDUM, J. H., and HAMEED, K. A., 1954, Drugs which antagonize 5-hydroxytryptamine, *Brit. J. Pharmacol.* **9:**240–248.

GADDUM, J. H., and PAASONEN, M. K., 1955, The use of some molluscan hearts for the estimation of 5-hydroxytryptamine, *Brit. J. Pharmacol.* **10:**474–483.

GADDUM, J. H., and PICARELLI, Z., 1957, Two kinds of tryptamine receptors, *Brit. J. Pharmacol.* **12:**323–328.

GARATTINI, S., and VALZELLI, L., 1965, *Serotonin*, Elsevier, Amsterdam.

GEARIEN, J. E., 1970, Cholinergics and anticholinesterases, in: *Medicinal Chemistry*, Part II, 3rd ed. (A. Burger, ed.), pp. 1296–1313, Wiley-Interscience, New York.

GEIGER, W. B., and ALPERS, H., 1964, Properties of an acetylated derivative of trimethylamine oxide, *Arch. Int. Pharmacodyn.* **148:**352–358.

GIESECKE, J., 1973, The crystal and molecular structure of apomorphine hydrochloride hydrate, *Acta Crystallog.* **B29:**1785–1791.

GILL, E. W., and RANG, H. P., 1966, An alkylating derivative of benzilylcholine with specific and long-lasting parasympatholytic activity, *Mol. Pharmacol.* **2:**284–297.

GLOWINSKI, J., 1970, Effects of amphetamine on various aspects of catecholamine metabolism in the central nervous system of the rat, in: *Amphetamines and Related Compounds* (E. Costa and S. Garattini, eds.), pp. 301–316, Raven Press, New York.

GOLDBERG, L. I., SONNEVILLE, P. F., and MCNAY, J. L., 1968, An investigation of the structural requirements for dopamine-like renal vasodilation: Phenylethylamines and apomorphine, *J. Pharmacol. Exp. Ther.* **163:**188–197.

GOODMAN, L. S., and GILMAN, A., 1970, *The Pharmacological Basis of Therapeutics*, 4th ed., Macmillan, New York.

GORDON, M., 1967, Phenothiazines, in: *Psychopharmacological Agents*, Vol. 11, (M. Gordon, ed.), pp. 1–198, Academic Press, New York.

GREEN, A. L., 1967, Activity correlations and the mode of action of aminoalkylphenothiazine tranquillizers, *J. Pharm. Pharmacol.* **19:**207–208.

GREENBERG, M. J., 1960, Structure–activity relationship of tryptamine analogues on the heart of *Venus mercenaria*, *Brit. J. Pharmacol.* **15:**375–388.

GUNN, J. A., and GURD, M. R., 1940, The action of some amines related to adrenaline: Cyclohexylalkylamines, *J. Physiol.* **97:**453–470.

GYERMEK, L., 1961, 5-Hydroxytryptamine antagonists, *Pharmacol. Rev.* **13:**399–439.

GYERMEK, L., 1966, Drugs which antagonize 5-hydroxytryptamine and related indolealkylamines, in: *5-Hydroxytryptamine and Related Indolealkylamines* (O. Eichler and A. Farah, eds.), pp. 471–528, Vol. 19 of *Handbook of Experimental Pharmacology*, Springer, Berlin.

GYERMEK, L., and BINDLER, E., 1962, Action of indole alkylamines and amidines on the inferior mesenteric ganglion of the cat, *J. Pharmacol. Exp. Ther.* **138:**159–164.

GYERMEK, L., and NADOR, K., 1957, The pharmacology of tropane compounds in relation to their steric structure, *J. Pharm. Pharmacol.* **9:**209–229.

GYERMEK, L., and UNNA, K. R., 1958, Relation of structure of synthetic muscarines and muscarones to their pharmacological action, *Proc. Soc. Exp. Biol. Med.* **98:**882–885.

HARMS, A. F., and NAUTA, W. T., 1960, The effects of alkyl substitution on drugs. 1. Substituted dimethylaminoethyl benzhydryl ethers, *J. Med. Pharm. Chem.* **2:**57–77.

HARRISON, D. C., 1971, *Circulatory Effects and Clinical Uses of Beta-Adrenergic Blocking Drugs*, Excerpta Medica, Amsterdam and London.

HAYLETT, D. G., and JENKINSON, D. H., 1972, Effects of noradrenaline on potassium efflux, membrane potential and electrolyte levels in tissue slices prepared from guinea-pig liver, *J. Physiol.* **225:**721–750.

HEBB, C. O., and KRNJEVIĆ, K., 1962, *Neurochemistry* (K. A. C. Elliot, I. H., Page, and J. H. Quastel, eds.), pp. 452–521, Thomas, Springfield, Ill.

HILEY, C. R., and BURGEN, A. S. V., 1974, The distribution of muscarinic receptor sites in the nervous system of the dog, *J. Neurochem.* **22:**159–162.

HILEY, C. R., YOUNG, J. M., and BURGEN, A. S. V., 1972, Labelling of cholinergic receptors in subcellular fractions from rat cerebral cortex, *Biochem. J.* **127:**86P.

HOLTON, P., and ING, H. R., 1949, Specificity of the trimethylammonium group in acetylcholine, *Brit. J. Pharmacol.* **4:**190–196.

HORN, A. S., and SNYDER, S. H., 1971, Chlorpromazine and dopamine: Conformational similarities that correlate with the antischizophrenic activity of phenothiazine drugs, *Proc. Natl. Acad. Sci.* **68:**2325–2328.

HORN, A. S., CUELLO, A. C., and MILLER, R. J., 1974, Dopamine in the mesolimbic system of the rat brain: Endogenous levels and the effects of drugs on the uptake mechanism and stimulation of adenylate cyclase activity, *J. Neurochem.* **22:**265–270.

HORNYKIEWICZ, O., 1966, Dopamine and brain function, *Pharmacol. Rev.* **18:**925–964.

HOWE, R., 1963, Structure–activity relationships of some β-adrenergic blocking agents, *Biochem. Pharmacol. Suppl.* **12:**85–86.

HUNT, C. C., and KUFFLER, S. W., 1950, Pharmacology of the neuromuscular junction, *Pharmacol. Rev.* **2:**96–120.

HUNT, R., and RENSHAW, R. R., 1925, On some effects of arsonium, stibonium, phosphonium and sulfonium compounds on the autonomic nervous system, *J. Pharmacol. Exp. Ther.* **25:**315–355.

HUNT, R., and RENSHAW, R. R., 1932, Thio and thiomethyl ammonium compounds, *J. Pharmacol. Exp. Ther.* **44:**151–169.

HUNT, R., and RENSHAW, R. R., 1933, Effects of some quaternary ammonium and analogous compounds on the autonomic nervous system, *J. Pharmacol. Exp. Ther.* **48:**51–66.

HUNT, R., and TAVEAU, R. de M., 1906, On the physiological action of certain cholin derivatives and new methods for determining cholin, *Brit. Med. J.* **2:**1788–1791.

HUNT, R., and TAVEAU, R. de M., 1909, On the relation between the toxicity and chemical constitution of a number of derivatives of choline and analogous compounds, *J. Pharmacol. Exp. Ther.* **1:**303–339.

HUTTRER, C. P., 1947, Chemistry of antihistamine substances, *Enzymologia* **12:**277–332.

IDSON, B., 1950, Antihistamine drugs, *Chem. Rev.* **47:**307–527.

ING, H. R., 1936, The curariform action of onium salts, *Physiol. Rev.* **16:**527–544.

ING, H. R., 1946, Synthetic substitutes for atropine, *Brit. Med. Bull.* **4:**91–95.

ING, H. R., 1949, The structure–action relationships of the choline group, *Science* **109:**264–266.

ING, H. R., 1956, Structure–action relationships of hypotensive drugs, in: *Hypotensive Drugs* (M. Harrington, ed.), pp. 7–22, Pergamon Press, Oxford.

ING, H. R., KOVDIK, P., and TUDOR-WILLIAMS, D. P. H., 1952, The structure–action relationships of the choline group, *Brit. J. Pharmacol.* **7:**103–116.

ISON, R. R., PARTINGTON, P., and ROBERTS, G. C. K., 1973, The conformation of catecholamines and related compounds in solution, *Mol. Pharmacol.* **9:**756–765.

JACOB, J., MARSZAK, I., BARDISA, L., MARSZAK-FLEURY, A., and EPSZTEIN, R., 1952, The relation of structure to activity in certain acetylcholine, ethylene and saturated derivatives of choline and acetylcholine. *Arch. Int. Pharmacodyn.* **91:**303–321.

JANSSEN, P. A. J., 1965, The evolution of the butyrophenones, haloperidol and trifluperidol from meperidine like 4-phenylpiperidines, *Int. Rev. Neurobiol.* **8:**221–263.

JANSSEN, P. A. J., 1967, Haloperidol and related butyrophenones, in: *Psychopharmacological Agents* (M. Gordon, ed.), pp. 199–248, Academic Press, New York.

JANSSEN, P. A. J., 1973, Structure–activity relationships (SAR) and drug design as illustrated with neuroleptic drugs, in: *Structure–Activity Relationships* (C. J. Cavalitto, ed.), pp. 37–73, *International Encyclopedia of Pharmacology and Therapeutics*, Pergamon Press, Oxford.

JANSSEN, P. A. J., NIEMEGEERS, C. J. E., and SCHELLEKENS, K. H. L., 1967, Is it possible to predict the clinical effects of neuroleptic drugs (major tranquillizers) from animal data? Part IV, *Arzneimittel-Forsch.* **17**:841–854.

JANSSEN, P. A. J., NIEMEGEERS, C. J. E., SCHELLEKENS, K. H. L., DRESSE, A., LENAERTS, F. M., PINCHARD, A., SCHAPER, W. K. A., VAN NUETEN, J. M., and VERBRUGGEN, F. J., 1968, Pimozide, a chemically novel, highly potent and orally long-acting neuroleptic drug, *Arzneimittel-Forsch.* **18**:261–279.

JANSSEN, P. A. J., NIEMEGEERS, C. J. E., SCHELLEKENS, K. H. L., LENAERTS, F. M., VERBRULGGEN, F. J., VAN NUETEN, J. M., MARSBOOM, R. H. M., HERIN, V. V., and SCHAPER, W. K. A., 1970, The pharmacology of fluspirilene (R6218), a potent, long acting and injectable neuroleptic drug, *Arzneimittel-Forsch.* **20**:1689–1698.

JARROUSSE, M. J., and REGNIER, M. T., 1951, Separation et activite physiologique des deux isomeres optiques du dimethylaminoethoxy-*p*-tolyphenylmethane, *Ann. Pharm. Franc.* **9**:321–325.

JONES, R. G., 1966, Chemistry of histamine and analogs: Relationship between structure and pharmacological activity, in: *Histamine and Anti-histamines*, Part 1 (O. Eichler and A. Farah, eds.), pp. 1–43, Vol. 18 of *Handbook of Experimental Pharmacology*, Springer, Berlin.

KAMENAR, B., PROUT, K., and GANELLIN, C. R., 1973, Crystal and molecular structure of the histamine H_2-receptor antagonist N-(4-imidazol-4-ylbutyl)-N'-methyl thiourea (burimamide), *J. Chem. Soc. (Perkin Trans.)* **11**:1734–1739.

KATZ, R., HELLER, S. R., and JACOBSON, A. E., 1973, A molecular orbital study of norepinephrine and 3,4-dihydroxyphenethylamine: A re-evolution of structure–activity relationships in norepinephrine, *Mol. Pharmacol.* **9**:486–494.

KEBABIAN, J. W., PETZOLD, G. L., and GREENGARD, P., 1972, Dopamine-sensitive adenylate cyclase in caudate nucleus of rat brain and its similarity to the "dopamine receptor," *Proc. Natl. Acad. Sci.* **69**:2145–2149.

KERKUT, G. A., 1973, Catecholamines in invertebrates, *Brit. Med. Bull.* **29**:100–104.

KERKUT, G. A., and WALKER, R. J., 1961, The effects of drugs on the neurones of the snail, *Helix aspersa*, *Comp. Biochem. Physiol.* **3**:143–160.

KIER, L. B., 1967, Molecular orbital calculation of preferred conformations of acetylcholine, muscarine and muscarone, *Mol. Pharmacol.* **3**:487–494.

KIER, L. B., 1968*a*, Preferred conformation of serotonin and a postulate on the nature of its receptor from molecular orbital calculations, *J. Pharm. Sci.* **57**:1188–1191.

KIER, L. B., 1968*b*, Molecular orbital calculations of the preferred conformations of histamine and a theory on its dual activity, *J. Med. Chem.* **11**:441–445.

KLEIN, D. F., and DAVIS, J. M., 1969, *Diagnosis and Treatment of Psychiatric Disorders*, Williams and Wilkins, Baltimore.

KOCH, M. H. J., 1973, 4-(4-Chloro-α,α,α-trifluoro-*m*-tolyl)-1-[4,4-bis-(*p*-fluorophenyl)butyl]-4-piperidinol (penfluridol), *Acta Crystallog.* **B29**:1538–1540.

KOCH, M. H. J., and GERMAIN, G., 1972, The crystal and molecular structure of 4'-fluoro-4-(1-[4-hydroxy-4-(4'-fluoro)-phenylpiperidinol])butyrophenone and its hydrochloride, *Acta Crystallog.* **B28**:121–125.

KOROLKOVAS, A., 1970, in: *Essentials of Molecular Pharmacology: Background for Drug Design*, Wiley, New York.

KOSHLAND, D. E., 1958, Application of a theory of enzyme specificity to protein synthesis, *Proc. Natl. Acad. Sci.* **44**:98–104.

KVAM, D. C., RIGGILO, D. A., and LISH, P. M., 1965, Effect of some new β-adrenergic blocking agents on certain metabolic responses to catecholamines, *J. Pharmacol. Exp. Ther.* **149**:183–192.

LAL, S., and SOURKES, T. L., 1972, Effects of various chlorpromazine metabolites on amphetamine induced stereotyped behaviour in the rat, *Eur. J. Pharmacol.* **17**:283–286.

LANDS, A. M., 1951, An investigation of the molecular configurations favorable for stimulation or blockade of the acetylcholine-sensitive receptors of visceral organs, *J. Pharmacol. Exp. Ther.* **102**:219–236.

LANDS, A.M., 1952a, The cardiovascular actions of 1-(3-aminophenyl)-2-aminoethanol and related compounds, *J. Pharmacol. Exp. Ther.* **104**:474–477.

LANDS, A. M., 1952b, The effect on blood pressure and toxicity of 1-(3-fluorophenyl)-2-aminoethanol and related compounds, *J. Pharmacol. Exp. Ther.* **106**:440–443.

LANDS, A. M., and BROWN, T. G., 1967, Sympathomimetic (adrenergic) stimulants, in: *Drugs Affecting the Peripheral Nervous System* (A. Burger, ed.), pp. 399–472, Dekker, New York.

LANDS, A. M., and CAVALLITO, C. J., 1954, An evaluation of the factors favorable for acetylcholine like stimulation by employing a series of quaternary ammonium alkyl sulfide and sulfoxide compounds, *J. Pharmacol. Exp. Ther.* **110**:369–384.

LANDS, A. M., and GRANT, J. I., 1952, The vasopressor action and toxicity of cyclohexylethylamine derivatives, *J. Pharmacol. Exp. Ther.* **106**:341–345.

LANDS, A. M., and LUDUENA, F. P., 1956, The cholinolytic action of substituted dialkylaminoalkanes and dialkylaminoalkanols, *J. Pharmacol. Exp. Ther.* **116**:177–190.

LANDS, A. M., and TAINTER, M. I., 1953, The effect of changes in molecular configuration on inhibitory sympathomimetic action, *Arch. Exp. Pathol. Pharmakol.* **219**:76–96.

LANDS, A. M., NASH, V. L., McCARTHY, H. M., GRANGER, H. R., and DERTINGER, B. L., 1947a, The pharmacology of N-alkyl homologues of epinephrine, *J. Pharmacol. Exp. Ther.* **90**:110–119.

LANDS, A. M., NASH, V. L., GRANGER, H. R., and DERTINGER, B. L., 1947b, The pharmacologic activity of N-methyl-β-cyclohexyl-isopropylamine HCl, *J. Pharmacol. Exp. Ther.* **89**:383–385.

LANDS, A. M., NASH, V. L., DERTINGER, B. L., GRANGER, H. R., and McCARTHY, H. M., 1948, The pharmacology of compounds structurally related to hydroxytryptamine, *J. Pharmacol. Exp. Ther.* **92**:369–380.

LANGER, S. Z., and RUBIO, M. C., 1973, Effects of the noradrenaline metabolites on the adrenergic receptors, *Naunyn Schmiedebergs Arch. Pharmakol.* **276**:71–88.

LARSEN, A. A., GOULD, W. A., ROTH, H. R., COMER, W. T., ULOTH, R. H., DUNGAN, K. W., and LISH, P. M., 1967, Sulfonanilides. 11. Analogs of catecholamines, *J. Med. Chem.* **10**:462–472.

LAVERTY, R., and SHARMAN, D. H., 1965, Modification by drugs of the metabolism of 3,4-dihydroxy phenylethylamine, noradrenaline and 5-hydroxytryptamine in the brain, *Brit. J. Pharmacol.* **24**:759–772.

LEHMANN, G., and RANDALL, L. O., 1948, Pharmacological properties of sympathomimetic diamines, *J. Pharmacol. Exp. Ther.* **93**:115–125.

LEONARD, F., and HUTTRER, C. P., 1950, *Histamine Antagonists*, Chemical Biological Coordination Center, National Research Council, Washington, D.C.

LEWIS, J. J., and MUIR, T. C., 1967, Drugs acting at nerve–skeletal muscle junctions, in: *Drugs Affecting the Peripheral Nervous System* (A. Burger, ed.), pp. 327–364, Dekker, New York.

LIQUORI, A. M., DAMIANI, A., and ELEFANTE, G., 1968a, Calculated minimum energy conformations of muscarine, *J. Mol. Biol.* **33**:439–444.

LIQUORI, A. M., DAMIANI, A., and DeCOEN, J. L., 1968b, Calculated minimum energy conformations of acetylcholine, *J. Mol. Biol.* **33**:445–450.

LOEW, E. R., 1947, Pharmacology of antihistamine compounds, *Physiol. Rev.* **27**:542–573.

LOEWI, O., 1921, Uber humorale Ubertragbarkeit der Herznervenwirkung. 1. Milleilung, *Pfluegers Arch. Ges. Physiol.* **189**:239–242.

MARSH, D. F., HOWARD, A., and HERRING, D. A., 1951, The comparative pharmacology of the isomeric nitrogen methyl substituted heptylamines, *J. Pharmacol. Exp. Ther.* **103**:325–329.

MARSZAK, I., OLOMUCKI, M., EPSZTEIN, R., and JACOB, J., 1954, Unsaturated amines. IX. Synthesis and parasympathomimetic properties of ethylenic quaternary ammonium salts, *Comp. Rend. Acad. Sci. Paris* **238**:166–168.

MATTHYSSE, S., 1973, Antipsychotic drug actions: A clue to the neuropathology of schizophrenia? *Fed. Proc.* **32**:200–205.

MAYER, S. E., and STULL, J. T., 1971, Cyclic AMP in skeletal muscle, *Ann. N.Y. Acad. Sci.* **185**:433–448.

MCDOWELL, J. J. H., 1969, The crystal and molecular structure of chlorpromazine, *Acta Crystallog.* **B25**:2175–2181.

MCGEER, E. G., MCGEER, P. L., and MCLENNAN, H., 1961, The inhibitory action of 5-hydroxytryptamine, gamma-aminobutyric acid (GABA) and some other compounds towards the crayfish stretch receptor neuron, *J. Neurochem.* **8**:36–49.

MCISAAC, W. M., and PAGE, I. H., 1958, New metabolites of serotonin in carcinoid urine, *Science* **128**:537.

MCNAY, J. L., MCDONALD, R. H., and GOLDBERG, L. I., 1965, Direct renal vasodilation produced by dopamine in the dog, *Circ. Res.* **16**:510–517.

MELVILLE, K. I., 1973, Antihistamine drugs, in: *Histamine and Antihistamines* (M. Schachter, ed.), pp. 127–171, *International Encyclopedia of Pharmacology and Therapeutics*, Pergamon Press, Oxford.

MILLER, R. J., and HILEY, C. R., 1974, Relation of anti-muscarinic properties of neuroleptics to drug induced parkinsonism, *Nature* **248**:596–597.

MILLER, R. J., and IVERSEN, L. L., 1974, Effect of psychoactive drugs on dopamine (3,4-dihydroxyphenethylamine)-sensitive adenylate cyclase activity in corpus striatum of rat brain, *Biochem. Soc. Trans.* **1**:90–93.

MOE, G. K., and FREYBURGER, W. A., 1950, Ganglionic blocking agents, *Pharmacol. Rev.* **2**:61–95.

MØLLER-NIELSEN, I., HOUGS, W., LASSEN, N., HOLM, T., and PETERSEN, P. V., 1962, Central depressant activity of some thiaxanthene derivatives, *Acta Pharmacol. Toxicol.* **19**:87–100.

MØLLER-NIELSEN, I., PEDERSEN, V., NYMARK, M., FRANCK, K. F., BOECK, V., FJALLAN, B., and CHRISTENSEN, A. V., 1973, The comparative pharmacology of flupenthixol and some reference neuroleptics, *Acta Pharmacol. Toxicol.* **33**:353–362.

NACHOD, F. C., and LANDS, A. M., 1953, Relationship between chemical structure and biological activity of compounds with atropine-like activity, *Trans. N.Y. Acad. Sci.* **16**:2–13.

NAUTA, W. T., REKKER, R. F., and HARMS, A. F., 1968, Diarylcarbinol ethers: Structure–activity relationships. A physico-chemical approach, in: *Proceedings of the Third International Pharmacology Meeting*, Vol. 7, pp. 305–325, Pergamon Press, New York.

NOGRADI, M., OLLIS, W. D., and SUTHERLAND, I. D., 1970, The conformational inversion of 2,3:6,7-dibenzo-derivatives of cycloheptatriene, tropone, heptafulvene, oxepin, thiepin and azepin, *Chem. Commun.* **1970**:158–160.

NYBACK, H., 1971, Regional disappearance of catecholamines formed from ^{14}C-tyrosine in rat brain: Effect of synthesis inhibitors and of chlorpromazine, *Acta Pharmacol. Toxicol.* **30**:372–384.

NYBACK, H., and SEDVALL, G., 1968, Effect of chlorpromazine on accumulation and disappearance of catecholamines formed from tyrosine-C^{14} in brain, *J. Pharmacol. Exp. Ther.* **162**:294–301.

NYBACK, H., and SEDVALL, G., 1972, Effect of chlorpromazine and some of its metabolites on synthesis and turnover of catecholamines formed from ^{14}C-tyrosine in mouse brain, *Psychopharmacologia* **26**:155–160.

OSBORNE, M., DETAR, R., and GABEL, L., 1962, Comparison between the autonomic pharmacology of 5-hydroxytryptamine and 5-acetyltryptamine (5-AT), *Fed. Proc.* **21**:324.

PATON, W. D. M., and ZAIMIS, E. J., 1952, The methonium compounds, *Pharmacol. Rev.* **4**:219–253.

PAULING, P., and PETCHER, T. J., 1973, Neuromuscular blocking agents: Structures and activity, *Chem. Biol. Interact.* **6**:351–365.

PEDERSON, L., HOSKINS, R. E., and CABLE, H., 1971, The preferred conformation of noradrenaline, *J. Pharm. Pharmacol.* **23**:216–218.

PERITI, P. F., 1970, On active conformation of histamine and analogues, *Pharmacol. Res. Commun.* **2**:309–318.

PETERSEN, P. V., and MØLLER-NIELSEN, I., 1964, Thioxanthene derivatives, in: *Psychopharmacological Agents*, Vol. 1 (M. Gordon, ed.), pp. 301–324, Academic Press, New York.

PHILLIS, J. W., and TEBECIS, A. K., 1967, The responses of thalamic neurones to iontophoretically applied monoamines, *J. Physiol.* **192**:715–745.

POST, M. L., KENNARD, O., and HORN, A. S., 1974, 2-Chloro-9-(w-dimethylaminopropylidene)thioxanthene, *Acta Crystallog* **B30**:1644–1646.

POWELL, C. E., and SLATER, I. H., 1958, Blocking of inhibitory adrenergic receptors by a dichloro analog of isoproterenol, *J. Pharmacol. Exp. Ther.* **122**:480–488.

PRATESI, P., LA MANNA, A., CAMPIGLIO, A., and GHISLANDI, V., 1958, The configuration of adrenaline and of its *p*-hydroxyphenyl analogue, *J. Chem. Soc.* **1958**:2069–2074.

PRATESI, P., LA MANNA, A., CAMPIGLIO, A., and GHISLANDI, V., 1959, The configuration of noradrenaline, *J. Chem. Soc.* **1959**:4062–4065.

PULLMAN, B., COURRIERE, P., and COUBEILS, J. L., 1971, Quantum mechanical study of the conformational and electronic properties of acetylcholine and its agonists muscarine and nicotine, *Mol. Pharmacol.* **7**:397–405.

PULLMAN, B., COUBEILS, J. L., COURRIERE, P., and GERVOIS, J. P., 1972, Quantum mechanical study of the conformation properties of phenethylamines of biochemical and medical interest, *J. Med. Chem.* **15**:17–23.

RANDRUP, A., and MUNKVAD, I., 1970, Biochemical anatomical and psychological investigations of stereotyped behavior induced by amphetamines, in: *Amphetamines and Related Compounds* (E. Costa and S. Garattini, eds.), pp. 695–713, Raven Press, New York.

RANDRUP, A., and SCHEEL-KRUGER, J., 1966, Diethyldithiocarbamate and amphetamine stereotype behaviour, *J. Pharm. Pharmacol.* **18**:752.

RANDRUP, A., MUNKVAD, I., and UDSEN, P., 1963, Adrenergic mechanisms and amphetamine induced abnormal behaviour, *Acta Pharmacol. Toxicol.* **20**:145–157.

REED, L. L., and SCHAEFER, J. P., 1973, The crystal and molecular structure of haloperidol, a potent psychotropic drug, *Acta Crystallog.* **B29**:1886–1890.

RENSHAW, R. R., and HOPKINS, C. T., 1929, Phosphoric acid ester derivatives of choline: Basis for the psychological activity of -onium compounds, *J. Am. Chem. Soc.* **51**:953–964.

RENSHAW, R. R., and HUNT, R., 1929, The pharmacological action of some homologues of betaine and choline esters, *J. Pharmacol. Exp. Ther.* **37**:309–337.

RENSHAW, R. R., DREISBACH, P. F., ZIFF, M., and GREEN, D., 1938, Thioesters of choline and β-methylcholine and their psychological activity: Onium compounds, *J. Am. Chem. Soc.* **60**:1765–1770.

ROBISON, G. A., BUTCHER, R. W., and SUTHERLAND, E. W., 1967, Adenylcyclase as an adrenergic receptor, *Ann. N.Y. Acad. Sci.* **139**:703–723.

ROBISON, G. A., BUTCHER, R. W., and SUTHERLAND, E. W., 1971, *Cyclic AMP*, p. 225, Academic Press, New York.

ROCHA, E SILVA, M., 1960, Influence of pH on the interaction of histamine with its receptors in the guinea pig ileum, *Arch. Int. Pharmacodyn.* **128**:355–374.

SAAVEDRA, J. M., BROWNSTEIN, M., and AXELROD, J., 1973, A specific and sensitive enzymatic-isotopic microassay for serotonin in tissues, *J. Pharmacol. Exp. Ther.* **186**:508–515.

SALLE, J., 1952, The pharmacology of fluroacetylcholine bromide, *Arch. Int. Pharmacodyn.* **91**:339–349.

SASTRY, B. V. R., PFEIFFER, C. C., and LASSLO, A., 1960, Relation between chemical constitution and biological response of D(−), L(+) and DL-lactoylcholines and related compounds, *J. Pharmacol. Exp. Ther.* **130**:346–355.

SCHAEFER, J. P., 1967, The structure of thiothixene, *Chem. Commun.* **1967**:743–744.

SCHEEL-KRUGER, J., 1972, Behavioural and biochemical comparison of amphetamine derivatives, cocaine, benztropine and tricyclic antidepressant drugs, *Eur. J. Pharmacol.* **18**:63–73.

SCHMIEDEBERG, O., and KOPPE, R., 1869, *Das Muscarine, das Giftige Alkaloid des Fliegenpilzes*, Vogel, Leipzig.

SCHUELER, F. W., 1953, The statistical nature of the intramolecular distance factor of the muscarinic moiety, *Arch. Int. Pharmacodyn.* **93**:417–426.

SCHUELER, F. W., and HANNA, C., 1951, The pharmacological activities of some hydrazonium analogs related to acetylcholine tetramethylammonium and tetraethylammonium, *Arch. Int. Pharmacodyn.* **88**:351–360.

SCHUELER, F. W., and KEASLING, H. H., 1951, Further studies on the RC (reversed carboxyl) analog of acetylcholine and some additional derivatives, *J. Pharmacol. Exp. Ther.* **103**:222–235.

SCOTT, K. A., and MAUTNER, H. G., 1967, Sulfur and selenium isologs related to acetylcholine and choline-1X, *Biochem. Pharmacol.* **16**:1903–1918.

SHADER, R. I., and DiMASCIO, A., 1970, *Psychotropic Drug Side Effects*, Williams and Wilkins, Baltimore.

SHEFTER, E., and TRIGGLE, D. T., 1970, Is there a unique conformation of cholinergic ligands responsible for muscarinic activity? *Nature* **227**:1354–1355.

SHEPPARD, H., BURGHARDT, C., and GREENGARD, P., 1973, The interaction of dopamine and its derivatives with the dopamine-sensitive adenylate cyclase of rat caudate nucleus, *Pharmacologist* **15**:231.

SIMONART, A., 1932, On the action of certain derivatives of choline, *J. Pharmacol. Exp. Ther.* **46**:157–193.

SIMONART, A., 1934, Contribution a l'etude des β alkyl cholines, *Arch. Int. Pharmacodyn.* **48**:328–332.

SIMPSON, T. R., JR., CRAIG, J. C., and KUMLER, W. D., 1967, Determination of the conformation of nicotine and some related compounds by nuclear magnetic resonance and dipole moments, *J. Pharm. Sci.* **56**:708–713.

SINGH GREWAL, R., 1952, The pharmacological actions of 6-methyladrenaline, *Brit. J. Pharmacol.* **7**:338–348.

SNYDER, S. H., 1972, Catecholamines in the brain as mediators of amphetamine psychosis, *Arch. Gen. Psychiat.* **27**:169–179.

SNYDER, S. H., GREENBERG, D., and YAMAMURA, H. I., 1974, Antischizophrenic drugs and brain cholinergic receptors: Affinity for muscarinic sites predicts extrapyramidal effects, *Arch. Gen. Psychiat.*, **31**:58–61.

SOUDIJN, W., and VAN WIJNGAARDEN, I., 1972, Localization of ^{3}H-pimozide in the rat brain in relation to its anti-amphetamine potency, *J. Pharm. Pharmacol.* **24**:773–780.

STEHLE, R. L., MELVILLE, K. I., and OLDHAM, F. K., 1936, Choline as a factor in the elaboration of adrenaline, *J. Pharmacol. Exp. Ther.* **56**:473–481.

STENLAKE, J. B., 1963, Some chemical aspects of neuromuscular block, in: *Progress in Medicinal Chemistry*, Vol. 3 (G. P. Ellis and G. B. West, eds.), pp. 1–51, Butterworth, London.

STOLL, H. C., 1948, Pharmacodynamic considerations of atropine and related compounds, *Am. J. Med. Sci.* **215**:577–592.

SWANSON, E. E., and CHEN, K. K., 1946, Comparison of pressor action of aliphatic amines, *J. Pharmacol. Exp. Ther.* **88**:10–13.

SWANSON, E. E., STELDT, F. A., and CHEN, K. K., 1945, Further observations on the pressor action of optical isomers of sympathomimetic amines, *J. Pharmacol. Exp. Ther.* **85**:70–73.

TAYLOR, D. B., and NEDERGUARD, O. A., 1965, Relation between structure and action of quaternary ammonium neuromuscular blocking agents, *Physiol. Rev.* **45**:523–554.

TESTA, B., and JENNER, P., 1973, Circular dichroic determination of the preferred conformation of nicotine and related chiral alkaloids in aqueous solution, *Mol. Pharmacol.* **9**:10–16.

TRENDELENBURG, U., 1956, The action of 5-hydroxytryptamine on the nictitating membrane and on the superior cervical ganglion of the cat, *Brit. J. Pharmacol.* **11**:74–80.

TRENDELENBURG, U., 1957, The action of morphine on the superior cervical ganglion and on the nictitating membrane of the cat, *Brit. J. Pharmacol.* **12**:79–85.

TRENDELENBURG, U., MUSKUS, A., FLEMING, W. W., and ALONSO DE LA SIERRA, B. G., 1962, Modification by reserpine of the action of sympathomimetic amines in spinal cats; a classification of sympathomimetic amines, *J. Pharmacol. Exp. Ther.* **138:**170–180.

TRIGGLE, D. J., 1970, Adrenergic hormones and drugs, in: *Medicinal Chemistry*, Vol. II (A. Burger, ed.), pp. 1235–1295, Wiley-Interscience, New York.

TRIGGLE, D. J., 1971, *Neurotransmitter–Receptor Interactions*, Academic Press, London.

TRIGGLE, D. J., 1972, Adrenergic receptors, *Ann. Rev. Pharmacol.* **12:**185–196.

TURTLE, J. R., and KIPNIS, D. M., 1967, An adrenergic receptor mechanism for the control of cyclic 3′,5′-adenosine monophosphate systems in tissue, *Biochem. Biophys. Res. Commun.* **28:**797–802.

UNGERSTEDT, U., 1971, Stereotaxic mapping of the monoamine pathways in the rat brain, *Acta Physiol. Scand. Suppl.* **376:**1–48.

URECH, E., MARXER, A., and MIESCHER, K., 1950, 2-Aminoalkyl-imidazoline, *Helv. Chim. Acta* **33:**1386–1407.

VANE, J. R., 1957, A sensitive method for the assay of 5-hydroxytryptamine, *Brit. J. Pharmacol.* **12:**344–349.

VANE, J. R., 1959, The relative activities of some tryptamine analogues on the isolated rat stomach strip preparation, *Brit. J. Pharmacol.* **14:**87–98.

VAN ROSSUM, J. M., 1962, Pharmacodynamics of parasympathetic drugs: Mechanism of action and structure action of tertiary ammonium salts, *Arch. Int. Pharmacodyn.* **140:**592–605.

VAN ROSSUM, J. M., and ARIENS, E. J., 1959, Pharmacodynamics of parasympathetic drugs: Structure–action relations in homologous series of quaternary ammonium salts, *Arch. Int. Pharmacodyn.* **118:**418–446.

WASER, P. G., 1961, Chemistry and pharmacology of muscarine, muscarone and some related compounds, *Pharmacol. Rev.* **13:**465–515.

WEISSMAN, A., KOE, K. B., and TENEN, S. S., 1966, Antiamphetamine effects following inhibition of tyrosine hydroxylase, *J. Pharmacol. Exp. Ther.* **151:**339–352.

WELCH, A. D., and ROEPKE, M. H., 1935, A comparative study of choline and certain of its analogues, *J. Pharmacol. Exp. Ther.* **55:**118–126.

WELSH, J. H., and TAUB, R., 1951, The significance of the carbonyl group and ether oxygen in the reaction of ACh with receptor substance, *J. Pharmacol. Exp. Ther.* **103:**62–73.

WERNER, L. H., and BARRETT, W. E., 1967, in: *Antihypertensive Agents* (E. Schlittler, ed.), pp. 331–392, Academic Press, New York.

WHITTAKER, V. P., 1963, in: *Handbook of Experimental Pharmacology*, Vol. 15 (G. B. Koelle, ed.), pp. 1–39, Springer, Berlin.

WILKINSON, S., 1961, The history and chemistry of muscarine, *Quart. Rev. Chem. Soc.* **15:**153–171.

WOODRUFF, G. N., 1971, Dopamine receptors: A review, *Comp. Gen. Pharmacol.* **2:**439–455.

WOODRUFF, G. N., and WALKER, R. J., 1969, The effect of dopamine and other compounds on the activity of neurones of *Helix aspersa*: Structure–activity relationships, *Int. J. Neuropharmacol.* **8:**279–289.

WOOLLEY, D. W., 1959, Highly potent antimetabolites of serotonin with little serotonin-like action, *Biochem. Pharmacol.* **1:**51–59.

WOOLLEY, D. W., and CAMPBELL, N. K., 1962, Serotonin-like and antiserotonin properties of psilocybin and psilocin, *Science* **136:**777–779.

WURZEL, M., 1959, A suggested mechanism for the action of choline esters on animal organs, inferred from a study of the effects of choline, β-methylcholine and thiocholine-esters, *Experientia* **15:**430–433.

YAMAMOTO, C., 1967, Pharmacologic studies of norepinephrine, acetylcholine and related compounds on neurons in Deiters' nucleus and the cerebellum, *J. Pharmacol. Exp. Ther.* **156:**39–47.

YAMAMURA, H. I., and SNYDER, S. H., 1974, Muscarinic cholinergic receptor binding in rat brain, *Prox. Natl. Acad. Sci.,* **71:**1725–1729.

YEH, B. K., McNAY, J. L., and GOLDBERG, L. I., 1969, Attenuation of dopamine renal and mesenteric vasodilation by haloperidol: Evidence of a specific dopamine receptor, *J. Pharmacol. Exp. Ther.* **168**:303–309.

ZIRKLE, C. L., and KAISER, C., 1970, Antipsychotic agents, in: *Medicinal Chemistry*, Vol. 11 (A. Burger, ed.), pp. 1410–1469, Wiley-Interscience, New York.

7

DENERVATION SUPERSENSITIVITY

S. Z. Langer

1. INTRODUCTION

It has been known for many years that surgical denervation of either cholinergically or adrenergically innervated organs leads to an increase in the responsiveness of the effector organ to the corresponding neurotransmitter and to chemically related agonists. This phenomenon was observed initially for catecholamines in the radial muscle of the denervated pupil (Budge, 1855; Langendorff, 1900) and for acetylcholine in the striated muscle of the tongue (Philipeaux and Vulpian, 1863). Since these early observations, considerable work has been carried out in this field, not only in the peripheral nervous system but also, more recently, in the central nervous system. In 1949, Cannon and Rosenblueth published a monograph in which, among other things, they formulated their "law of denervation," which states that surgical denervation causes supersensitivity of all the distal elements in the functional chain of neurons, including the effectors, to the action of chemical agents and nerve impulses. In addition, Cannon and Rosenblueth (1949) stated that denervation supersensitivity is greater for the links that immediately follow the cut neurons and that supersensitivity decreases progressively for the more distal elements.

The mechanisms involved in the development of supersensitivity after denervation of skeletal muscle are mainly related to the spread of the

S. Z. Langer ● Instituto de Investigaciones Farmacológicas, Consejo Nacional de Investigaciones, Científicas y Técnicas, Buenos Aires, Argentina

nicotinic cholinergic receptors outward from the end-plate region (Thesleff, 1960; Creese *et al.*, 1971). On the other hand, in adrenergically innervated smooth muscle such as the nictitating membrane of the cat two types of supersensitivity can be clearly distinguished after surgical denervation (Trendelenburg, 1963*a*, 1966; Langer and Trendelenburg, 1966; Langer *et al.*, 1967). One component is the prejunctional type of supersensitivity, which develops rapidly during the first days after denervation and has a high degree of specificity for norepinephrine and other sympathomimetic amines. The second component is the postjunctional type of supersensitivity, which develops slowly with time and appears to be due to changes at the level of the effector organ. The postjunctional component of denervation supersensitivity lacks agonist specificity.

In effector organs such as salivary glands which are innervated by both cholinergic and adrenergic fibers, the development of denervation supersensitivity follows a different pattern depending on whether the cholinergic or the sympathetic innervation is removed. Adrenergic denervation leads to the development of both the prejunctional and the postjunctional components of supersensitivity in a manner and with a time course similar to those described for the cat nictitating membrane (Stefano *et al.*, 1974). On the other hand, cholinergic denervation of salivary glands leads to a postjunctional type of supersensitivity which develops slowly as a function of time, is nonspecific, and is of moderate magnitude (Emmelin, 1961, 1965).

In addition to the examples discussed for denervation supersensitivity in the peripheral nervous system, this phenomenon has been studied in the central nervous system (Stavraky, 1961; Sharpless, 1964, 1969; Dominic and Moore, 1969; Kalisker *et al.*, 1973).

2. QUANTITATIVE METHODS IN THE STUDY OF SUPERSENSITIVITY

In studies of changes in sensitivity of effector organs to agonists, full dose–response curves rather than responses to single doses should be employed (Trendelenburg, 1963*b*). When full dose–response curves are determined, the degree of supersensitivity can be measured accurately by the magnitude of their horizontal shift to the left. Supersensitivity is defined precisely as a decrease in the amount or concentration of the agonist required to elicit a given biological response: contraction of a smooth or striated muscle, secretion of saliva, etc. The importance of studies based on full dose–response curves and the shortcomings in analysis of vertical responses to single doses or concentrations of the agonists are thoroughly discussed in an excellent review by Trendelenburg (1963*b*).

In most instances, denervation supersensitivity leads to a horizontal shift to the left in the dose–response curve without changes in the maximal responses (Fleming *et al.*, 1973). However, it has been reported that for norepinephrine, in addition to the shift to the left in the dose–response curve, an increase in the maximum development of tension is observed after surgical denervation in the rat vas deferens (Wakade and Krusz, 1972), in the cat spleen capsule (Granata and Langer, 1973), and in the cat nictitating membrane (Langer, 1974). While the horizontal shift to the left is the most important parameter in the quantitative determination of the degree of supersensitivity, one should be alerted to the possibility that the maximal response to the effector organ can be increased after denervation. While the significance of increases in maximal responses is still obscure, it appears to be related to the development of the postjunctional component of denervation supersensitivity (Langer, 1974). Table 1 shows the pD_2 values and the maximum development of tension to norepinephrine and to methoxamine in normal and in denervated nictitating membranes. An increase in maximal response was observed both for norepinephrine and for methoxamine, although the prejunctional component of denervation supersensitivity developed only for norepinephrine (Table 1). In addition, the time course of the increase in maximal responses coincided with the temporal sequence for the development of the postjunctional component of denervation supersensitivity.

Differences in baseline values between denervated and control tissues can lead to underestimates of the actual degree of supersensitivity on the one hand and to an apparent decrease in the maximal response on the other (Langer, 1966a). In the denervated nictitating membrane of the cat, *in vivo*, there is a sustained contraction or tone which increases the baseline values of

TABLE 1

Effects of Surgical Denervation on pD_2 Values and on the Maximal Responses to $(-)$-Norepinephrine and to Methoxamine in the Medial Smooth Muscle of the Cat Nictitating Membrane

Experimental group	n^a	$pD_2{}^b$	Tension[c] (g)
Norepinephrine, controls	41	5.15 ± 0.03	19.8 ± 0.51
Norepinephrine, DEN[d] 3 days	30	6.84 ± 0.08^e	23.8 ± 1.22
Norepinephrine, DEN 7 days	12	7.13 ± 0.16^e	29.7 ± 1.47^f
Methoxamine, controls	14	5.27 ± 0.08	19.9 ± 1.08
Methoxamine, DEN 3 days	8	5.26 ± 0.08	21.6 ± 1.58
Methoxamine, DEN 7 days	5	5.39 ± 0.12	24.8 ± 1.24^f

[a] Number of experiments.
[b] Mean negative log molar ED_{50} (mean value $\pm$ SEM).
[c] Maximum development of tension (mean values $\pm$ SEM).
[d] Surgical denervation.
[e] $p < 0.001$ compared with the corresponding controls.
[f] $p < 0.05$ compared with the corresponding controls.

the supersensitive membrane but not of the normal contralateral membrane. The tone developed by the denervated membrane is due to its supersensitivity to circulating catecholamines (Langer, 1966a; Langer et al., 1967). For accurate determinations of supersensitivity, these differences in baseline values between control and denervated tissues have to be taken into account (Langer, 1966a; Langer et al., 1967). Otherwise, the actual increase in sensitivity to the agonist is underestimated. Figure 1 shows the difference in the magnitude of decentralization and of denervation supersensitivity to synephrine obtained under conditions of tone (A) and with the appropriate correction (B).

Another parameter which has received attention only recently is the slope of the dose–response curve. Use of the measurement of horizontal shifts of dose–response curves as an accurate estimate of the degree of supersensitivity is based on the assumption that the shift in the dose–response curve to the left is of a parallel nature. However, in the cat nictitating membrane the slope of the dose–response to norepinephrine is significantly decreased after surgical denervation (Langer and Trendelenburg, 1969). As shown in Table 2, the shift to the left is more pronounced when determined at the level of the ED_{20} compared to the ED_{50} or the ED_{80}. In fact, there is nearly a full log unit difference when the shift to the left obtained by denervation is determined at the level of the ED_{20} rather than at

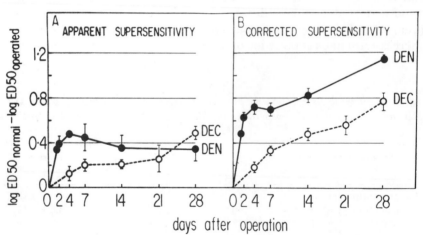

FIG. 1. Underestimation of supersensitivity to synephrine due to the presence of tone in the nictitating membrane of the cat. Ordinate: increase in sensitivity to synephrine after decentralization (DEC) and after denervation (DEN) of the nictitating membrane. 0, No change in sensitivity; 1, tenfold increase in sensitivity. Abscissa: days after the operation. ●, Denervated nictitating membranes; ○, decentralized nictitating membranes. (A) Apparent supersensitivity obtained in untreated spinal cats (without correction for tone). (B) Corrected supersensitivity (after correction for tone). Note the pronounced difference between apparent (A) and corrected (B) values for supersensitivity to synephrine. From Langer (1966a).

the level of the ED_{80} (Table 2). When the dose–response curves to norepine-phrine are shifted to the left by exposure to cocaine, a concomitant decrease in the slope of the dose–response curve is obtained in the cat nictitating membrane (Fig. 2). Since cocaine reproduces the prejunctional component of denervation supersensitivity in adrenergically innervated organs, these results support the view that the decrease in the slope of the dose–response curve to norepinephrine after surgical denervation of the cat nictitating membrane is related to the prejunctional component of denervation supersensitivity (Langer and Trendelenburg, 1969). However, changes in slopes of dose–response curves have also been described for different agonists, and in connection with the postjunctional component of super-sensitivity (Trendelenburg et al., 1970; Westfall, 1970). There is no doubt that a great deal of additional attention should be given to studies of slopes of dose–response curves and of maximal responses in the quantitative analysis of supersensitivity. As mentioned earlier, supersensitivity results in a complete shift to the left in the dose–response curve for the agonist whether the shift is completely parallel or there is a concomitant decrease in the slope.

Supersensitivity should not be confused with the increased responsive-ness of a tissue due to the additive effects of two agonists. These additive effects may result in apparent potentiation of the responses which are obtained for low doses of one of the agonists. Additive effects result in dose–responses which are convergent: there is a shift to the left in the range

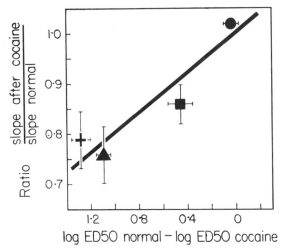

FIG. 2. Effects of cocaine on the slope of the dose–response curve to norepinephrine in the isolated nictitating membrane of the cat. Ordinate: ratio "slope after cocaine/slope in absence of cocaine." Abscissa: degree of cocaine-induced supersensitivity in muscles obtained from reser-pine-pretreated cats. Cocaine doses: ●, 2.6×10^{-8} M; ■, 2.6×10^{-7} M; ▲, 2.6×10^{-6} M; +, 2.6×10^{-5} M. Note the decrease in the slope of the dose–response curve with increases in sensitivity to (−)-norepinephrine. From Langer and Trendelenburg (1969).

TABLE 2

Effects of Surgical Denervation on Slopes of Dose–Response Curves to Norepinephrine in the Cat Nictitating Membrane[a]

Experimental group	n[b]	ED_{20}	ED_{50}	ED_{80}	Slope	Δ_{20}	Δ_{50}	Δ_{80}
Norepinephrine, controls	41	6.16 ± 0.09	5.15 ± 0.03	4.48 ± 0.03	37.2 ± 1.92			
Norepinephrine, DEN[d] 3 days	30	8.40 ± 0.13[e]	6.84 ± 0.08[e]	5.83 ± 0.08[f]	24.7 ± 0.98[f]	$+2.24$	$+1.69$	$+1.35$

[a] $ED_{20,50,80}$. Mean negative log molar concentration for responses of 20, 50, or 80% of maximum $\pm$ SEM.
$\Delta_{20,50,80}$. Difference in $ED_{20,50,80}$ from the corresponding controls (plus sign indicates shift to the left in the dose–response curve).
[b] Number of experiments.
[c] Slope of the dose–response curve [$60/(\log ED_{80} - \log ED_{20})$].
[d] Surgical denervation.
[e] $p < 0.001$ compared with the corresponding controls.
[f] $p < 0.05$ compared with the corresponding controls.

of low concentrations and thereafter the dose–response curves are superimposed. A typical example of such a misinterpretation is provided by the report that metanephrine potentiates the responses of the cat nictitating membrane to norepinephrine and epinephrine (Bacq and Renson, 1961). The study by Bacq and Renson (1961) was based on responses to single doses, and both metanephrine and the catecholamines are agonists on the α-receptors of the nictitating membrane. Consequently, additive effects could not be distinguished from true supersensitivity. A subsequent study with complete dose–response curves (Langer *et al.*, 1967) revealed that the interaction between metanephrine and norepinephrine was only that of additive effects and did not represent true potentiation or supersensitivity.

3. SURGICAL AND PHARMACOLOGICAL DENERVATION

the surgical procedure, which consists of transection of postganglionic nerves or removal of the corresponding ganglion where the cell body of the postganglionic neuron is located. In addition, chemical denervation of adrenergic nerves can be produced with 6-hydroxydopamine (Tranzer and Thoenen, 1967; Thoenen and Tranzer, 1968) or by immunosympathectomy (Levi-Montalcini and Booker, 1960; Levi-Montalcini and Angeletti, 1962). Uptake of 6-hydroxydopamine by adrenergic nerves is an essential step for the subsequent degeneration of the nerve endings. Inhibition of neuronal uptake by imipramine or related drugs can prevent the degeneration of adrenergic nerve endings induced by 6-hydroxydopamine (Stone *et al.*, 1964; Malmfors and Sachs, 1968). In general, chemical sympathectomy with 6-hydroxydopamine does not lead to the destruction of the whole neuron since it affects mainly the adrenergic nerve terminals. In contrast to the effects of surgical denervation on the peripheral sympathetic system, several weeks after the administration of 6-hydroxydopamine there is a progressive recovery in the endogenous norepinephrine stores (Thoenen and Tranzer, 1968; Haeusler *et al.*, 1969; Perec *et al.*, 1973) which is due to the appearance of newly formed adrenergic nerve endings (Tranzer *et al.*, 1969). The destruction of adrenergic nerve endings by 6-hydroxydopamine is related to the ability of this agent to accumulate in the sympathetic neuron and its susceptibility to nonenzyamtic oxidation. The latter leads to the formation of quinones and their melanin-like polymers, which are responsible for the irreversible alterations of various biological structures (Breese, Chap. 7, Vol. 1).

Immunosympathectomy is based on the discovery that a specific antiserum to the mouse salivary gland nerve growth factor can be prepared that destroys the sympathetic ganglia of newborn animals (Levi-Montalcini and Cohen, 1960). It is of interest that not all the sympathetic ganglia are equally susceptible to the antiserum. For instance, the peripheral sympathetic ganglia innervating the male and female sex organs are resistant to the antiserum (Vogt, 1964; Levi-Montalcini and Angeletti, 1966). In addition, immunosympathectomy does not affect the adrenergic neurones in the central nervous system. In adult animals the effect of the antiserum is much less pronounced than in newborn animals. This is probably because sympathetic neurons are more sensitive to the antiserum at a critical stage in their development.

While surgical denervation is still the method of choice for study of the effects of removing the sympathetic innervation from many organs, this procedure is possible only in tissues where the innervation is easily accessible. Both chemical sympathectomy and immunosympathectomy are very useful tools for the destruction of adrenergic nerves in organs in which the innervation is complex or not easily accessible. However, it should be stressed that neither immunosympathectomy nor chemical sympathectomy leads to a complete destruction of the adrenergic nervous system. While chemical sympathectomy with 6-hydroxydopamine can be achieved at any age, it produces only a temporary denervation in adult animals because there is a slow but progressive regeneration of nerve endings from the undamaged proximal part of the neuron. Immunosympathectomy, on the other hand, implies a permanent destruction of the adrenergic neurons involved. However, this procedure can be applied only at certain ages: prenatally or both pre- and postnatally. In addition, there are particular patterns of susceptibility to immunosympathectomy for the adrenergic neurons from different organs (Thoenen, 1972).

6–Hydroxydopamine, administered either directly into the brain or intraventricularly, is a powerful tool for the destruction of adrenergic and dopaminergic neurons in the central nervous system (Ungerstedt, 1968; Bloom et al., 1969; Uretsky and Iversen, 1969). In contrast to the results obtained in the periphery, in the central nervous system there is no evidence of any recovery from the effects of 6-hydroxydopamine for a period of up to 75 days (Uretsky and Iversen, 1970). These results are compatible with the view that in the brain not only the nerve terminals but also the cell bodies are damaged by 6-hydroxydopamine (Breese, Chap. 7, Vol. 1).

In addition to the methods discussed, there are a number of procedures which lead to the development of a type of postjunctional supersensitivity but do not result in the degeneration of nerve endings or in the destruction of the postganglionic neuron. These procedures include (1) chronic decentralization or chronic preganglionic denervation, which leaves the postganglionic neuron intact but disconnects the effector organ from the continuous influence of the central nervous system; (2) chronic prevention of the release of the neurotransmitter, by use of reserpine or adrenergic neuron blockers for norepinephrine and botulinum toxin for acetylcholine; (3) chronic blockade of the receptors of the effector organ by the administration of drugs; and (4) chronic ganglionic blockade.

4. SUPERSENSITIVITY AFTER DENERVATION OF SYMPATHETICALLY INNERVATED ORGANS

4.1. Events During Degeneration of Adrenergic Nerves

4.1.1. Transient Period of Activity in Denervated Organs

It is well known that denervation of sympathetically innervated tissues leads to the loss of the norepinephrine stores in the effector organ (Cannon and Lissák, 1939; von Euler and Purkhold, 1951; Burn and Rand, 1959; Kirpekar et al., 1962; Smith et al., 1966; Brimijoin et al., 1970). The loss of norepinephrine during the process of degeneration of adrenergic nerve endings results in a transient period of activity in the denervated effector organ which coincides with the time course of the decline in the stores of the neurotransmitter. This transient period of activity has been observed in many adrenergically innervated tissues of several species (Table 3). In the smooth muscle of the cat nictitating membrane, the transient contraction starts approximately 22 h after surgery (Langer, 1966b). The development of the degeneration contraction coincides with the time course of the loss of endogenous norepinephrine stores in the nictitating membrane (Smith et al.,

TABLE 3

Transient Period of Activity Observed in Sympathetically Denervated Effector Organs During Loss of Neurotransmitter from Degenerating Nerve Endings

Species and tissue	Transient response	References
Rabbit eye	Reduction in intraocular pressure	Linner and Prijot (1955), Langham and Taylor (1960)
Cat salivary glands	Salivary secretion	Coats and Emmelin (1962)
Cat nictitating membrane	Contraction	Langer (1966b)
Rat periorbital muscle	Contraction	Lundberg (1969, 1970)
Rabbit ear artery	Fall in skin temperature	Emmelin and Ohlin (1969), Bárány and Treister (1970)
Chicken expansor secundariorum	Contraction	Geffen and Hughes (1972)
Cat heart	Transient episodes of tachycardia	Osorio et al. (1972)
Rat submaxillary gland	Salivary secretion	Stefano et al. (1974)

1966). The contraction, which lasts about 10 h (Langer, 1966b), subsides when the norepinephrine stores in the tissue have fallen to less than 10% of the control values (Smith *et al.*, 1966). The relationship between the loss of endogenous norepinephrine and the development of the degeneration contraction in the cat nictitating membrane is shown in Fig. 3. The appearance of the degeneration contraction is prevented when the endogenous stores of the transmitter are depleted by pretreatment with reserpine (Langer, 1966b). In addition, the administration of α-receptor

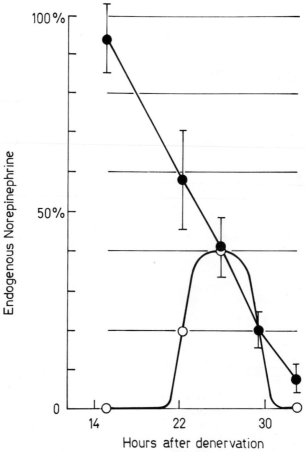

FIG. 3. Time course of the loss of endogenous norepinephrine and the development of the degeneration contraction after surgical denervation of the cat nictitating membrane. Ordinate: endogenous norepinephrine levels in the denervated smooth muscle of the nictitating membrane as percent of the contralateral control membrane. Abscissa: hours after removal of the superior cervical ganglion. ●, Endogenous norepinephrine levels in the nictitating membrane; ○, transient contraction of the denervated nictitating membrane during the degeneration of adrenergic nerve endings. From Langer (1966b) and Smith *et al.* (1966).

blocking agents such as phentolamine antagonizes the degeneration contraction of the nictitating membrane (Langer, 1966*b*). Degeneration contraction of the cat nictitating membrane can also be observed after chemical
denervation with 6-hydroxydopamine (Wagner and Trendelenburg, 1971).
Similar results have been reported for the periorbital smooth muscle of the
rat by Lundberg (1971).

4.1.2. Time Course of Degeneration in Adrenergic Nerves

After surgical denervation of sympathetically innervated organs, the
endogenous norepinephrine levels remain unchanged for a period varying
from 10 to 36 h (Fig. 3). Thereafter, there is a rapid fall in the endogenous
norepinephrine stores, which are completely lost within the following
10–20 h (Weiner *et al.*, 1962; Benmiloud and von Euler, 1963; Eakins and
Eakins, 1964; Malmfors and Sachs, 1965; Sears *et al.*, 1966; Smith *et al.*,
1966; Brimijoin *et al.*, 1970; Stefano *et al.*, 1974).

Histochemical and electron microscopic studies carried out in the cat
nictitating membrane during degeneration of adrenergic nerves revealed
that the number of granular vesicles and the intensity of fluorescence of
adrenergic nerves declined in parallel with the endogenous norepinephrine
content (Van Orden *et al.*, 1967). As discussed above, the loss of the
transmitter during the degeneration of adrenergic nerves coincides with the
development of a transient period of activity in the denervated organ. While
there is an obvious causal relationship between the loss of endogenous
norepinephrine and the transient response of the effector organ, there is
another factor involved in this phenomenon. As shown in Fig. 4, during the
period in which the neurotransmitter is lost the presynaptic component of
denervation supersensitivity to norepinephrine develops rapidly. Consequently, the increase in sensitivity to the neurotransmitter, which is due to
the progressive loss of the ability to take up norepinephrine by adrenergic
nerve endings (Fig. 4), contributes to the development of the transient
period of activity in the sympathetically denervated effector organ. As
shown in Fig. 4, there is a good correlation between the time course of the
development of the presynaptic component of denervation supersensitivity
and the gradual loss of the ability to take up and retain [^{3}H]norepinephrine
in the cat nictitating membrane (Langer *et al.*, 1967). A similar correlation
between the development of supersensitivity to norepinephrine and the
decline in neuronal uptake of the exogenous amine was obtained after
denervation of the cat spleen (Brimijoin *et al.*, 1970).

As will be discussed in subsequent sections of this chapter, hyperactivity of the effector organ leads to a decrease in sensitivity to the neurotransmitter. During the degeneration of adrenergic nerves, prolonged exposure of
the denervated effector organ to the transmitter should result in a transient
period of subsensitivity. This temporary decrease in sensitivity to

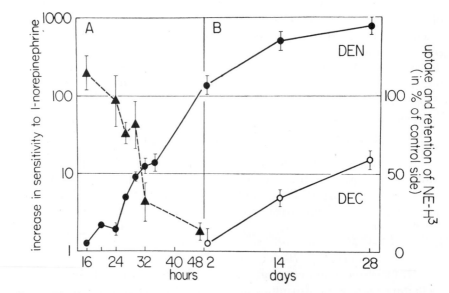

FIG. 4. Time course of development of supersensitivity to (−)-norepinephrine after denerva-tion (DEN) or decentralization (DEC) of the nictitating membrane of the cat. Ordinate: increase in sensitivity to (−)-norepinephrine after DEN (●) or after DEC (○) (log scale, left side of graph) and uptake and retention of (±)-[^{3}H]norepinephrine (▲) in percent of control side (right side of graph). Abscissa: hours (A) and days (B) after the operation. Note that supersensitivity to norepinephrine develops rapidly during the second postoperative day and follows the time course of decline and loss in the ability of the nictitating membrane to take up and retain (±)-[^{3}H]norepinephrine. From Langer et al. (1967).

norepinephrine is difficult to demonstrate when at the same time the sensitivity to norepinephrine increases by a hundred-fold in the course of only 24 h (Fig. 4). However, this phenomenon can be observed if similar experiments are carried out with an amine which is not taken up by adrenergic nerves, such as methoxamine. Under these experimental condi-tions, subsensitivity to methoxamine can be observed during the develop-ment of the degeneration contraction in the cat nictitating membrane (Trendelenburg et al., 1970). This transient decrease in the sensitivity to methoxamine appears to be due to the hyperactivity of the smooth muscle of the nictitating membrane during the degeneration of the adrenergic nerves.

It is well known that after chronic denervation of sympathetically innervated organs the activity of the enzymes involved in the synthesis and metabolic degradation of norepinephrine is reduced or even completely lost. Tyrosine hydroxylase, the rate-limiting enzyme in the synthesis of norepinephrine, disappears completely after denervation (Sedvall and Kopin, 1967; Nagatsu et al., 1969; Rubio and Langer, unpublished observa-tions). Similar results have been obtained for dopamine β-hydroxylase

(Fischer *et al.*, 1964). On the other hand, the activity of aromatic L-amino acid decarboxylase is reduced but not entirely abolished by denervation (Andén *et al.*, 1964). With regard to monoamine oxidase, a reduction of the activity after denervation is observed in tissues with a dense adrenergic innervation, such as the nictitating membrane (Jarrot and Langer, 1971) and the vas deferens (Jarrott, 1971*a*). Yet, in other organs, e.g., the heart, the reduction in monoamine oxidase activity following denervation is not significant (Potter *et al.*, 1965). The second metabolic enzyme involved in the degradation of norepinephrine, catechol-*O*-methyltransferase, appears to be present predominantly in extraneuronal tissues (Potter *et al.*, 1965; Jonason, 1969). However, there is more recent evidence indicating that at least a small fraction of tissue catechol-*O*-methyltransferase activity is associated with adrenergic nerve endings, because sympathetic denervation leads to a significant decrease in the activity of the enzyme (Jarrott and Langer, 1971; Jarrott, 1971*b*). In support of this view, Langer *et al.*(1972) found that the [³H]normetanephrine formed during the spontaneous efflux of radioactivity from the intact smooth muscle of the cat nictitating membrane originated through the activity of presynaptic catechol-*O*-methyltransferase.

In contrast to the information on the effects of *chronic* sympathetic denervation on the activities of the enzymes involved in the synthesis and metabolic degradation of norepinephrine, very little is known about changes in the activities of these enzymes *during* the degeneration of adrenergic nerves. Studies carried out in the cat nictitating membrane indicate that tyrosine hydroxylase activity begins to decline 24 h after surgical denervation (Rubio and Langer, unpublished observations). The activity of tyrosine hydroxylase in this tissue is still 40% of the control values 48 h after the operation, at a time when the endogenous stores of norepinephrine are already totally depleted (Fig. 3). Finally, 3 days after denervation the activity of tyrosine hydroxylase is completely lost (Rubio and Langer, unpublished observations). When similar studies were carried out for monoamine oxidase, it was found that the onset in the decline of the activity of this enzyme after denervation could already be detected 18 h after denervation and a maximum reduction to 50% of the contralateral control values was obtained as soon as 36 h after the operation (Rubio and Langer, unpublished observations). It is likely that the early decline in monoamine oxidase activity is partly responsible for the release of the neurotransmitter toward the receptors as unmetabolized norepinephrine during the degeneration of adrenergic nerves. Stefano *et al.*, (1974) have reported evidence compatible with this view in the rat submaxillary gland. In addition, it seems that monoamine oxidase plays some role both in the onset and in the duration of the transient period of activity observed in the denervated effector organ during the degeneration of the adrenergic nerves. In the cat nictitating membrane, inhibition of monoamine oxidase delays the onset and prolongs the duration of the degeneration contraction (Wagner and Trendelenburg,

1971). Similar results were reported after inhibition of monoamine oxidase in the denervated rat submaxillary gland.

The administration of colchicine delays the onset of the degeneration contraction in the rat periorbital smooth muscle (Lundberg, 1970). Similar results were obtained in the same preparation with other mitotic inhibitors: vinblastine and vincristine (Lundberg, 1972). It is of interest that the local application of these mitotic inhibitors to the superior cervical ganglion results in the appearance of a degeneration contraction in the rat periorbital muscle (Lundberg, 1972).

Adrenergic neuron blocking agents also delay the onset of the transient period of activity which occurs in denervated organs during the degeneration of adrenergic nerve endings (Benmiloud and von Euler, 1963; Langer, 1966b; Lundberg, 1969; Hennemann and Trendelenburg, 1970; Treister and Bárány, 1970). Pluchino et al. (1970) clearly demonstrated that the adrenergic neuron blocking agent β-TM10 does not affect the rate of degeneration of the nerve endings in the nictitating membrane. Consequently, the effects of the adrenergic neuron blocking agents might be due to a delay in the leakage of the neurotransmitter from the degenerating nerve endings: a greater degree of degeneration would be required before the norepinephrine is lost from the nerve terminals (Emmelin and Trendelenburg, 1972). Several agents antagonize the delaying effects of bretylium: desipramine (Lundberg, 1970) and indirectly acting sympathomimetic amines (Lundberg, 1969).

4.2. Prejunctional Component of Denervation Supersensitivity

Use of the term "prejunctional" or "presynaptic" was introduced by Trendelenburg (1963a, 1966) to distinguish this component from the second component of denervation supersensitivity, which is postjunctional or postsynaptic. The postjunctional component of denervation supersensitivity is due to an increase in the sensitivity of the responding cells of the effector organ. In the prejunctional type of supersensitivity, there is no change in the sensitivity of the responding cells of the effector organ. The loss of uptake of norepinephrine which results from the degeneration of adrenergic nerves increases the concentration of the agonist reaching the receptors of the effector organ and leads to an enhanced response. However, no change occurs in the relationship between the concentration of the agonist in the biophase and the magnitude of the response of the effector organ. The absence of the neuronal uptake mechanism for sympathomimetic amines eliminates the concentration gradient which normally develops for the agonist between the medium and the vicinity of the receptors (Langer and Trendelenburg, 1969; Trendelenburg, 1972). Consequently, a given concentration of norepinephrine will reach a higher level at the receptors of the denervated tissue compared to that in the same tissue with intact innervation. The absence of the main inactivating mechanism for norepinephrine (neuronal uptake) appears to be the most important factor in the prejunctional component of denervation supersensitivity.

4.2.1. Time Course of Development and the Role of Neuronal Uptake

As shown in Fig. 4, the prejunctional component of denervation supersensitivity develops rapidly between the first and the second post-operative day. In approximately 24 h, the sensitivity of the nictitating membrane to norepinephrine increases approximately a hundred-fold. The prejunctional or cocaine-like component develops simultaneously with the progressive decline in neuronal uptake of norepinephrine and the degeneration of adrenergic nerve endings (Langer et al., 1967; Van Orden et al., 1967). The prejunctional component of denervation supersensitivity appears to be causally related to the loss of the neuronal uptake mechanism since a strict correlation was obtained between the time course of the development of supersensitivity and that of the reduction in the ability of the tissue to take up and store [^{3}H]norepinephrine (Langer and Trendelenburg, 1966; Smith et al., 1966; Langer et al., 1967). Parallel morphological studies showed that the degeneration of adrenergic nerve endings also took place between the first and the second postoperative day (Van Orden et al., 1967). A similar correlation between the development of prejunctional supersensitivity and the loss in neuronal uptake of exogenous norepinephrine was reported in the cat spleen (Brimijoin et al., 1970). An additional piece of evidence for the causal relationship between the prejunctional component of denervation supersensitivity and the loss of the neuronal uptake mechanism was provided by Pluchino et al. (1970), who delayed the loss of endogenous norepinephrine from the denervated nictitating membrane by the administration of β-TM10. Under these conditions, the progression of morphological degeneration of nerve endings as well as the development of supersensitivity to norepinephrine proceeded in spite of the delay in the loss of the neurotransmitter.

The prejunctional component of denervation supersensitivity is also known as "cocaine-like" because of its resemblance to the supersensitivity induced by cocaine, which is due to the ability of this agent to inhibit neuronal uptake of norepinephrine (Trendelenburg et al., 1970, 1972; Granata and Langer, 1973). As observed for cocaine, the magnitude of the prejunctional component of denervation supersensitivity is directly related to the affinity of the agonist for the neuronal uptake mechanism. For instance, the degree of supersensitivity to norepinephrine 48 h after denervation is a hundred-fold while that for epinephrine is ten-fold (Langer et al., 1967). This difference corresponds well with the rates of uptake of these two amines in the normal smooth muscle of the nictitating membrane (Draskóczy and Trendelenburg, 1970). In addition, for an amine such as methoxamine which is not taken up by adrenergic nerve endings there is no prejunctional component of denervation supersensitivity (Trendelenburg *et al.*, 1970; see also Table 1). Cocaine does not produce supersensitivity to sympathomimetic amines which are not taken up by adrenergic nerves: methoxamine (Trendelenburg *et al.*, 1970) and isoproterenol (Granata and Langer, 1973). Further support for a causal relationship between inhibition of neuronal uptake of norepinephrine and cocaine-induced supersensitivity was obtained by Muscholl (1961), who reported in the rat a correlation between the degree of inhibition of uptake produced by cocaine and the magnitude of the potentiation of the pressor response to norepinephrine. In addition, cocaine fails to increase the sensitivity to norepinephrine in denervated tissues (Langer *et al.*, 1967; Granata and Langer, 1973). Finally, when a large number of drugs which share the property of inhibiting neuronal uptake of norepinephrine were studied it was found that they all induce supersensitivity to this amine (Trendelenburg, 1966).

The presence of a postjunctional effect in the potentiation obtained with cocaine has been postulated by Kasuya and Goto (1968) and by Kalsner and Nickerson (1969). However, the evidence available indicates quite clearly that the potentiation induced by cocaine is predominantly due to a prejunctional site of action of the drug (Trendelenburg, 1972; Trendelenburg *et al.*, 1972; Granata and Langer, 1973).

4.2.2. Characteristics of Prejunctional Supersensitivity in Individual Tissues

Some of the differences in the magnitude of the prejunctional type of supersensitivity to norepinephrine between tissues are related to the following parameters (Trendelenburg, 1972): (1) the width of the synaptic gap or neuromuscular distance; (2) the density of adrenergic innervation, as indicated by the endogenous norepinephrine content per gram of tissue; and (3) the symmetry of innervation. In tissues such as the vas deferens and the nictitating membrane, the synaptic gap is rather narrow: around 200–300Å (Merrillees *et al.*, 1963; Van Orden *et al.*, 1967; Esterhuizen *et al.*, 1968). In such tissues, the neuronal uptake of norepinephrine plays a very important role in the removal of the agonist from the vicinity of the receptors. As the width of the synaptic gap increases, the role of neuronal uptake in regulating the concentration of the agonist at the receptor sites decreases progressively. In support of this view, there is a good correlation between the size of the neuromuscular interval and the degree of cocaine-induced supersensitivity: as the width of the synaptic gap increases, the degree of cocaine-induced supersensitivity to norepinephrine decreases (Verity, 1971).

The importance of another factor, the density of innervation, can be demonstrated by taking as an example the two smooth muscles of the cat nictitating membrane: the medial and the inferior. The endogenous norepinephrine content of the medial muscle is almost twice of that of the inferior (Trendelenburg *et al.*, 1969). The more densely innervated medial muscle is less sensitive to norepinephrine than the inferior muscle, but this difference in sensitivity to norepinephrine disappears once the prejunctional component of denervation supersensitivity has developed (Trendelenburg *et al.*, 1969). Consequently, for sympathomimetic amines which are taken up by adrenergic nerve endings the sensitivity appears to be inversely related to the density of innervation. However, Trendelenburg (1972) clearly demonstrated that the density of innervation is not the *main* factor in determining the sensitivity of the tissue to norepinephrine because the degree of supersensitivity obtained after either cocaine or surgical denervation is not related to the norepinephrine content of various organs from different species.

With regard to the symmetry of innervation, it is well known that in arterial smooth muscle the nerve endings are arranged asymmetrically: they are located only along the adventitiomedial border (Ehinger *et al.*, 1967; Verity and Bevan, 1968). When norepinephrine is administered into the lumen of a blood vessel, it reaches the site of action before it has access to the sites of neuronal uptake, and as a result the potentiation by cocaine or by denervation is only two-fold. On the other hand, when norepinephrine is administered extraluminally the agonist reaches the sites of uptake before it has access to the site of action. Under these conditions, supersensitivity to norepinephrine induced by either cocaine or denervation is much more pronounced, reaching nearly tenfold. Studies of this nature were carried out in the perfused ear artery of the rabbit (De La Lande and Waterson, 1967; De La Lande *et al.*, 1967) and in the tail artery of the rat (Bonaccorsi *et al.*, 1970).

4.3. Postjunctional Component of Denervation Supersensitivity

4.3.1. Time Course of Development and Lack of Specificity

In contrast to the rapid development of the prejunctional component of denervation supersensitivity—approximately a hundredfold in 24 h (Langer *et al.*, 1967)—the postjunctional component of denervation supersensitivity develops gradually and increases slowly as a function of time (Fig. 4). In studies in which the tone of the denervated cat nictitating membrane *in vivo* was eliminated to avoid underestimating the degree of supersensitivity (Langer, 1966a) it was found that the postjunctional component of denervation supersensitivity increased steadily with time up to 4 wk after surgical denervation (Langer *et al.*, 1967). A similar time course was obtained when the supersensitivity developed by decentralization was studied under similar experimental conditions (Langer *et al.*, 1967). Tsai and Kuhn (1974) have determined the time course of development of supersensitivity after denervation and decentralization of the cat nictitating membrane *in vivo*, employing infusions of norepinephrine instead of injections of the agonists. Under these experimental conditions, they found that both types of supersensitivity reached their maximum within 7 days after the operation. The difference between the time course of development of supersensitivity obtained by Langer *et al.* (1967) and that reported by Tsai and Kuhn (1974) may be due to the fact that injections of norepinephrine were employed to determine the dose–response curves in the experiments carried out by Langer *et al.* (1967). Tsai and Kuhn (1974) determined dose–response curves based on the measurement of steady-state responses to infusions of norepinephrine.

The slow development as a function of time is a typical characteristic of the postjunctional component of denervation supersensitivity. A similar time course for the development of supersensitivity is obtained with other procedures which produce the postjunctional type of increase in sensitivity: decentralization (Langer *et al.*, 1967), chronic treatment with reserpine (Fleming and Trendelenburg, 1961; Westfall and Fleming, 1968a,b; Kasuya *et al.*, 1969; Westfall, 1970), and use of adrenergic neuron blockers or chronic ganglionic blockade (Trendelenburg and Weiner, 1962). The postjunctional component of supersensitivity can also be observed after chemical sympathectomy with 6-hydroxydopamine. These studies have been carried out in the rat salivary glands (Perec *et al.*, 1973).

In the cat nictitating membrane, the postjunctional component of denervation supersensitivity reveals, in addition to the shift to the left in the dose–response curve, an increase in the maximum development of tension (Langer, 1974). This increase in the maximal response of the effector organ, in connection with the development of the postjunctional component of denervation supersensitivity (Table 1), is an interesting phenomenon that deserves further investigation.

In contrast to the high degree of specificity in the prejunctional type of supersensitivity which develops early after surgical or chemical denervation, the postjunctional component of denervation supersensitivity is nonspecific in nature (Trendelenburg, 1963b, 1966; Langer, 1966a; Langer *et al.*, 1967; Fleming *et al.*, 1973). The postjunctional component of denervation supersensitivity develops not only for the chemical transmitter and related substances but also for other unrelated agonists which act through the stimulation of different receptors. In addition, it is important that the postjunctional supersensitivity developed to the natural transmitter is of approximately the same magnitude as that obtained for agents which activate different types of receptors or even for ions such as K^+, Ca^{2+}, or Ba^{2+} which do not act through traditional drug receptors (Seidemahel *et al.*, 1966; Langer *et al.*, 1967; Westfall and Fleming, 1968a; Westfall, 1970; Morrison and Fleming, 1971; Westfall *et al.*, 1972).

It has been suggested that the changes related to postjunctional supersensitivity in smooth muscle are the result of an increase in the concentration of receptors (Langer and Trendelenburg, 1968; Bito and Dawson, 1970). The decrease in effectiveness of phenoxybenzamine in blocking responses to norepinephrine after chronic denervation or chronic decentralization of the cat nictitating membrane is compatible with the view that these procedures result in an increase in the population of spare receptors (Langer and Trendelenburg, 1968; Waud, 1968). In addition, it is of interest that the postjunctional type of supersensitivity does not alter the pA_2 or K_b value of phentolamine (Green and Fleming, 1967; Taylor and Green, 1971).

Another hypothesis to account for the mechanism of postjunctional supersensitivity was proposed by Fleming (1963). According to this author, postjunctional supersensitivity is the consequence of a physiological change in the smooth muscle, beyond the level of the receptors, such as an alteration in membrane permeability or in the contractile mechanism. In connection with this hypothesis, it has been reported that 1 wk after decentralization or denervation of the guinea pig vas deferens there is a significant reduction in the resting membrane potential (Fleming, 1972).

4.3.2. Characteristics of Postjunctional Supersensitivity in Individual Tissues

In the cat nictitating membrane, the magnitude of postjunctional supersensitivity for several agonists is approximately the same in spite of the different procedures employed: surgical denervation, decentralization, chronic neuronal blockade, chronic ganglionic blockade, or chronic administration of reserpine (Fleming et al., 1973). It is of interest that while the postjunctional component of denervation supersensitivity can be obtained for all the agonists which stimulate the smooth muscle of the nictitating membrane, the situation is different for agents which have inhibitory effects on this effector organ. Isoproterenol relaxes the partially contracted nictitating membrane through the activation of adrenergic β-receptors (Smith, 1963; Langer and Trendelenburg, 1966). However, neither denervation nor decentralization increases the sensitivity of the nictitating membrane to the inhibitory effects of isoproterenol (Smith, 1963; Pluchino and Trendelenburg, 1968). Yet when the β-receptors are blocked the presence of supersensitivity to the α-stimulatory effects of isoproterenol can be demonstrated after chronic decentralization (Pluchino and Trendelenburg, 1968). Consequently, in the cat nictitating membrane the postjunctional component of denervation supersensitivity can be demonstrated for many agents which have direct stimulant actions on this smooth muscle: sympathomimetic amines, 5-hydroxytryptamine, acetylcholine, and barium. However, sensitivity is not increased to the inhibitory β-effects of isoproterenol.

The denervated nictitating membrane of the cat can be reinnervated by cholinergic fibers from the hypoglossal nerve (Vera *et al.*, 1957). Recent studies have demonstrated that the cholinergic reinnervation of the chronically denervated nictitating membrane does not reduce the prejunctional component of denervation supersensitivity to norepinephrine (Langer and Osorio, 1973; Osorio and Langer, 1973). However, the development of cholinergic reinnervation reduces or abolishes the postjunctional component of denervation supersensitivity to norepinephrine and to acetylcholine (Langer and Osorio, 1973; Osorio and Langer, 1973). These results support the view that prolonged inactivity of the effector organ is the main factor in the development of the postjunctional component of denervation supersensitivity.

It is of interest that for the cat nictitating membrane the postjunctional component of denervation supersensitivity and also decentralization supersensitivity have been obtained *in vivo* (Langer, 1966a; Seidemahel *et al.*, 1966; Langer *et al.*, 1967) but could not be demonstrated when similar experiments were carried out *in vitro* (Tsai *et al.*, 1968). Failure to demonstrate the postjunctional component of supersensitivity under *in vitro* conditions has been reported in other tissues as well (Green and Fleming, 1968; Haeusler and Haefely, 1970). The trauma and changes in ion balance during the isolation procedure may be the reason (Westfall and Fleming, 1968a,c; Fleming *et al.*, 1973). However, it has been demonstrated (Langer, 1974) that even under *in vitro* conditions the postjunctional component of denervation supersensitivity can be obtained in the medial muscle of the cat nictitating membrane for norepinephrine and for methoxamine as an increase in the maximum development of tension in chronically denervated tissues (Table 1).

In the guinea pig vas deferens, the presence of the postjunctional type of supersensitivity has been demonstrated after denervation, decentralization, and chronic reserpine administration (Westfall, 1970; Westfall *et al.*, 1972). Similar results have been obtained for the denervated vas deferens of the rat (Kasuya *et al.*, 1969; Birmingham *et al.*, 1970).

Pretreatment with reserpine enhances the sensitivity of the vascular smooth muscle to directly acting sympathomimetic amines (Burn and Rand, 1958; Fleming and Trendelenburg, 1961; Brody and Dixon, 1964; Van Zwieten *et al.*, 1965; Hudgins and Fleming, 1966). Interestingly enough, in rabbit aortic strips the supersensitivity obtained by chronic administration of reserpine is associated with an increase in the maximum response to acetylcholine (Taylor and Green, 1971). Supersensitivity to the chronotropic effects of drugs has been observed after pretreatment with reserpine (Fleming and Trendelenburg, 1961; Westfall and Fleming, 1968a,b). However, after denervation by neural ablation (Dempsey and Cooper, 1968) or by heterotopic transplantation of the heart (Osorio *et al.*, 1974) postjunctional supersensitivity to the cardiac inotropic effects of sympathomimetic amines was not observed. Under these experimental conditions, supersensitivity was obtained for the inotropic effects of norepinephrine but not for those of isoproterenol. Similar results were observed in the cat heart after chemical sympathectomy with 6-hydroxydopamine (Haeusler *et al.*, 1969): the supersensitivity obtained for the chronotropic effect was only of a prejunctional nature.

In the pineal gland after chronic surgical denervation there is an increase in the sensitivity of adenylate cyclase to norepinephrine (Weiss and Costa, 1967) and to sodium fluoride as well (Weiss, 1969).

Deguchi and Axelrod (1973) have reported that in the pineal gland of the rat surgical sympathetic denervation results in a greater induction of serotonin *N*-acetyltransferase and higher elevation of cyclic AMP in the pineal cells in response to isoproterenol. A similar effect can be obtained by depletion of the norepinephrine stores through the administration of reserpine (Deguchi and Axelrod, 1973). Since the repeated administration of isoproterenol to the denervated or reserpine-treated rats prevented the development of superinduction, these authors concluded that the responsiveness of the postsynaptic β-adrenoceptor in the pineal gland is conditioned by prior exposure to norepinephrine: repeated exposure to large concentrations of catecholamines causes subsensitivity, while a decrease in norepinephrine results in supersensitivity (Deguchi and Axelrod, 1973).

5. SUPERSENSITIVITY AFTER DENERVATION OF CHOLINERGICALLY INNERVATED ORGANS

5.1. Events During Degeneration of Cholinergic Nerves

5.1.1. Transient Period of Activity in Denervated Organs

As described already for sympathetically innervated organs, after section of the postganglionic parasympathetic nerves and other cholinergic nerves a transient period of activity has been observed in the denervated effector organ, coinciding with the loss of endogenous acetylcholine from degenerating nerves. In cholinergically denervated salivary glands, a paroxysmal secretion of saliva has been observed in the parotid glands starting 24–36 h after denervation (Emmelin and Strömblad, 1958; Ohlin, 1963; Nordenfelt, 1964; Emmelin, 1967, 1968). This phenomenon, called "degeneration secretion" by Emmelin and Strömblad (1958), is abolished when atropine or other muscarinic blocking agents are administered. If the salivary gland is previously sensitized by parasympathetic decentralization, the degeneration secretion obtained after parasympathetic denervation starts earlier, reaches a higher level, and lasts much longer than in the gland which has not been sensitized. During the development of degeneration secretion, it has been reported that the administration of a parasympathomimetic agent such as acetylcholine, methacholine, or carbachol accelerates the salivary flow, or may start a period of secretion (Emmelin, 1968). In addition. the administration of physostigmine, a cholinesterase inhibitor, may either provoke the onset of degeneration secretion in the denervated salivary gland or accelerate considerably the established flow (Emmelin, 1967). The evidence available clearly indicates that the degeneration secretion obtained after parasympathetic denervation in different salivary glands from several species is due to the loss of acetylcholine from degenerating cholinergic nerve endings. During the period in which degeneration secretion is observed, there is a progressive decrease in the choline acetyltransferase activity of the denervated salivary gland (Nordenfelt, 1967). On the other hand, the reduction in acetylcholinesterase activity during degeneration secretion is rather small since the time course in the decline of this enzyme after denervation is considerably slower (Nordenfelt, 1967). In several cholinergically innervated organs it has been reported that after denervation there is a similar time course for the disappearance of endogenous acetylcholine and of choline acetyltransferase from degenerating presynaptic nerve terminals (Feldberg, 1943; Hebb and Waites, 1956; Nordenfelt, 1964). In general, it appears that the degeneration secretion in salivary glands starts earlier the shorter the length of the nerve which remains connected to the effector organ (Emmelin and Malm, 1965; Emmelin, 1968). It is likely that the difference in the time of the onset of the degeneration secretion according to the site of section of the postganglionic nerve is related to axonal transport.

Studies of the degeneration of the cholinergic nerves which innervate the sweat glands of the cat foot pad were carried out by Reas and Trendelenburg (1967). These authors found that the development of denervation supersensitivity to muscarinic agents was preceded by a period of subsensitivity apparently caused by loss of acetylcholine from the degenerating nerves. In connection with the leakage of acetylcholine from degenerating nerves, a transient period of excessive sweating has been reported in patients 3–4 days after sympathetic ganglionectomy (Greenhalgh et al., 1971). This phenomenon may be due to the degeneration activity in the denervated sweat glands.

5.1.2. Changes in Sensitivity During Degeneration of Cholinergic Nerves

As it will be discussed in more detail below, supersensitivity after denervation of cholinergically innervated organs develops gradually. In contrast to the time course of supersensitivity after sympathetic denervation, the increase in sensitivity to acetylcholine is rather small during the first few days after denervation. In addition, a period of subsensitivity has been described, coinciding with the loss of endogenous acetylcholine from degenerating cholinergic nerves (Emmelin, 1964a,b; Reas and Trendelenburg, 1967). It appears that this transient period of subsensitivity is due to the stimulation of the effector organ by the neurotransmitter acetylcholine, which leaks from the degenerating nerve endings toward the receptors. This is similar to the short period of subsensitivity to methoxamine observed during the degeneration contraction of the cat nictitating membrane (Trendelenburg *et al.*, 1970), and this phenomenon can be attributed to stimulation of the effector organ by norepinephrine which is lost from degenerating nerve endings.

5.2. Time Course of Development of Supersensitivity and Pharmacological Characteristics

In cholinergically innervated organs, there is no evidence for the presence of a prejunctional type of supersensitivity similar to that observed in sympathetically innervated tissues. Both in salivary glands and in sweat glands the development of supersensitivity to acetylcholine after denervation is related to the prolonged inactivity of the effector organ (Emmelin *et al.*, 1952: Emmelin, 1961; Reas and Trendlenburg, 1967). In support of this view, it was reported that denervation supersensitivity of sweat glands developed rapidly as soon as synaptic transmission failed. In addition, prolonged pretreatment with a ganglionic blocking agent, chlorisondamine, led to a similar degree of supersensitivity as with surgical denervation (Reas and Trendelenburg, 1967). Similar results were obtained in innervated salivary glands of cats, supporting the view that prolonged inactivity of the effector organ leads to the development of supersensitivity (Emmelin, 1961).

In the denervated sweat glands of the cat, the degree of supersensitivity to acetylcholine, which is hydrolyzed by cholinesterase, was equal to that of pilocarpine, which is not a substrate for cholinesterase (Reas and Trendelenburg, 1967). These results are not compatible with the view that changes in cholinesterase activity are responsible for the development of denervation supersensitivity.

In general, supersensitivity in exocrine glands is induced by any procedure which interrupts for a certain time the contact between the transmitter and the effector organ (Emmelin, 1961, 1965). Under these experimental conditions, the supersensitivity develops slowly and is nonspecific. It is of interest that subsensitivity of the effector organ is obtained when the amount of the transmitter that reaches the receptors is increased by the chronic administration of a cholinesterase inhibitor or of a muscarinic agent (Emmelin, 1964b; Reas and Trendelenburg, 1967; Bito *et al.*, 1967;

McPhillips, 1969; Perrine and McPhillips, 1970). These changes in the sensitivity of salivary glands are reversible after discontinuation of the pharmacological procedure which induced either supersensitivity or sub-sensitivity. Yet both types of changes in sensitivity are slow to develop and slow to disappear (Fleming et al., 1973).

The results discussed so far are compatible with the view that the sensitivity of an effector organ is inversely related to the concentration of the neurotransmitter to which the receptors of the effector are exposed (Emme-lin, 1964b; Bito et al., 1971; Deguchi and Axelrod, 1973; Fleming et al., 1973). Consequently supersensitivity and subsensitivity would be opposite expressions of the same basic phenomenon. It is possible that both the absence and the excess of the neurotransmitter may lead to changes in the conformation or the availability of receptor sites for the physiological or pharmacological response of the effector organ.

Denervation of skeletal muscle leads to a very pronounced increase in sensitivity to cholinergic agents. This type of supersensitivity is postjunction-al in nature and it is due to the spread to nicotinic cholinergic receptors outward from the end-plate region (Thesleff, 1960; Creese et al., 1971). In addition, the denervated skeletal muscle responds to drugs which do not cause a contraction of the normally innervated muscle: caffeine (Gutman and Sandow, 1965), 5-hydroxytryptamine, histamine, and bradykinin (Alonso de Florida et al., 1965a,b). Within a few days after denervation, there are several changes in the electrical properties of skeletal muscle cells: the resting membrane potential decreases (Klaus et al., 1960; Thesleff, 1963; Redfern and Thesleff, 1971), and there is a decrease in the rate of rise and an increase in the duration of the action potential (Hubbard, 1963; Albuquerque and Thesleff, 1968; Redfern and Thesleff, 1971). It is of interest that in the denervated skeletal muscle the decrease in resting membrane potential is fully developed by the time at which the spread of receptors is just beginning (Redfern and Thesleff, 1971). With the develop-ment of denervation supersensitivity in skeletal muscle, there is a progres-sive resistance of the action potential to tetrodotoxin (Redfern et al., 1970; Albuquerque and Warnick, 1972). In addition, there is a decrease in potassium permeability (Klaus et al., 1960) and an increase in sodium permeability (Creese et al., 1968). Some of the changes induced by denerva-tion of skeletal muscle depend on the synthesis of new proteins. In support of this view, Grampp et al. (1972) reported that actinomycin D, in a dose which reduces the incorporation of uridine into skeletal muscle, inhibited the development of extrajunctional cholinergic receptors and tetrodotoxin-resistant action potentials after denervation of mouse skeletal muscle. The results obtained by Grampp et al. (1972) are compatible with the view that under normal conditions the motor nerve cell exerts a regulatory influence on the expression of the genome in the muscle cell.

6. SUPERSENSITIVITY IN THE CENTRAL NERVOUS SYSTEM

In contrast to the extensive literature available on denervation supersensitivity in the periphery, information on supersensitivity or subsensitivity in the central nervous system is rather scarce. Several examples of supersensitivity in the central nervous system are discussed in a review by Sharpless (1969). Supersensitivity of the temperature-regulating center in the hypothalamus can be produced by chronic administration of scopolamine. This phenomenon develops slowly and can be reversed when the treatment is discontinued. There are several instances in which interruption of afferent pathways or surgical isolation of neurons in the central nervous system produces supersensitivity to acetylcholine (Stavraky, 1961). Since this type of supersensitivity develops slowly and is nonspecific, it appears to resemble the postjunctional type of supersensitivity described in peripheral structures. In addition, chronic surgical isolation of cortical neurons results in the slow development of a greatly prolonged afterdischarge following repetitive stimulation (Sharpless, 1964).

Prolonged treatment with α-methyltyrosine, an inhibitor of catecholamine synthesis, leads to the development of supersensitivity to the behavioral effects of amphetamine and ephedrine (Dominic and Moore, 1969). Under these experimental conditions, the decrease in the amount of the transmitter appears to be responsible for the increase in the sensitivity of the postjunctional neurons. A long-lasting reduction in the brain levels of norepinephrine and dopamine has been obtained after the administration of 6-hydroxydopamine directly into the brain (Ungerstedt, 1968) or intraventricularly (Bloom et al., 1969; Burkard et al., 1969; Uretsky Iversen, 1969, 1970). Under these experimental conditions, neither γ-aminobutyric acid nor 5-hydroxytryptamine is significantly reduced. Further evidence for degeneration of catecholamine-containing neurons in the central nervous system after the intraventricular administration of 6-hydroxydopamine was obtained by Bell et al. (1970). These authors found a rapid decrease in tyrosine hydroxylase activity, [^{3}H]norepinephrine uptake, and norepinephrine content in the rat hypothalamus after the intraventricular administration of 6-hydroxydopamine. The supersensitivity that develops in the central dopaminergic receptors after the administration of 6-hydroxydopamine was studied by Ungerstedt (1971). Unilateral degeneration of the nigrostriatal dopaminergic system was obtained by the intracerebral injection of 6-hydroxydopamine. Under these conditions, the denervated striatum was more sensitive to dopaminergic stimulating agents (L-dopa and apomorphine) than the innervated striatum (Ungerstedt, 1971). In these experiments, supersensitivity to the dopaminergic receptor agonists developed gradually and did not follow the time course of the degeneration of the dopaminergic nerve endings, which is complete within 24–48 h (Hökfelt and Ungerstedt, 1969; Ungerstedt, 1971). This type of supersensitivity of the central dopaminergic receptors appears to be post-junctional in nature because of its slow development and because it is observed for agonists such as apomorphine which are not substrates for the membrane uptake mechanism in dopaminergic nerves (Ungerstedt, 1971).

The properties of the catecholamine-sensitive adenylate cyclase were studied in the rat cerebral cortex after degeneration of adrenergic nerve terminals induced by intraventricular administration of 6-hydroxydopamine (Kalisker et al., 1973). An early effect was found which was attributed to the destruction of adrenergic nerve terminals by 6-hydroxydopamine: potentiation of the increase in cyclic AMP content induced by norepinephrine but not by isoproterenol. In addition, Kalisker et al. (1973) found a late-developing increase in responsiveness which was observed both for norepinephrine and for isoproterenol. While the early effects were attributed to the loss of presynaptic catecholamine uptake sites, the late-developing component appeared to be similar to the postjunctional type of supersensitivity observed in the periphery after denervation. It is of interest that in these experiments cocaine potentiated the effects of norepinephrine on slices from control rats but did not potentiate the increase in cyclic AMP content induced isoproterenol (Kalisker et al., 1973). Thus cocaine reproduced the prejunctional component of denervation supersensitivity also in the central nervous system.

7. CLINICAL IMPLICATIONS OF SUPERSENSITIVITY AND SUBSENSITIVITY

Several of the phenomena discussed in this chapter have important clinical implications. A few examples will be mentioned, to stress the applications of research carried out in this field.

It is well known that organ transplantation involves sympathetic dener-vation and leads to the development of denervation supersensitivity of the transplanted organ and its blood vessels. Denervation supersensitivity of the prejunctional type has been reported by Osorio et al. (1974) after heterotopic heart transplant in the cat. In addition, Osorio et al. (1972) reported transient periods of tachycardia during the first 48 h following experimental heart transplant. This phenomenon is probably related to the transient period of activity described in several denervated organs during the degeneration of the nerve endings. At the level of the neuroeffector synapse in the cardiovascular system, Green and Robson (1965) suggested that the tolerance which develops to prolonged treatment with some antihypertensive agents such as adrenergic neuron blocking agents may involve the development of supersensitivity to catecholamines.

In the iris, repeated topical application of diisopropylfluorophosphate (DFP) or echothiophate leads to a progressive decrease in the effectiveness of these agents in producing miosis (Bito *et al.*, 1967). The subsensitivity produced by the local administration of cholinesterase inhibitors is quite marked, and both carbachol and pilocarpine lose their ability to constrict the pupil a few days after the administration of DFP or echothiophate. This phenomenon can be of importance in the treatment of glaucoma.

During the third and fourth days after sympathectomy, sweating and a fall in the temperature of the preganglionically sympathectomized extremity is observed (Smithwick, 1940). In addition, it has been reported that in some patients a transient decrease in blood flow is observed a few days after postganglionic sympathectomy (Barcroft and Walker, 1949). This phenomenon may justly be called degeneration vasoconstriction (Emmelin and Trendelenburg, 1972).

It appears that after myocardial infarction norepinephrine released locally from damaged or degenerating adrenergic nerve endings results in a high incidence of arrhythmias (Emmelin and Trendelenburg, 1972; Taylor *et al.*, 1970; Day and Bacaner, 1971). In connection with this possibility, it is of interest that chronic cardiac denervation or pretreatment with reserpine is effective in preventing the arrhythmias which normally appear in the dog heart after coronary artery ligation (Ebert *et al.*, 1970). Also in support of this view, the antiarrhythmic effects of bretylium after myocardial infarction appear to be related to the ability of this drug to delay the leakage of the neurotransmitter from the degenerating nerve endings (Benmiloud and von Euler, 1963; Langer, 1966*b*; Pluchino *et al.*, 1970).

Of great interest is the possibility that supersensitivity may play a role in the mechanism of clinical epilepsy: certain neurons might become supersensitive to stimuli as a result of partial isolation through some pathological process. These supersensitive neurons would overreact to stimuli, leading to convulsions (Stavraky, 1961).

The development of tolerance and the withdrawal syndrome observed with many drugs acting on the central nervous system may be related to disuse supersensitivity (Sharpless, 1969). This possibility opens a very interesting field for additional work in connection with the phenomenon of tolerance and addiction which develops with the chronic use of some depressants of the central nervous system.

The postsynaptic type of supersensitivity which develops for the central dopaminergic receptors after degeneration of the nigrostriatal dopaminergic system (Ungerstedt, 1971) is probably an important reason for the effectiveness of L-dopa therapy against Parkinson's disease. In patients with Parkinson's disease, the dopamine formed from exogenously administered

L-dopa would act on supersensitive central dopaminergic receptors, leading to a marked improvement in the symptoms of this disease.

These examples of the clinical implications of supersensitivity and subsensitivity stress the importance of these changes at the level of effector organs in the periphery and in the central nervous system. It is likely that further studies of changes in the responsiveness of effector organs to drugs in relation to the phenomena of supersensitivity and subsensitivity may help clarify several problems of clinical significance in therapeutics.

8. REFERENCES

ALBUQUERQUE, E. X., and THESLEFF, S., 1968, A comparative study of membrane properties of innervated and chronically denervated fast and slow skeletal muscles in the rat, *Acta Physiol. Scand.* **73**:471–480.

ALBUQUERQUE, E. X., and WARNICK, J. E., 1972, The pharmacology of batrachotoxin. IV. Interactions with tetrodotoxin on innervated and chronically denervated rat skeletal muscle, *J. Pharmacol. Exp. Ther.* **180**:683–697.

ALONSO DE FLORIDA, F., DEL CASTILLO, J., GONZALEZ, C. C., and SANCHEZ, V., 1965a, Anaphylactic reaction of denervated skeletal muscle in the guinea-pig, *Science* **147**:1155–1156.

ALONSO DE FLORIDA, F., DEL CASTILLO, J., GONZALEZ, C. C., and SANCHEZ, V., 1965b, On the pharmacological and anaphylactic responsiveness of denervated skeletal muscle of the guinea-pig, *Brit. J. Pharmacol.* **25**:610–620.

ANDÉN, N., HÄGGENDAL, E., MAGNUSSON, J., and ROSENGREN, T., 1964, The time course of the disappearance of noradrenaline and 5-hydroxytryptamine in the spinal cord after transection, *Acta Physiol. Scand.* **62**:115–118.

BACQ, Z. M., and RENSON, J., 1961, Actions et importance physiologique de la metanephrine et de la normetanephrine, *Arch. Int. Pharmacodyn.* **130**:385–402.

BÁRÁNY, E. H., and TREISTER, G., 1970, Time relations of degeneration mydriasis and degeneration vasoconstriction in the rabbit ear after sympathetic denervation: Effect of bretylium, *Acta Physiol. Scand.* **80**:79–92.

BARCROFT, H., and WALKER, A. J., 1949, Return of tone in blood vessels of the upper limb after sympathectomy, *Lancet* **1**:1035–1039.

BELL, L. J., IVERSEN, L. L., and URETSKY, N. J., 1970, Time course of the effects of 6-hydroxydopamine on catecholamine containing neurons in rat hypothalamus and striatum, *Brit J. Pharmacol.* **40**:790–799.

BENMILOUD, M., and VON EULER, U. S., 1963, Effects of bretylium, reserpine, guanetidine and sympathetic denervation on the noradrenaline content of the rat submaxillary gland, *Acta Physiol. Scand.* **59**:34–42.

BIRMINGHAM, A. T., PATERSON, G., and WÓJCICKI, J., 1970, A comparison of the sensitivities of innervated and denervated rat vasa deferentia to agonist drugs, *Brit. J. Pharmacol.* **39**:748–754.

BITO, L. Z., and DAWSON, M. J., 1970, The site and mechanism of the control of cholinergic sensitivity, *J. Pharmacol. Exp. Ther.* **175**:673–684.

BITO, L. Z., HYSLOP, K., and HYNDMAN, J., 1967, Antiparasympathomimetic effects of cholinesterase inhibitor treatment, *J. Pharmacol. Exp. Ther.* **157**:159–169.

BITO, L. Z., DAWSON, M. J., and PETRINOVIC, L., 1971, Cholinergic sensitivity: Normal variability as a function of stimulus background, *Science* **172**:583–585.

BLOOM, F., GROPPETTI, A., REVUELTA, A., and COSTA, E., 1969, Biochemical and fine structural effects of 6-hydroxydopamine on rat central nervous system after intracisternal injection (abst.), in: *Proceedings of the Fourth International Congress of Pharmacology, Basle.* pp. 218–219.

BONACCORSI, A., JESPERSEN, J., and GARATTINI, S., 1970, The influence of desipramine on the sensitivity and accumulation of noradrenaline in the isolated tail artery of the rat, *Eur. J. Pharmacol.* **9:**124–127.

BRIMIJOIN, S., PLUCHINO, A., and TRENDELENBURG, U., 1970, On the mechanism of supersensitivity to norepinephrine in the denervated cat spleen, *J. Pharmacol. Exp. Ther* **175:**503–513.

BRODY, M. J., and DIXON, R. L., 1964, Vascular reactivity in experimental diabetes mellitus, *Cir. Res.* **14:**494–501.

BUDGE, J. L., 1855, *Ueber die Bewegung der Iris: Für Physiologen und Artze*, Vieweg, Braunschweig.

BURKARD, W. P., JALFRE, M., and BLUM, J., 1969, Effect of 6-hydroxydopamine on behaviour and cerebral amine in rats, *Experientia* **25:**1295–1296.

BURN, J. H., and RAND, M. J., 1958, Noradrenaline in artery walls and its dispersal by reserpine, *Brit. Med. J.* **1:**903–908.

BURN, J. H., and RAND, M. J., 1959, The cause of the supersensitivity of smooth muscle to noradrenaline after sympathetic denervation, *J. Physiol.* **147:**135–143.

CANNON, W. B., and LISSÁK, K., 1939, Evidence for adrenaline in adrenergic neurons, *Am. J. Physiol.* **125:**765–777.

CANNON, W. B., and ROSENBLUETH, A., 1949, *The Supersensitivity of Denervated Structures*, Macmillan, New York.

COATS, D. A., and EMMELIN, N., 1962, The short-term effects of sympathetic ganglionectomy on the cat's salivary secretion, *J. Physiol.* **162:**282–288.

CREESE, R., EL-SHAFIE, A. L., and VRBOVÁ, G., 1968, Sodium movements in denervated muscle and the effects of actinomycin A, *J. Physiol.* **197:**279–294.

CREESE, R., TAYLOR, D. B., and CASE, R., 1971, Labeled decamethonium in denervated skeletal muscle, *J. Pharmacol. Exp. Ther.* **176:**418–422.

DAY, H., and BACANER, M., 1971, Use of bretylium tosylate in the management of acute myocardial infarction, *Am. J. Cardiol.* **27:**177–189.

DEGUCHI, T., and AXELROD, J., 1973, Supersensitivity and subsensitivity of the β-adrenergic receptor in pineal gland regulated by catecholamine transmitter, *Proc. Natl. Acad. Sci.* **70:**2411–2414.

DE LA LANDE, I. S., and WATERSON, J. G., 1967, Site of action of cocaine on the perfused artery, *Nature* **214:**313–314.

DE LA LANDE, I. S., FREWIN, D., and WATERSON, J. G., 1967, The influence of sympathetic innervation on vascular sensitivity of noradrenaline, *Brit. J. Pharmacol.* **31:**82–93.

DEMPSEY, P. J., and COOPER, T., 1968, Supersensitivity of the chronically denervated feline heart, *Am. J. Physiol.* **215:**1245–1249.

DOMINIC, J. A., and MOORE, K. E., 1969, Supersensitivity to the central stimulant actions of adrenergic drugs following discontinuation of a chronic diet of α-methyltyrosine, *Psychopharmacologia* **15:**96–101.

DRASKÓCZY, P. R., and TRENDELENBURG, U., 1970, Intraneuronal and extraneuronal accumulation of sympathomimetic amines in the isolated nictitating membrane of the cat, *J. Parmacol. Exp. Ther.* **174:**290–306.

EAKINS, K. E., and EAKINS, H. M. T., 1964, Adrenergic mechanisms and the outflow of aqueous humour from the rabbit eye, *J. Pharmacol. Exp. Ther.* **144:**60–65.

EBERT, P. A., VANDERBEEK, R. B., ALLGOOD, R. J., and SABISTON, D. C., Jr., 1970, Effect of chronic cardiac denervation on arrhythmias after coronary artery ligation, *Cardiovasc. Res.* **4:**141–147.

EHINGER, N., FALCK, B., and SPORRONG, B., 1967, Adrenergic fibers to the heart and to peripheral vessels, *Bibl. Anat.* **8:**35–45.

EMMELIN, N., 1961, Supersensitivity following "pharmacological denervation," *Pharmacol. Rev.* **13:**17–37.

EMMELIN, N., 1962, Submaxillary and sublingual secretion in cats during degeneration of post-ganglionic parasympathetic fibres, *J. Physiol.* **162:**270–281.

EMMELIN, N., 1964a, Influence of degenerating nerve fibers on the responsiveness of salivary gland cells, *J. Physiol.* **171**:132–138.

EMMELIN, N., 1964b, Action of acetylcholine on the responsiveness of effector célls, *Experientia* **20**:275.

EMMELIN, N., 1965, Action of transmitters on the responsiveness of effector cells, *Experientia* **21**:57–65.

EMMELIN, N., 1967, Parotid secretion after cutting the auriculotemporal nerve at different levels, *J. Physiol.* **188**:44–45P.

EMMELIN, N., 1968, Degeneration activity after sympathetic denervation of the submaxillary gland and the eye, *Experientia* **24**:44–45.

EMMELIN, N., and MALM, L., 1965, Development of supersensitivity as dependent on the length of degenerating nerve fibers, *Quart. J. Exp. Physiol.* **50**:142–145.

EMMELIN, N., and OHLIN, P., 1969, Skin temperature of the rabbit ear during degeneration of its sympathetic nerve supply, *Quart. J. Exp. Physiol.* **54**:207–210.

EMMELIN, N., and STRÖMBLAD, B. C. R., 1957, Sensitation of the submaxillary gland above the level reached after section of the chorda tympani, *Acta Physiol. Scand.* **38**:319–330.

EMMELIN, N., and STRÖMBLAD, B. C. R., 1958, A "paroxysmal" secretion of saliva following parasympathetic denervation of the parotid gland, *J. Physiol.* **143**:506–514.

EMMELIN, N., and TRENDELENBURG, U., 1972, Degeneration activity after parasympathetic or sympathetic denervation, *Rev. Physiol.* **66**:148–211.

EMMELIN, N., JACOBSOHN, D., and MUREN, A., 1952, Effects of prolonged administration of atropine and pilocarpine on the submaxillary gland of the cat, *Acta Physiol. Scand.* **24**:128–143.

ESTERHUIZEN, A. C., GRAHAM, J. D. P., LEVER, J. D., and SPRIGGS, T. L. B., 1968, Catecholamine and acetylcholinesterase distribution in relation to noradrenaline release: An enzyme histochemical and autoradiographic study on the innervation of the cat nictitating membrane, *Brit. J. Pharmacol.* **32**:46–56.

FELDBERG, W., 1943, Synthesis of acetylcholine in sympathetic ganglia and cholinergic nerves, *J. Physiol.* **101**:432–445.

FISCHER, F. E., MUSACCHIO, J., KOPIN, I. J., and AXELROD, J., 1964, Effects of denervation on the uptake and β-hydroxylation of tyramine in the rat salivary gland, *Life Sci.* **3**:413–419.

FLEMING, W. W., 1963, Changes in sensitivity of the cat's nictitating membrane to norepinephrine, acetylcholine and potassium, *Biochem. Pharmacol. Suppl.* **12**:202.

FLEMING, W. W., 1972, Altered resting membrane potential (RMP) of supersensitive smooth muscle cells (abst.), in: *Proceedings of the Fifth International Congress of Pharmacology, San Francisco.* p. 70.

FLEMING, W. W., McPHILLIPS, J. J., and WESTFALL, D. P., 1973, Postjunctional supersensitivity and subsensitivity of excitable tissues to drugs, *Rev. Physiol* **68**:56–119.

FLEMING, W. W., and TRENDELENBURG, U., 1961, Development of Supersensitivity to norepinephrine after pretreatment with reserpine, *J. Pharma. Exp. Ther.* **133**:41–51.

GEFFEN, L. B., and HUGHES, C. C., 1971, Degeneration of sympathetic nerves *in vitro* and development of smooth muscle supersensitivity to noradrenaline, *J. Physiol.* **221**:71–84.

GRAMPP, J. B., HARRIS, J. B., and THESLEFF, S., 1972, Inhibition of denervation changes in the skeletal muscle by blockers of protein synthesis, *J. Physiol.* **221**:743–754.

GRANATA, A. R., and LANGER, S. Z., 1973, Effects of cocaine or denervation on responses of isolated strips of cat spleen to (−)-noradrenaline and (−)-isoprenaline, *Brit. J. Pharmacol.* **46**:667–675.

GREEN, A. F., and ROBSON, R. B., 1965, Adrenergic neurone blocking agents: Tolerance and hypersensitivity to adrenaline and noradrenaline, *Brit. J. Pharmacol.* **25**:497–506.

GREEN, R. D., and FLEMING, W. W., 1967, Agonist–antagonist interactions in the normal and supersensitive nictitating membrane of the spinal cat. *J. Pharmacol. Exp. Ther.* **156**:207–214.

GREEN, R. D., and FLEMING, W. W., 1968, Analysis of supersensitivity in the isolated spleen of. the cat, *J. Pharmacol. Exp. Ther.* **162**:254–262.

GREENHALGH, R. M., ROSENGARTEN, D. S., and MARTIN, P., 1971, Role of sympathectomy for hyperhydrosis, *Brit. Med. J.* **1**:332–334.

GUTMAN, E., and SANDOW, A., 1965, Caffeine-induced contracture and potentiation of contraction in normal and denervated rat muscle, *Life Sci.* **4**:1149–1156.

HAEUSLER, G., and HAEFELY, W., 1970, Pre- and postjunctional supersensitivity of the mesenteric artery preparation from normotensive and hypertensive rats, *Naunyn-Schmiedebergs Arch. Pharmakol.* **266**:18–33.

HAEUSLER, G., HAEFELY, W., and THOENEN, H., 1969, Chemical sympathectomy of the cat with 6-hydroxydopamine, *J. Pharmacol. Exp. Ther.* **170**:50–61.

HEBB, C. O., and WAITES, G. M. H., 1956, Choline acetylase in antero- and retrograde degeneration of a cholinergic nerve, *J. Physiol.* **132**:667–671.

HENNEMANN, H. M., and TRENDELENBURG, U., 1970. Effect of the adrenergic neurone blocker β-TM10 on the depletion of noradrenaline induced by denervation or reserpine, *Naunyn-Schmiedebergs Arch. Pharmakol.* **265**:363–371.

HÖKFELT, T., and UNGERSTEDT, U., 1969, Electron and fluorescence microscopical studies on the nucleus caudatus putamen of the rat after unilateral lesions of ascending nigroneo-striatal dopamine neurons, *Acta Physiol. Scand.* **76**:415.

HUBBARD, S. J., 1963, The electrical constants and the component conductances of frog skeletal muscle after denervation, *J. Physiol.* **165**:443–456.

HUDGINS, P. M., and FLEMING, W. W., 1966, A relatively non specific supersensitivity in aortic strips resulting from pretreatment with reserpine, *J. Pharmacol. Exp. Ther.* **153**:70–80.

JARROTT, B., 1971a, Occurrence and properties of monoamine oxidase in adrenergic neurons, *J. Neurochem.* **18**:7–16.

JARROTT. B., 1971b, Occurrence and properties of catechol-*O*-methyltransferase in adrenergic neurons, *J. Neurochem.* **18**:17–27.

JARROTT, B., and LANGER, S. Z., 1971. Changes in monoamine oxidase and catechol-*O*-methyltransferase activities after denervation of the nictitating membrane of the cat, *J. Physiol.* **212**:549–559.

JONASON, J., 1969, Metabolism of dopamine and noradrenaline in normal atrophied and postganglionically sympathectomized rat salivary glands *in vitro*, *Acta Physiol. Scand.* **76**:299–311.

KALISKER, A., RUTLEDGE, C. O., and PERKINS, J. P., 1973, Effect of nerve degeneration by 6-hydroxydopamine on catecholamine-stimulated adenosine 3'-5'-monophosphate formation in rat cerebral cortex, *Mol. Pharmacol.* **9**:619–629.

KALSNER, S., and NICKERSON, M., 1969, Disposition of norepinephrine and epinephrine in vascular tissue, determined by the technique of oil immersion, *J. Pharmacol. Exp. Ther.* **165**:152–165.

KASUYA, Y., and GOTO, K., 1968, The mechanism of supersensitivity to norepinephrine induced by cocaine in rat isolated vas deferens, *Eur. J. Pharmacol.* **4**:355–362.

KASUYA, K., GOTO, K., HASHIMOTO, H., WATANABE, H., MUNAKATA, H., and WATANABE, M., 1969, Non specific denervation supersensitivity in the rat vas deferens *in vitro*, *Eur. J. Pharmacol.* **8**:177–184.

KIRPEKAR, S. M., CERVONI, P., and FURCHGOTT, R. F., 1962. Catecholamine content of the cat nictitating membrane following procedures sensitizing it to norepinephrine, *J. Pharmacol. Exp. Ther.* **135**:180–190.

KLAUS, W., LÜLLMANN, H., and MUSCHOLL, E., 1960, Der Kalium-Flux des normalen und denervierten Rattenszwerchfells, *Pflügers Arch. Ges. Physiol.* **271**:761–775.

LANGENDORFF, O., 1900, Der Deutung der "paradoxen" Pupilleberweiterung, *Klin. Mbl. Augenheilk.* **38**:823–827.

LANGER, S. Z., 1966a, Presence of tone in the denervated and in the decentralized nictitating membrane of the spinal cat and its influence on determinations of supersensitivity, *J. Pharmacol. Exp. Ther.* **154**:14–34.

LANGER, S. Z., 1966b, The degeneration contraction of the nictitating membrane in the unanesthetized cat, *J. Pharmacol. Exp. Ther.* **151**:66–72.

LANGER, S. Z., 1974, Increase in the maximal responses to the agonists during the development of the postsynaptic component of denervation supersensitivity, *Acta Physiol. Latinoam.* **24:**166–167.

LANGER, S. Z., and OSORIO, M. L., 1973, Reinervación colinérgica de la membrana nictitante de gato, *Medicina* **33:**602–603.

LANGER, S. Z., and TRENDELENBURG, U., 1966, The onset of denervation supersensitivity, *J. Pharmacol. Exp. Ther.* **151:**73–86.

LANGER, S. Z., and TRENDELENBURG, U., 1968, Decrease of effectiveness of phenoxybenzamine after chronic denervation and chronic decentralization of the nictitating membrane of the pithed cat, *J. Pharmacol. Exp. Ther.* **163:**290–299.

LANGER, S. Z., and TRENDELENBURG, U., 1969, The effect of a saturable uptake mechanism on the slopes of dose–response curves for sympathomimetic amines and on the shifts of dose–response curves elicited by a surmountable antagonist, *J. Pharmacol. Exp. Ther.* **167:**117–142.

LANGER, S. Z., DRASKÓCZY, P. R., and TRENDELENBURG, U., 1967, Time course of the development of supersensitivity to various amines in the nictitating membrane of the pithed cat after denervation and decentralization, *J. Pharmacol. Exp. Ther.* **157:**255–273.

LANGER, S. Z., STEFANO, F. J. E., and ENERO, M. A., 1972, Pre- and postsynaptic origin of the norepinephrine metabolites formed during transmitter release elicited by nerve stimulation, *J. Pharmacol. Exp. Ther.* **183:**90–102.

LANGHAM, M. E., and TAYLOR, C. B., 1960, The influence of superior cervical ganglionectomy on intraocular dynamics, *J. Physiol.* **152:**447–458.

LEVI-MONTALCINI, R., and ANGELETTI, P. U., 1962, Noradrenaline and monoamine oxidase content in immunosympathectomized animals, *Pharmacol. Rev.* **18:**619–628.

LEVI-MONTALCINI, R., and ANGELETTI, P. U., 1966, Immunosympathectomy, *Pharmacol. Rev.* **18:**619–628.

LEVI-MONTALCINI, R., and BOOKER, B., 1960, Destruction of sympathetic ganglia in mammals by antiserum to a nerve-growth protein, *Proc. Natl. Acad. Sci.* **42:**384–391.

LEVI-MONTALCINI, R., and COHEN, S., 1960, Effects of the extract of the mouse submaxillary salivary glands on the sympathetic system of mammals, *Ann. N.Y. Acad. Sci.* **85:**324–341.

LINNER, E., and PRIJOT, E., 1955, Cervical sympathetic ganglionectomy and aqueous flow, *Arch. Ophthalmol.* **54:**831–833.

LUNDBERG, D., 1969, Adrenergic neuron blockers and transmitter release after sympathetic denervation studied in the conscious rat, *Acta Physiol. Scand.* **75:**415–426.

LUNDBERG, D., 1970, Bretylium and the degeneration contraction of the sympathetically innervated periorbital smooth muscle in the rat, *Acta Physiol. Scand.* **79:**411–422.

LUNDBERG, D., 1971, Studies on 6-hydroxydopamine in conscious rats, in: *6-Hydroxydopamine and Catecholamine Neurons* (T. Malmfors and H. Thoenen, eds.), pp. 225–237, North-Holland, Amsterdam.

LUNDBERG, D., 1972, Effects of colchicine, vinblastine and vincristine on degeneration transmitter release after sympathetic denervation studied in the conscious rat, *Acta Physiol. Scand.* **85:**91–98.

MALMFORS, T., and SACHS, C., 1965, Direct studies on the disappearance of the transmitter and changes in the uptake–storage mechanisms of degenerating adrenergic nerves, *Acta Physiol. Scand.* **64:**211–223.

MALMFORS, T., and SACHS, C., 1968, Degeneration of adrenergic nerves produced by 6-hydroxydopamine, *Eur. J. Pharmacol.* **3:**89–92.

MCPHILLIPS, J. J., 1969, Subsensitivity of the rat ileum to cholinergic drugs, *J. Pharmacol. Exp. Ther.* **166:**249–254.

MERRILLEES, N. C. R., BURNSTOCK, G., and HOLMAN, M. E., 1963, Correlation of fine structure and physiology of the innervation of smooth muscle in the guinea-pig vas deferens, *J. Cell. Biol.* **19:**529–550.

MORRISON, J. M., and FLEMING, W. W., 1971, Supersensitivity of decentralized and denervated nictitating membranes to barium, *Proc. Soc. Exp. Biol.* **131:**196–199.

MUSCHOLL, E., 1961, Effect of cocaine and related drugs on the uptake of noradrenaline by heart and spleen, *Brit. J. Pharmacol.* **16**:352–359.

NAGATSU, T., RUST, L. A., and DEQUATTRO, V., 1969, The activity of tyrosine hydroxylase and related enzymes of catecholamine biosynthesis and metabolism in dog kidney—Effects of denervation, *Biochem. Pharmacol.* **18**:1441–1446.

NORDENFELT, I., 1963, Choline acetylase in normal and denervated salivary glands, *Quart, J. Exp. Physiol.* **48**:67–79.

NORDENFELT, I., 1964, Choline acetylase in salivary glands of the rabbit, dog and rat after sympathetic denervation, *Acta Univ. Lund. Sect. II* **10**:1–7.

NORDENFELT, I., 1965, Choline acetylase in salivary glands of the cat after sympathetic denervation, *Quart. J. Exp. Physiol.* **50**:57–61.

NORDENFELT, I., 1967, Metabolism of transmitter substances in salivary glands, in: *Secretory Mechanisms of Salivary Glands* (L. Schneyer and C. A. Schneyer, eds.), pp. 142–145, Academic Press, New York.

OHLIN, P., 1963, Secretion of saliva in the rabbit after postganglionic parasympathetic denervation, *Experientia* **19**:156.

OSORIO, M. L., and LANGER, S. Z., 1973, Persistencia de la supersensibilidad a las catecolaminas en la membrana nictitante de gato crónicamente desnervada luego de su reinervación colinérgica por el nervio hipogloso, *Acta Physiol. Latinoam.* **23**:192 (Suppl. 3).

OSORIO, M. L., OSORIO, Z. I. G., and LANGER, S. Z., 1972, Taquicardia precoz y transitoria en el transplante experimental del corazón: Su relación con la pérdida del neurotransmisor adrenérgico, *Medicina* **32**:710–711.

OSORIO, M. L., STEFANO, F. J. E., and LANGER, S. Z., 1974, Heterotopic heart transplant in the cat: An experimental model for the study of the development of sympathetic denervation and of allograft rejection, *Naunyn-Schmiedebergs Arch. Pharmakol.* **283**:389–407.

PEREC, C. J., STEFANO, F. J. E., and BARRIO-RENDO, M. A., 1973, Long-lasting supersensitivity after 6–hydroxydopamine in the submaxillary gland of the rat, *J. Pharmacol. Exp. Ther.* **186**:220–229.

PERRINE, S. E., and MCPHILLIPS, J. J., 1970, Specific subsensitivity of the rat atrium to cholinergic drugs, *J. Pharmacol. Exp. Ther.* **175**:496–502.

PHILIPEAUX, J. M., and VULPIAN, A., 1863, Note sur une modification physiologique qui se produit dans le nerf lingual par suite de l'abolition temporaire de la motricité dans le nerf hypoglasse du memme coté, *Compt. Rend. Acad. Sci Paris* **56**:1009–1011.

PLUCHINO, S., and TRENDELENBURG, U., 1968, The influence of denervation and of decentralization on the alpha and beta effects of isoproterenol on the nictitating membrane of the pithed cat, *J. Pharmacol. Exp. Ther.* **163**:257–265.

PLUCHINO, S., VAN ORDEN, L. S., III, DRASKÓCZY, P. R., LANGER, S. Z., and TRENDELENBURG, U., 1970, The effect of beta-TM10 on the pharmacological, biochemical and morphological changes induced by denervation of the nictitating membrane of the cat, *J. Pharmacol. Exp. Ther.* **172**:77–90.

POTTER, L. T., COOPER, T., WILLMAN, V. L., and WOLFE, D. E., 1965, Synthesis, binding, release and metabolism of norepinephrine in normal and transplanted dog hearts, *Circ. Res.* **16**:468–481.

REAS, H. W., and TRENDELENBURG, U., 1967, Changes in the sensitivity of the sweat glands of the cat after denervation, *J. Pharmacol. Exp. Ther.* **156**:126–136.

REDFERN, P., and THESLEFF, S., 1971. Action potential generation in denervated rat skeletal muscle. I. Quantitative aspects, *Acta Physiol. Scand.* **81**:557–564.

REDFERN, P., LUNDH, H., and THESLEFF, S., 1970, Tetrodotoxin resistant action potentials in denervated rat skeletal muscle, *Eur. J. Pharmacol.* **11**:263–265.

SEARS, M. L., and BÁRÁNY, E. H., 1960, Outflow resistance and adrenergic mechanisms, *Arch. Ophthalmol.* **64**:839–848.

SEARS, M. L., MIZUNO, K., CINTRON, C., ALTER, A., and SHERK, T., 1966, Changes in outflow facility and content of norepinephrine in iris and ciliary processes of albino rabbits after cervical ganglionectomy, *Invest. Ophthalmol.* **5**:312–318.

SEDVALL, G. C., and KOPIN, I. J., 1967, Influence of sympathetic denervation and nerve impulse activity of tyrosine hydroxylase in the rat submaxillary gland, *Biochem. Pharmacol.* **16**:39–46.

SEIDEMAHEL, R. J., PATIL, P. N., TYE, A., and LAPIDUS, J. B., 1966, The effects of norepinephrine isomers on various supersensitivities of the cat nictitating membrane, *J. Pharmacol. Exp. Ther.* **153**:81–89.

SHARPLESS, S. K., 1964, Reorganization of function in the nervous system, use and disuse, *Ann. Rev. Physiol.* **26**:357–388.

SHARPLESS, S. K., 1969, Isolated and deafferented neurons: Disuse supersensitivity, in: *Basic Mechanisms of the Epilepsies* (H. H. Japser, A. A. Ward, and A. Pope, eds.), Little, Brown, Boston.

SMITH, C. B., 1963, Relaxation of the nictitating membrane of the spinal cat by sympathomimetic amines, *J. Pharmacol. Exp. Ther.* **142**:163–170.

SMITH, C. B., TRENDELENBURG, U., LANGER, S. Z., and TSAI, T. H., 1966, The relation of retention of norepinephrine-H^3 to the norepinephrine content of the nictitating membrane of the spinal cat during development of denervation supersensitivity, *J. Pharmacol. Exp. Ther.* **151**:87–94.

SMITHWICK, R. H., 1940, Surgical intervention on the sympathetic nervous system for peripheral vascular disease, *Arch. Surg.* **40**:286–306.

STAVRAKY, G. W., 1961, *Supersensitivity Following Lesions of the Nervous System*, University of Toronto Press, Toronto.

STEFANO, F. J. E., PEREC, C. J., and TUMILASCI, O., 1974, Changes in neuronal uptake metabolism and sensitivity to norepinephrine during the degeneration secretion in the rat submaxillary gland, *J. Pharmacol. Exp. Ther.* **191**:403–417.

STONE, C. A., PORTER, C. C., STAVORSKI, J. M., LUDDEN, C. T., and TOTATO, J. A., 1964, Antagonism of certain effects of catecholamine-depleting agents by antidepressant and related drugs, *J. Pharmacol. Exp. Ther.* **144**:196–204.

TAYLOR, J., and GREEN, R. D., 1971, Analysis of reserpine-induced supersensitivity in aortic strips of rabbits, *J. Pharmacol. Exp. Ther.* **177**:127–135.

TAYLOR, S. H., SAXTON, C., DAVIES, P. S., and STOKER, J. B., 1970, Bretylium tosylate in prevention of cardiac disrhythmias after myocardial infarction, *Brit. Heart J.* **32**:326–396.

THESLEFF, S., 1960, Supersensitivity of skeletal muscle produced by botulinum toxin, *J. Physiol.* **151**:598–607.

THESLEFF, S., 1963, Spontaneous electrical activity in denervated rat skeletal muscle, in: *The Effect of Use and Disuse on Neuromuscular Functions* (E. Gutmann and P. Honik, eds.), Elsevier, Amsterdam.

THOENEN, H., 1972, Surgical, immunogical and chemical sympathectomy: Their application in the investigation of the physiology and pharmacology of the sympathetic nervous system, in: *Catecholamines* (H. Blaschko and E. Muscholl, eds.), pp. 813–844, Springer, Berlin.

THOENEN, H., and TRANZER, J. P., 1968, Chemical sympathectomy by selective destruction of adrenergic nerve endings with 6-hydroxydopamine, *Naunyn-Schmiedebergs Arch. Pharmakol Exp. Pathol.* **261**:271–288.

TRANZER, J. P., and THOENEN, H., 1967, Ultramorphologische Veränderungen der sympathischen Nervenendigungen der Katze nach Vorbehandlun mit 5- und 6-Hydroxy-Dopamin, *Naunyn-Schmiedebergs Arch. Pharmakol. Exp. Pathol.* **257**:343–344.

TRANZER, J. P., SNIPES, R. L., and RICHARDS, J. G., 1969, Recent developments on the ultrastructural aspect of adrenergic nerve endings in various experimental conditions, *Prog. Brain Res.* **31**:33–46.

TREISTER, G., and BÁRÁNY, E. H., 1970, The effect of bretylium on the degeneration mydriasis and intraocular pressure decrease in the conscious rabbit after unilateral cervical ganglionectomy, *Invest. Ophthalmol.* **9**:343–353.

TRENDELENBURG, U., 1963a, Time course of changes in sensitivity after denervation of the nictitating membrane of the spinal cat, *J. Pharmacol. Exp. Ther.* **142**:335–342.

TRENDELENBURG, U., 1963*b*, Supersensitivity and subsensitivity to sympathomimetic amines, *Pharmacol. Rev.* **15**:225–276.

TRENDELENBURG, U., 1966, Mechanisms of supersensitivity and subsensitivity to sympathomimetic amines, *Pharmacol. Rev.* **18**:629–640.

TRENDELENBURG, U., 1972, Factors influencing the concentrations of catecholamines at the receptors, in: *Catecholamines* (H. Blaschko and E. Muscholl, eds.), pp. 726–761, Springer, Berlin.

TRENDELENBURG, U., and WEINER, N., 1962, Sensitivity of the nictitating membrane after various procedures and agents, *J. Pharmacol. Exp. Ther.* **136**:152–161.

TRENDELENBURG, U., DRASKÓCZY, P. R., and PLUCHINO, S., 1969, The density of adrenergic innervation of the cat's nictitating membrane as a factor influencing the sensitivity of the isolated preparation to *l*-norepinephrine, *J. Pharmacol. Exp. Ther.* **166**:14–25.

TRENDELENBURG, U., MAXWELL, R. A., and PLUCHINO, S., 1970, Methoxamine as a tool to assess the importance of intraneuronal uptake of *l*-norepinephrine in the cat's nictitating membrane, *J. Pharmacol. Exp. Ther.* **172**:91–99.

TRENDELENBURG, U., GRAEFE, K. H., and ECKERT, E., 1972, The prejunctional effect of cocaine on the isolated nictitating membrane of the cat, *Naunyn-Schmiedeberg's Arch. Pharmakol.* **275**:69–82.

TSAI, T. H., and KUHN, W. L., 1974, Sensitivity of the nictitating membrane of the pithed cat to infusions of *l*-norepinephrine after denervation or decentralization, *J. Pharmacol. Exp. Ther.* **188**:630–639.

TSAI, T. H., DENHAM, S., and MCGRATH, W. R., 1968, Sensitivity of the isolated nictitating membrane of the cat to norepinephrine and acetylcholine after various procedures and agents, *J. Pharmacol. Exp. Ther.* **164**:146–157.

UNGERSTEDT, U., 1968, 6-Hydroxydopamine induced degeneration of central monoamine neurons, *Eur. J. Pharmacol.* **5**:107–110.

UNGERSTEDT, U., 1971, Postsynaptic supersensitivity after 6-hydroxydopamine induced degeneration of the nigro-striatal dopamine system, *Acta Physiol. Scand. Suppl.* **367**:69–93.

URETSKY, N. J., and IVERSEN, L. L., 1969, Effects of 6-hydroxydopamine on noradrenaline-containing neurons in the rat brain, *Nature* **221**:557–559.

URETSKY, N. J., and IVERSEN, L. L., 1970, Effects of 6-hydroxydopamine on catecholamine-containing neurons in the rat brain, *J. Neurochem.* **173**:269–278.

VAN ORDEN, L. S., III, BENSCH, K. G., LANGER, S. Z., and TRENDELENBURG, U., 1967, Histochemical and fine structural aspects of the onset of denervation supersensitivity in the nictitating membrane of the spinal cat, *J. Pharmacol. Exp. Ther.* **157**:274–283.

VAN ZWIETEN, P. A., WIDHALM, S., and HERTTING, G., 1965, Influence of cocaine and of pretreatment with reserpine on the pressor effect and the tissue uptake of injected *dl*-catecholamines-2-H^3, *J. Pharmacol. Exp. Ther.* **149**:50–56.

VON EULER, U. S., and PURKHOLD, A., 1951, Effect of sympathetic denervation on the noradrenaline and adrenaline content of the spleen, kidney and salivary glands in the sheep, *Acta Physiol. Scand.* **24**:212–217.

VERA, C. L., VIAL, J. D., and LUCO, J. V., 1957, Reinnervation of nictitating membrane of the cat by cholinergic fibers, *J. Neurophysiol.* **20**:365–373.

VERITY, M. A., 1971, Morphological studies of vascular neuroeffector apparatus, in: *Proceedings of a Symposium on the Physiology and Pharmacology of Vascular Neuroeffector Systems*, Interlaken, 1969, pp. 2–12, Karger, Basel.

VERITY, M. A., and BEVAN, J. A., 1968, Fine structural study of the terminal effector plexus, neuromuscular and intermuscular relationships in the pulmonary artery, *J. Anat.* **103**:49–63.

VOGT, M., 1964, Sources of noradrenaline in the "immunosympathectomized" rat, *Nature* **204**:1315–1316.

WAGNER, K., and TRENDELENBURG, U., 1971, Development of degeneration contraction and supersensitivity in the cat's nictitating membrane after 6-hydroxydopamine, *Naunyn-Schmiedebergs Arch. Pharmakol.* **270**:215–236.

WAKADE, A. R., and KRUSZ, J., 1972, Effect of reserpine, phenoxybenzamine and cocaine on neuromuscular transmission in the vas deferens of the guinea pig, *J. Pharmacol. Exp. Ther.* **181:**310–317.

WAUD, D. R., 1968, On the estimation of receptor occlusion by irreversible competitive pharmacological antagonists, *Biochem. Pharmacol.* **17:**649–653.

WEINER, N., PERKINS, M., and SIDMAN, R. L., 1962, Effect of reserpine on noradrenaline content of innervated and denervated brown adipose tissue of the rat, *Nature* **193:**137–138.

WEISS, B., 1969, Effects of environmental lighting and chronic denervation on the activation of adenyl cyclase of rat pineal gland by norepinephrine and sodium fluoride, *J. Pharmacol. Exp. Ther.* **168:**146–152.

WEISS, B., and COSTA, E., 1967, Adenylcyclase activity in rat pineal gland: Effects of chronic denervation and norepinephrine, *Science* **156:**1750–1751.

WESTFALL, D. P., 1970, Nonspecific supersensitivity of the guinea-pig vas deferens produced by decentralization and reserpine treatment, *Brit. J. Pharmacol.* **39:**110–120.

WESTFALL, D. P., and FLEMING, W. W., 1968a, The sensitivity of the guinea-pig pacemaker to norepinephrine and calcium after pretreatment with reserpine, *J. Pharmacol. Exp. Ther.* **164:**259–269.

WESTFALL, D. P., and FLEMING, W. W., 1968b, Sensitivity changes in the dog heart to norepinephrine and calcium after pretreatment with reserpine, *J. Pharmacol. Exp. Ther.* **159:**98–106.

WESTFALL, D. P., and FLEMING, W. W., 1968c, Reserpine-induced supersensitivity in perfused rabbit hearts, *Pharmacologist* **10:**218.

WESTFALL, D. P., McCLURE, D. C., and FLEMING, W. W., 1972, The effects of denervation, decentralization and cocaine on the response of the smooth muscle of the guinea-pig vas deferens to various drugs, *J. Pharmacol. Exp. Ther.* **181:**328–338.

INDEX